D1234353

# Practicing Desire

# Practicing Desire

## Homosexual Sex in the Era of AIDS

Gary W. Dowsett

*Stanford University Press, Stanford, California*

1996

Stanford University Press
Stanford, California
© 1996 by the Board of Trustees of the
Leland Stanford Junior University
Printed in the United States of America

CIP data are at the end of the book

Stanford University Press publications are distributed exclusively by
Stanford University Press within the United States, Canada, Mexico,
and Central America; they are distributed exclusively by
Cambridge University Press throughout the rest of the world.

This study is dedicated to the late Peter Charlton—actor, writer, gay man, model PLWHA, and friend—and his muse, the greatest diva of them all.

# Acknowledgments

My thanks first go to the men who participated in this study. They gave their time and opened their lives that other gay men might learn from them and survive the HIV epidemic. Colleagues at the National Centre for HIV Social Research at Macquarie University, Sydney, were ever supportive and helpful. During 1991–92 the research was supported by a Commonwealth AIDS Research Grants Committee Postgraduate Scholarship. The Humanities Research Centre at the Australian National University, Canberra, provided warm support and much-needed time and space for working on the manuscript during my time there in 1993 as a Visiting Fellow. Members of the Sociology Department at Macquarie University were always helpful. I owe a special debt of gratitude to Bob Connell and Rosemary Pringle for their unfailing support and guidance. My thanks also to Stanford University Press, and particularly Andrew Lewis, for expert help.

To Vonnie Santo and Neal Fitzgerald I owe the extent to which I remained calm throughout this study. Phil Stevenson, Rolf Petherbridge, and the late Tim Carrigan were patient and loyal friends—thanks, girls. Donizetti and Rossini brought peace and order in tumultuous times. The gay communities of Australia were constantly inspirational as they struggled with many of the issues I was writing about; they deserve more praise than this country will ever give them.

Finally, to Graeme Skinner, my partner, whose unfailing love, assistance, wisdom, and caring form the center of my life, I offer my thanks, although no thanks are adequate.

I am grateful to Michael Hurley and Jan Hutchinson for permission to quote from their book, *Two Timing* (Sydney: Local Consumption Publications, 1991), and to Robert Peters for permission to quote his poem "The First Kiss," in *The Male Muse*, ed. Ian Young (Trumansburg, N.Y.: The Crossing Press, 1973). Peters, the prolific poet, dramatist, critic, novelist, and actor, lives in Southern California and recently retired after 30 years of teaching at the University of California. His *Poems Selected and New: 1967-1991* was published by Asylum Arts Press.

Thanks also to Kerry Bashford for permission to quote "Time Likes His Toes Sucked," by Kurt Joseph Schranzer, in *Pink Ink*, ed. Kerry Bashford (Sydney: Wicked Women Publications, 1991), and to Antler for permission to quote from his poem "What Every Boy Knows," in *The Son of the Male Muse*, ed. Ian Young (Trumansburg, N.Y.: The Crossing Press, 1983). Antler, from Milwaukee, is the author of *Factory* (City Lights) and *Last Words* (Ballantine). A winner of the Walt Whitman Award, the Witter Bynner Prize, and a Pushcart Prize, his poetry appears in many anthologies, including *Gay and Lesbian Poetry of Our Time, Gay Roots: Twenty Years of Gay Sunshine, Erotic by Nature*, and *Heartpieces: Wisconsin Poets Against AIDS*.

Permission was sought to quote from "Himn" by Laurence Collinson in his *Hovering Narcissus* (London: Grandma Press; Melbourne: Overland, 1977), but no reply was received. Permission was also sought from Jim Eggeling to quote "Aphorism," in *The Male Muse*, ed. Ian Young (Trumansburg, N.Y.: The Crossing Press, 1973), but The Crossing Press were unable to trace him.

Aspects of an earlier version of the argument in Chapter 3 were published in the *Australian Journal of Social Issues* 35, no. 3 (1990): 186-98, and in *AIDS in Australia*, ed. Eric Timewell, Victor Minichiello, and David Plummer (Sydney: Prentice-Hall, 1992), reproduced with permission. Chapter 4 is an expanded version of "Working-Class Masculinity, Gay Community and the Masculine Sexual (Dis)order," originally published in *Revue sexologique* 2, no. 2 (1994): 75-105, included with permission. Some of the material on methodology discussed in Chapter 2 was published in "What Is Sexuality: A Bent Answer to a Straight Question," *Meanjin* 55, no. 1 (1996): 16-30. A short, early version of the sexed bodies discussion in Chapter 5 appeared in *Australian Sexual Cultures*, ed. Jill Matthews (Sydney: George Allen & Unwin, 1996).

# Contents

# Tables

# Note on Textual Conventions

In quotations from research participants, ellipses (. . .) will be used only to indicate that text has been excised or skipped. A dash (—) is used to indicate sudden breaks in speech patterns and syntax or for parenthetical statements. Brackets enclose authorial comment or explanation, to include the indication of certain undercurrents in the interview, for example [pause], [laughter], [very quiet]. Parentheses within such quotations enclose the interviewer's questions or interpolated interviewer comment within the respondent's reply. All emphases in quoted matter are original unless otherwise stated.

As he grew up he had been faced with the choice
all homosexuals must make between sticking to the
rules—perhaps for a lifetime—or making sense of
life by following the irrational, often painful truths
revealed within themselves. Curiosity, scepticism
and doubt are second nature to those who choose
the second path.

—David Marr, *Patrick White: A Life*

# Starting Points

In December 1987 five hundred gay men and lesbians gathered in Amsterdam for an international scientific conference. It was a remarkable event, bringing together academics, activists, and writers who were working on the various tasks and undertakings loosely called "gay and lesbian studies." The conference released a number of volumes of pre-conference readings covering the varied intellectual terrain that occupies the attention of the international gay and lesbian intelligentsia. Some of these papers were collected in *Homosexuality, Which Homosexuality? Essays from the International Scientific Conference on Gay and Lesbian Studies* (Altman et al. 1989).

In February 1992, again in Amsterdam, a few hundred gay and lesbian academics, activists, health professionals, and public servants gathered for the Second European Conference on Homosexuality and HIV, "HIV Policy, Prevention, Care, and Research: A Gay and Lesbian Perspective." Again a large number of papers were presented and discussed. (Publication of some of these papers in an edited collection similar to *Homosexuality, Which Homosexuality?* was even planned.)

There the similarity ends.

These two conferences form the parentheses of this study. I was unable to attend the first, having only returned to academia in mid-1986 to coordinate a series of research projects investigating the sexual and social responses of homosexually active men in Sydney and other parts of New South Wales, Australia, to the human immunodeficiency virus (HIV) epidemic and its consequence for many infected with the virus, Acquired Immune Deficiency Syndrome (AIDS). The conference, while of immense interest to anyone such as myself interested in social theory, homosexuality, sexual politics, and gay liberation, seemed too "academic" in the face of the hard and urgent HIV/AIDS work we were engaged in. It seemed a luxury at the time; but now I regret not attending.

I did attend the second conference and delivered a paper. This conference offered the possibility of making useful connections between the still urgent practical concerns of HIV/AIDS and developments in social theory on homosexuality, which had continued since the first conference and to a considerable degree been stimulated by it.

The time between these conferences had been filled for me, in part, by this study, as one of a number of ongoing investigations of homosexuality, HIV/AIDS, and social theory that colleagues and I have undertaken. A second major preoccupation has been the development of an ongoing relationship between social HIV/AIDS research and the gay communities in Australia fighting to stop the HIV epidemic. This was done in the belief that social research, *when grounded in social theory AND pursued through empirical inquiry*, was and still is able to offer gay communities, public health officials, health professionals, and people living with HIV or AIDS (PLWHAs) the best possible advice on strategies for preventing the sexual transmission of HIV between men. Although the earliest work of the team with which I was involved for over eight years focused on preventing sexual transmission of HIV through education, the scope of this work has grown well beyond that singular concern to include other transmission and prevention issues and to investigate the needs of people infected with and affected by the virus.

The 1987 conference was not unconcerned with HIV/AIDS, but had as its focus the heated debate between "essentialism" and "social constructionism." This debate seemed to go to the heart of the sexual identities upon which much gay liberation politics had been constructed and which had offered such a significant challenge to social theory and political thought in the West since the early 1970's. The range of approaches was indeed very large: psychological modeling (Schippers 1989); the use of gender as a broad social-structural category (Odijk 1987); cross-cultural and historical searches for the existence of homosexually active persons throughout history (Vicinus 1989); considerable recasting and reworking of psychoanalysis (Fletcher 1989; de Kuyper 1987); reexaminations of pedophilia (van Naerssen 1987; Sandfort 1987). These are just some examples.

The second conference was vitally concerned with HIV/AIDS. The four thematic strands in its title engendered presentations, lively discussions, and workshops covering the vast range of issues that had emerged as a result of the HIV epidemic. These were interspersed with plenaries on subjects deemed especially significant. Yet Simon Watney, noted British cultural theorist, reported that

Questions of sexual identity are absolutely central to our ability to design and implement effective education strategies. Yet the shocking paradox of the [conference] . . . was the evidence that a powerful and perhaps central strand of the northern European post–Gay Liberation lesbian and gay politics is hopelessly unable to acknowledge, let alone confront, the catastrophe that already surrounds us. (1992: 45)

Many attending the conference witnessed this profound failure in gay and lesbian theory and politics to deal with the lives of gay men (and lesbians) as they are currently being lived, facing the extraordinary pain, exhaustion, and loss of nearly fifteen years of struggle with HIV/AIDS.

Yet the first conference had offered so much, particularly on the issue of identity, and there had been a strong link between theory, politics, and HIV/AIDS in a number of papers. Watney himself, leading the charge in a powerful piece, "AIDS: The Cultural Agenda," (1987a), and Australian gay writer Dennis Altman, in his paper "AIDS and the Reconceptualisation of Homosexuality" (1989), offered incisive and sophisticated analyses of the social framing of the HIV epidemic. Altman pointed also to a resurgence in gay liberation politics as a result of HIV/AIDS. Beyond HIV/AIDS, these writers and others exemplified the challenging heights to which gay and lesbian intellectual work had risen in the twenty years since the publication of Mary McIntosh's (1968) seminal essay "The Homosexual Role."

Yet the second conference was almost bereft of theoretically informed work, and the political edge of the entire debate was dulled by a complacent acceptance of terms of reference that positioned homosexuality as merely an accepted cultural variant, that is, a minority in the diversifying social fabric of the postindustrial social democracies of northwestern Europe. It certainly appeared that "Integration = Death"! The desperate situation of gay men and lesbians in eastern and southern Europe, let alone homosexually active men and women in the developing world, was almost ignored in a dangerously inward-looking Eurocentric focus. Furthermore, a critique of political and social responses to HIV/AIDS in many of the European countries represented at the conference was almost nonexistent. A plenary session on "Mainstreaming," that is, the integration of services for gay men within general population services, as opposed to a strategy of separate gay service provision, was, to be polite about it, completely "other-worldly" to the delegates from disintegrating countries of central and eastern Europe.

ᔋ

What had happened to the promise of 1987? Where were the theorists and activists (for they are often the same people), and why had the intellectual ferment ensuing from the 1987 conference failed to affect so many of the gay and lesbian health professionals, bureaucrats, and activists of 1992? Many were still struggling on. Watney himself represented *par excellence* what had happened: the pervasive frustration, anger, and exhaustion evident in much of his commentary reveal the dilemmas of producing an activist- or intellectual-generated response to the epidemic, and of witnessing in despair an often pain- and panic-driven politics of HIV/AIDS pragmatism, which unwittingly undercuts the larger and longer-term agenda of the project of sexual liberation—a project that still occupies the attention of many gay and lesbian intellectuals and activists.

On the one hand, there was a disturbing lack of connection between the theoretical and the political work done over the past twenty years: an ignoring of the intimate connection between gay liberationist-inspired social theory and politics in, for example, the recognition of relations between sexuality and the state and the determination of HIV/AIDS policy activism. On the other, there was evidence that a kind of "grand theory" in gay and lesbian studies, fortified with exciting attempts to universalize "sexuality" and capture an ontological hegemony within social theory, had lost touch with the oppression and subjugation under which many homosexually active men and women live and was not speaking to those engaged in HIV/AIDS work. In short, a worrisome gap was appearing between theory and practice.

A contributing factor to this gap has been the advent of theoretical approaches, often loosely called *postmodern* or *poststructuralist*, that question many of the frameworks of thought that have supported the sexual liberation project for a long time. This challenge appeared at a time when the political, social, and sexual dilemmas produced by HIV were emerging. Dave Sargent (1983) in his essay "Reformulating (Homo)sexual Politics: Radical Theory and Practice in the Gay Movement" surveyed the work of Mieli, Foucault, Deleuze and Guattari, Hocquenghem, and Weeks, among others, and hoped that "a more thorough consideration of various Feminisms and other radical theories might lead to a deconstruction of the Gay Movement as we've come to know it—toward a radically different reformulation of (homo)sexual politics" (p. 164). Sargent's death from AIDS in early 1985 not only robbed Australia of a key gay intellectual and activist, but highlighted the political dangers of deconstruction: the need for strong gay communities to respond to the HIV epidemic, and to its particular form in Australia, was crystal clear.

It is important to remember the speed with which the HIV epidemic overtook the gay communities of Australia in advance of much of Europe and Great Britain. (As Watney noted at the 1992 conference, Britain and much of Europe have yet to experience an "AIDS epidemic"; they are currently experiencing an epidemic of "HIV infection." Australia, like the United States, has already experienced the horror of AIDS.) The tension between these largely European-inspired theoretical advances, with their challenge to deconstruct gay identity, politics, and, inevitably, communities, and an epidemic shaped much more like that experienced by gay communities in the United States at that time, particularly in New York and San Francisco, presented Australian gay activists and intellectuals with a very different problem and much less leisure in which to deal with it.

The Australian gay communities have responded to HIV/AIDS magnificently (see Chapter 3), making Australia one of the few places on the planet where it can be said with some confidence that the epidemic is under control. The gay communities have grown enormously, not least in infrastructure, since the early 1980's. For example, the AIDS Council of New South Wales, the gay community AIDS service organization that coordinates gay communities' responses to HIV/AIDS in Sydney and the rest of New South Wales, has over seventy-five full-time staff and a number of others who work on fixed-term projects. Its annual budget is nearly AU$5.9 million (AIDS Council of New South Wales 1994).

In contrast, the late Michaël Pollak, one of the key intellectuals writing on HIV/AIDS in France, had reported on the devastating effects of the disorganized French gay community's failure to mobilize a collective response to the epidemic (1989). Similarly, the French delegate at the 1992 conference pleaded desperately for assistance in fighting what Watney referred to as France's "genocide-by-negligence" (1992: 46), a consequence of the deconstruction of gay community partly in response to the intellectual developments of the 1970's and 1980's.

Cindy Patton (1990) succinctly analyzes the failure of the gay HIV/AIDS "professionals" in community-based organizations in the United States to recognize the consequences of their creeping (no, galloping) bureaucratization and their steady incorporation into mainstream public health, a process increasingly at odds with the goals of even the minority-style gay liberation politics of that country. This accusation has been leveled at various times at Australian gay community AIDS service organizations as well. There appears to be a growing danger that gay communities might follow one trajectory in modern feminism by producing, for the few, certain career paths, for the rest, cul-de-sac "minority" status in postindustrial pluralism (Yeatman 1990).

Another area of concern at the 1992 conference was the swag of differences between lesbians and gay men, and the positioning of HIV/AIDS in that long-standing debate. Again the contrast between the two conferences is illuminating. The sophistication of lesbian theory in 1987, exemplified in work such as Monique Wittig's "On the Social Contract" (1989) and Martha Vicinus's "The Historical Roots of the Modern Lesbian Identity" (1989), gave way to a claim for the inclusion of lesbians centrally in HIV prevention campaigns. An alleged neglect of lesbians was contrasted to the "overwhelming" efforts directed toward gay men. The irony of this poorly thought through claim, which confuses sexual identities and HIV-related transmission vectors, was that the speaker came from the United Kingdom, where, as Watney reported (1992: 46), the amount of money spent on prevention among gay men (70 percent of AIDS cases) was at that time less than 5 percent of the HIV/AIDS education budget! Moreover, many of the eastern European countries represented at the conference had *no* funding or infrastructure at all to fight their (largely male-to-male sexually transmitted) epidemics. Here was another set of theorists failing miserably to comprehend the enormity of the problem facing gay men in the West.

The theoretical sophistication of the international, emergent gay intelligentsia has often been at odds with the urgent need to fight an epidemic in practice; yet the very urgency of this need has often produced a sketchy and shortsighted politics of pragmatism that is in danger of undercutting gains made by and for gay men and lesbians over the past twenty years.

All in all, the time between these two conferences proved to be one of remarkable change in gay communities around the world. Anyone living, working, and being (homo)sexually active within them could not help but witness the turmoil: the uncertainty concerning goals and directions; the increasing distance between theory and practice; the paradox contained in gay sex itself as a consequence of the HIV epidemic; the epistemological crisis produced by this paradox; the desperate need for informed action given the enormous growth and increased sophistication of modern (and postmodern) gay life.

It is this apparent failure of theory and practice which the current study addresses. One of its aims is to investigate the gay liberation project itself, to test out in the practices of gay men's daily lives the applicability of the essentialist/social constructionist debate mapped so convincingly in 1987. At that conference the sides in this debate were firm and clear; they no longer are. Those who gathered in Amsterdam in 1987 demonstrated extraordinary political and intellectual solidarity, despite different positions on the issues under debate and argument between gay men and lesbians about the various branches of feminism that have always so profoundly affected (homo)sexual politics and theory. By 1992 the liberation project was either seen to have been achieved, or largely forgotten and neglected; yet it was still so urgently needed, particularly in eastern Europe.

My own concerns as a gay man, an intellectual worker, an activist on the Left (increasingly broadly defined), and someone who worked full-time in HIV/AIDS for eight years were stimulated by the first conference, to the point that I grew anxious about the remarkable, largely successful response of the Sydney gay community to the epidemic. My concern grew from an early recognition, for example, of the limitations of a particular conceptualization of the HIV epidemic generated within gay communities, and of the consequent truncation of the preventive education programs it produced. There was a discernible smugness about *"the* gay community"—what it was, what it had done and could do, and who was "in" it or not. My concern has risen anew with the more recent development of HIV politics manifested in the advent of an "HIV identity" (Dowsett 1992), an "HIV community" (Duffin 1990), an "HIV career" (Ariss, Carrigan, and Dowsett 1992), and their effects on gay communities.

I found myself, very early on, questioning whether there *was* a "gay community" in Sydney; then whether there were actually "gay communi*ties*" in Sydney; and soon thereafter, whether "membership" in gay community/ies was even possible—was it in fact a fiction? The essentialism/social constructionism debate, in which I had previously found myself squarely on the constructionist side of the binary, was fast becoming a waste of time, a diversion. Apart from the minor irritation of seeing too frequently in the gay press and hearing at meetings such absurdities as "Well, the way I construct my sexuality . . ." when referring to everything from fur coats to feral lovers, the heat the binary generated was not so much useless as unnecessary. Something was *certainly* being constructed, but I had doubts about what it was.

As research findings began to accumulate on the changes in the sexual behavior of gay men worldwide in response to HIV/AIDS, it was becoming clear in Australia very early on that sexual identity was related in crucial ways to prevention of HIV infection, but that the axis of analysis of the essentialist/social constructionist binary was largely irrelevant to that relationship. HIV/AIDS activist-educators, trying to reach all homosexually active men regardless of how they comprehended their sexuality, could no longer rely on this discursive finery, this simplistic binary, for the strategic educational advice they needed.

More recently, others have begun simply to bypass the binary itself (for example, Sedgwick 1990) for a more pressing concern: returning the original challenge of sexual liberation to the forefront of our minds. It seemed to me that some of these early or basic liberationist principles might prove important to HIV prevention, particularly among the newly homosexual and those who do not identify with a gay community.

Despite the discursive sophistication of the identity debate, I was increasingly convinced that what was needed was a clear investigation of how men come to both the practices and meanings of male-to-male sex acts. Surely their *experiences* would inform the formation of identity, the intellectual debate, and, I hoped, the educational thinking needed in HIV prevention programs.

A second concern grew from noticing that the terms of the debate on essentialism/social constructionism were cast almost entirely abstractly/deductively/rhetorically; not a skerrick of empirical work was being done to investigate the *living* of gay lives to find out how these powerful concepts of sex, sexuality, sexual identity, gay community, and so on, were enacted and embodied. The metaphysics and the metonymy were there; the people and their practices were not. In particular, I was struck by this in much of the important intellectual work on homosexuality done during the 1980's (for example, Gay Left Collective 1980; Fernbach 1981; Plummer 1981; Altman 1982; Weeks 1985, 1990). My desire for a dose of real persons is no crude claim for empiricism, nor is it an act of reification; it is a recognition that empirical investigation might throw light on social processes in ways that would illuminate debate and link it again to politics.

This absence of experience and persons was nowhere more obvious than when it came to sex itself—to the actual sexual action going on all around us in (and beyond) the gay communities. I later read with instant recognition Carole Vance's keynote address delivered at the 1987 conference in which she warned, "To the extent that social construction theory grants that sexual acts, identities and even desire are mediated by cultural and historical factors, the object of the study—sexuality—becomes evanescent and threatens to disappear" (1989: 21). We were witnessing in the HIV epidemic the most extraordinary changes in gay men's sexual behavior, their ways of having sex, and the meanings and the amount of sex they were having, all of which was being directly influenced by their own efforts. Yet sex itself, the meanings and sensations of sex, was almost entirely absent from the discussions.

In the course of this investigation into sex as practice I came up against the same inhibitions in myself I recognized elsewhere in gay intellectual work concerning how to represent sex as practice in language. The participants in this study had no difficulty in describing their sex lives in graphic detail; nor do I find any difficulty in doing the same. Yet I found myself adopting clinical terms for sex, for example, "penis," "oral-genital sex," and "oral-anal contact," derived largely from the etiquette of "scientific" HIV/AIDS discourse. The men I interviewed talked of "dicks," "sucking," and "rimming"; as do I. Was I to censor them and myself in this study? My central purpose was to investigate sex as it is experienced by homosexually active men. Therefore I have refused to render the language of (homo)sex (and by extension [homo]sex itself) as a descent from proper academic manners either by translating it into sterile jargon or wrapping it in inverted commas. At times, a fuck is simply that—a fuck; and in this study it is important to say so.

This became more urgent on the issue of anal intercourse between men. The use of the words "penetration" and "penetrate" brought with it considerable baggage from discussions of heterosexual sex, baggage that obscured the radically different intentions, sensations, meanings, and context associated with that sexual activity for gay men. "Fucking" and "being fucked," as more appropriate terms, not only describe exactly how the men in this study think and talk about anal intercourse, they do not automatically collapse into the taken-for-granted analogue that penetrator/penetrated *equals* active/passive or powerful/powerless—a collapse I seriously wanted to avoid.

The 1987 conference almost entirely neglected sex, deserving the epithet flung at gay activists (now almost apocryphal, and from another time and place) as being "gay only from the neck up"! Therefore, this study also focuses on sex, on coming to sex, on *doing* sex. It investigates the process of enacting homosexuality.

This neglect of sex is ironic when one considers that the social construction of anything implies, first, the presence of sociality, and, second, the existence of a means, a mechanism, an action wherein construction occurs. The focus of much of the theoretical work at that conference was remarkably abstract; the concern was with *being* homosexual (or gay or lesbian), not *doing* homosexual, and was individualist rather than collective.

On this theme, the legacy of psychoanalysis has been, perhaps, excessively influential. Psychoanalysis renders sexuality as essentially a psychic and intrapsychic process (leaving aside the profoundly sociocultural reading of Freud available in, for example, "Civilisation and Its Discontents" and the clearer focus on the body in the "Three Essays on the Theory of Sexuality"). Indeed, as revealed in the controversies generated by J. M. Masson (1984), the curious lack of action or practice in the formation of sexual desire in psychoanalysis has tended to support a concentration on sexuality as a largely consciousness-focused individual achievement. This is not to be read as a repudiation of Freudian thought or a denial of consciousness, but as a claim for the addition of physical experience to the mix. A second consequence is that the *social* becomes merely an antonym for the *natural* in the conventional binaries nature/nurture and organic/cultural. Rarely is it rendered in terms of its complexity, as both social and natural, as both embodied and psychic, and as an activity engaged in with others.

This study pursues the collective and experiential sexual construction of homosexuality in the lives of the men who volunteered to open their sexual histories and practices to scrutiny. Within that collective activity the viability of gay community and the sexual liberation project itself is evaluated. In *States of Desire* (1986), which inspired part of the present study, Edmund White began such an evaluation. In that book there is a focus on the construction of male homosexual lives as "gay" in various cities of the United States, and its most important feature to my mind was the clearly different lives enacted within the vastly different sexual possibilities available in the diverse cities White visited. Frances Fitzgerald's updating of the situation in San Francisco in *Cities on a Hill* (1987, see "The Castro") pointed to the profound and visible effects of the HIV epidemic. (See also Altman 1982 and Weeks 1990.)

My more modest attempt here is to subject to evaluation the Sydney gay community, Australia's largest and most visible, known worldwide as one of the great gay cities, "the gateway to gay and lesbian Australia, brash and frivolous to some, paradise for the rest" (Cribb and Herbert 1991: 35). It is most famous nowadays for its annual Gay and Lesbian Mardi Gras and the accompanying month-long cultural and sporting festival.

It is this community which is hardest hit by HIV/AIDS in Australia, and many of the men in this study are either infected with HIV or affected closely by the epidemic among their lovers, friends, and relatives. Two of the infected men have died since I interviewed them, several are ill or are experiencing various deteriorations of their immune systems. The rest are well or uninfected. Part of the interest in the study was to find out how these men came to be infected and how they dealt with their infection sexually and socially. Another obvious concern was how to do prevention programs better, how to make sure as many homosexually active lives are saved as possible. Although this book did not start as an HIV/AIDS study primarily and although it takes HIV/AIDS in stride as a fact of life before, during, and after the five years of investigation between the two Amsterdam conferences, HIV/AIDS has ultimately claimed a central place in it.

To assess the gap between theory and practice in the context of HIV/ AIDS, and to explore the issues outlined above, I conducted a series of interviews with twenty men over a period of three years (see Chapter 2 for a discussion of methodology). These men tell their own tales and thereby demand that the *social process of being homosexual be recognized as a historically constructed sexual and collective practice.* By way of introduction to their contribution I would first like you to meet someone very important—a quite ordinary Australian gay man named Barney Sherman, who embodies many of the themes of this study.

## Barney Sherman

Barney Sherman is an orphan, born in 1932 in a Salvation Army hostel and adopted out in babyhood. He did know his biological mother's name, but never traced her and knew nothing about her. The only child of his adoptive parents, he retained a fondness for his strong adoptive mother. However, fondness was something he never felt for his adoptive father, an alcoholic whom mother and son left when Barney was ten. For most of her adult life, his mother ran a series of mixed businesses, pubs, and "residentials" (private hotels or guest houses) in various cities and towns. Barney was forever moving around, somewhat friendless, and eventually ended up in a Catholic boarding school to stabilize his education. Later his mother moved him to a "private" college in Sydney (probably a technical college of some sort), which he attended until age fifteen when he left school for a short period to work as a wool grader. Later, being "mechanically minded," Barney took up an apprenticeship. At some stage during his late adolescence Barney moved north, following his mother, and lived in boarding houses while she worked in country towns. At age nineteen Barney returned to Sydney on his own and eventually found his feet in electrical work.

By the time of my first interview with him, Barney was a small businessman running a relatively thriving electrical repair shop in inner Sydney. He was proud of his work and the success he had made. Barney was then fifty-six. He rarely attended any inner-city gay community functions and there was little evidence of a substantial gay friendship network, although he reported having lots of male friends and frequented a local working-class gay pub. In response to my opening question, Barney indicated things were going fine: he was "eating well, drinking well, smoking well." He immediately added that he had a lover, M, living with him. M was a younger man, about thirty and getting chubby, unemployed owing to "family reasons," and a classic bottle blond. An ex-lover, P, was also living with them.

Barney indicated that this caused friction, but he found being fought over delightful.

His very next sentence stunned me: "The association with the police is terrific. No troubles there; because I'm tied up with community activities with the police." This referred to his involvement with Neighbourhood Watch, something he did as an openly gay man. He owned a modest house and ran his business from a room built over the garage, stuffed with computing equipment and software, littered with obsolete paperwork, cigarette butts overflowing the ashtrays, and gadgetry everywhere. Barney's passion was computers; he owned at least four, and he was connected to the gay bulletin boards available in Sydney. He gave me a printout from his latest access, which contained notices about safe sex and a couple of very explicit amateur pornographic stories.

This smoothly flowing life changed for Barney in 1986; he discovered he was HIV antibody positive. This came as a shock, since he had previously tested negative to HIV a number of times. At the first interview this diagnosis had made little impact on his life, apart from producing some changes in his sex practices.

The second interview took place in early 1992, nearly four years after the first. Barney, nearing sixty, had become the centerpiece of this study, his life history offering many of the starting points from which the rest of the investigation unfolded. The Barney of 1992 was far less cocky and self-assured. The ex-lover of long standing, P, had just died from an AIDS-related condition, but not before accidentally burning Barney's house down.

Barney was no longer working much—the odd job here and there with a few customers paying "on the black" (off the books). He was on the Invalid Pension and intended to rent out a room in his newly repaired house to help make ends meet. The computers lay idle, and the gay bulletin boards went unread. He was not watching pornography much, partly because his collection and his audiovisual equipment had been destroyed in the fire. He had dropped out of Neighbourhood Watch and did not go to gay bars at all. He was increasingly bitter about other people's petty behavior, drink prices in gay bars, and "lazy coppers" in Neighbourhood Watch. All in all it was picture of a life in decline, and the moments of the deliciously wicked Barney with the glint in his eye so prominent in the first interview were few and far between.

Barney is not just a gay man with HIV; he is also a self-employed worker with HIV. The loss of income as a result of his illness has been significant. His work history is unremarkable for a man of his generation. There were efforts at some sort of social mobility through schooling and a trade apprenticeship. Barney got his "ticket" (trade certificate) and succeeded in operating a small business. He made one stab at the big time, forming a partnership with an engineer, but it did not work out. There is a hint that Barney just never quite comprehended how big money is made.

He did succeed in setting himself up in a business much as his mother had done. It is important to remember that people like Barney are simply workers who work for themselves. Barney had stated his income as being under AU$6,000 in the first interview, which tells more about how he ran the company than about his actual take-home pay. He was not classically working class in that he owned capital and ran his own company; but he was also its only employee. Barney settled for this. He lacked ambition beyond his pride in the reliability of service and the quality of his workmanship. His income was only marginally protected from the ups and downs of the job market, and a recession could easily wreck a small business like his. His office was hardly an investment property accumulating capital gains through tax exemptions. In short Barney never really escaped his working-class origins.

However, it was not just in his working life that Barney had a distinct working-class style. There was a distinctly working-class texture in his yarn-spinning, his principles about doing the right thing, and in his sexuality.

### Sexuality

Barney's first remembered sexual experiences occurred at age three or four in bed with a cousin on a farm while the adults were off milking. This went on for four years or so: ". . . just fondling and playing around, I suppose, which is natural amongst boys." A little later he was caught in sex play with a maid's young daughter at the hotel his mother managed. This drew a classic maternal response:

Mum caught me—"Come inside here." Went inside. She got a big knife out and chased me round the kitchen table and she said: "I'll cut it off! I'll cut it off!"

(Did she really? [asks the incredulous interviewer].)

Yes, you know, when you look back on it, more to frighten me, you know, so I wouldn't do it again, kind of thing. But it didn't stop me. We found another spot to do it.

And do so he did, but with boys. Barney had only one other close shave with heterosexual sex. He had one girlfriend in late adolescence, a girl with twelve siblings. Barney used to have sex with her brother while he was going out with her.

Barney became somewhat of a sexual servant at his boarding school. One prefect used him regularly for interfemoral sex; another demanded that Barney masturbate him. There were also circle jerks behind the boarding house and later at the college. There was no open talk of sex, however, in any way. More startling was the schoolmaster who started by rubbing himself up against Barney's backside, eventually doing so with his penis exposed and with Barney's pants on the floor. This occurred quite often but never led to intercourse.

There were similar post-school experiences: a boarder (now a heterosexual policeman) masturbating into a "frenchy" (condom) while fondling Barney; being "screwed" by an army man in a cubicle in the dressing sheds at a beach pavilion; being "groped" and "sucked" by adults in cinemas in the city; a regular session with an old man who would take Barney for a drive: "All he wanted to do was suck me off—that suited me fine"; a foreman at his first job who would "flip me off" (masturbate him) during the lunch hour behind the wool bales.

These incidents did not just happen accidentally to Barney: "I used to go looking for it." Indeed, he seems to have been preoccupied with finding places where such things could happen. He was a loner with few friends or mates, which made possible his private searches for sex. He was never paid for sex: "I was never commercial," and he had little connection with any homosexual subculture, but was undoubtedly obtaining sex within that context. It was to be Barney's move north a little later that changed the character of his sex life.

Barney had what might be counted as a first "affair" in this new town with a man he met at church. It was not a "relationship"—a distinction he insisted on; it was just that they were both "horny." They were boarding in the same house and used to go to the park across the road for sex, none of it anal intercourse. But he met other boys through the church choir, and he "screwed" them. It was all "hush hush." There were no bars, dance halls, or pubs that he knew of, so he just met men as he was walking around. Barney also soon found the local *beat* and would cycle there for sex.[1] He told a wonderful story about a Salvation Army man whom he would "screw the arse off" and who would then preach to Barney about God.

---

[1] "Beats": an Australian term for places such as parks, public toilets, changing sheds, railway station restrooms, and so on, where men can meet other men for casual sexual activity. Called "tearooms" in the United States and "cottages" in Great Britain.

"Coming out" in its original sense—joining society—occurred at age nineteen when Barney moved back to Sydney's eastern suburbs, leaving his mother behind. Soon he was living in a household of three homosexual men, having parties for "poofters," and going to the few pubs for homosexual men at Kings Cross (in those days the main "red light" district in Sydney). Many of the men had drag names—"Bubbles," "Scheherazade"—but not Barney. The Trocadero (a famous wartime and postwar dance club) was in action in the city, and he went there with his first lover. This was the social and sexual context of Barney's twenties and thirties and represents the classic Sydney "camp" homosexual subculture of the era, described by Wotherspoon (1991), centered around certain venues and parts of the city, and soon to be challenged by the rise of gay liberation (Carrigan 1981).

Barney certainly did not consider himself "gay": " 'Gay' wasn't here in Sydney then, it was all 'camp,' which I think is a better word than 'gay.' " Barney's use of the terms does not contain the magnificence of Weeks's characterization of homosexual as "sexual preference" and gay as "a subversively political way of life" (1985: 198). Nor is it of the character of Cohen and Dyer's (1980) distinction between "traditional gay male culture" and "radical gay male culture," or "gay" versus "queer." True, the sophisticated discourse of gay liberation developing during Barney's heyday in the 1970's saw homosexuality as a challenge to the sexual order (see Altman 1979). But for Barney: "It's not our choice of sex we want. It's the choice of person we wish to love."

In this conceptualization he points to the relational character of homoeroticism, something many men in this study emphasized. Being gay is simply a personal and emotional state. His memories of Oxford Street,[2] which had become the heart of the inner-Sydney gay community during the 1970's, were of its social and sexual character, not of its burgeoning gay politics.

Barney knew all the well-known bars of those days, and in 1979 he and friends started their own club just off Oxford Street, a nonlicensed, BYO (bring-your-own alcohol) nightclub with amateur drag shows. It was not a success. This marked the end of Barney's active participation in the *gay community*, which was then overtaking the older homosexual subculture. Bars were not the only attraction of gay life, though. He was a member of

---

[2] Oxford Street, Darlinghurst, is an inner-city boulevard that has become synonymous with Sydney's gay community precinct or quarter. It houses bars, sex-on-premises venues, shops, restaurants, and so on, most with declared gay connections, and is the site of the Gay and Lesbian Mardi Gras Parade.

an inner-suburban social club, at one point doing the lighting for their drag shows (no frocks for him); but he left over a dispute about the honesty of the committee's financial dealings.

In the inner-Sydney gay community of the late 1980's, Barney was on the fringe. He was very cross with a local gay hotel, muttering darkly about the rhetoric of "brothers and sisters" yet being ripped off by gay venues in general. Repeating the classic working man's complaint, he railed against the price of a "middy" (an average glass of beer) at gay venues when compared with the local RSL (a returned soldiers club).

The deterioration in Barney's connections with the gay community and his own gay social networks was even more marked by the second interview. I asked with whom he spent time? His answer: "I spend it more with square [heterosexual] people at the moment. Speaking about square people — since I became crook there are these squares up in [nearby suburb] and they have been excellent to me. They've been better than gay friends." These "square" friends know he is gay, and Barney still takes the odd opportunity to confront them with his sexuality, remarking on men's bums, for example, in a bit of fun. But this is all tinged with resentment at gays for somehow not being there for him in his troubles.

Barney was never strongly attached to the newer gay community. His participation had been decreasing unwittingly over the previous decade. Yet he still thought himself someone who had contributed to and was still *in* the gay community, someone who was owed something — something undefinable. Unfortunately, Barney's memory of his contribution to the community and its memory of him are two different things, and he now felt unfairly excluded. This exclusion he was resenting so strongly had begun to occur socially and sexually well before he contracted HIV:

(What about parties or any of the events in the gay community like Mardi Gras and things like that?)

Oh, Mardi Gras I may go to and see the parade, but as far as those parties are concerned at the Showground and what for have you, no, they can stick them right up their bum.

(You don't like them?)

No, no. You go there, the music is that loud and the place is full of drugs, you know, who wants that!

(You don't like that sort of scene?)

No.

(What about the men though, is that an attraction?)

Oh, yeah, but what's the good of me looking at something young and, say, that looks nice, and they look at me and, say, well I don't want to bloody know you. So I've got a problem.

(What do you think it is?)

Age. Definitely age.

(You're fifty-nine now, aren't you?)

Yeah, I'll be sixty this year.

(You don't feel it and don't look it though, eh?)

No.

(But, is it a problem in the gay community, do you think, for older men?)

What? Age? Oh yeah, definitely, because once you get over thirty-five now nobody wants to know you and, ah, the only ones that want to know you are someone who wants to take you home and rip you off or something.

A combination of factors has produced this estrangement: his age and diminishing sexual attractiveness; his critique of changes in gay culture (dance parties, drugs, youth and beauty); bad faith among so-called gay "brothers and sisters" (drink prices, financial misdealing, bitchiness); the difference between gay community rhetoric and gay community practice; and so on. Finally, when he needed assistance with his illness, Barney found there was little about.

◡

Barney's first relationship (with P) lasted thirteen years. At the time of the first interview he was in his second relationship (with M). It had been going about two years, and they had been living together for one year. There had also been a number of short affairs over the years, each lasting a few weeks. At the time of the first interview M did the domestic labor in lieu of rent. M's domestic "role" seemed to carry over into anal sex. "She loves it, being screwed!" said Barney with wicked laughter—the gender of the pronoun being a revealing moment of campery, a declaration of who is on "top," and a hint of the character of Barney's attitude to sex.

Barney reckoned he has had over 3,000 sex partners, and that he has fucked 75 percent of them, 25 percent have sucked him, 20 percent have fucked him, and he has sucked "a few. I was never, no never, a big sucker: basically butch." He liked his men smooth-skinned, with penises large enough "so you can grab a hold of them." He used pornography, some of which turned him on, but he disliked the muscle men dominating gay magazines: "They don't do a bloody thing to me," offering in this comment another moment in his exclusion from emergent gay community culture; as he aged and *his* gayness became dated, the hegemonic gay object choice evolved away from him.

Barney has done the beats (though never at night) throughout his life, reckoning that there were about a hundred or so in Sydney at one time; but many are now closed down. Every public toilet was a beat, he said. He stopped doing them because of HIV/AIDS. He had been questioned by police on a beat on one occasion years ago, and charged with indecent assault. He received a bond and was angry that this conviction was not expunged from his record when homosexuality was legalized in New South Wales in 1984. Barney also told of letting himself be fucked by coppers patrolling the beats in those days to avoid being run in. This was not uncommon, he suggested, and certainly corroborates the repeated complaints made by gay liberation activists about the use of good-looking police as *agents provocateurs* on beats, and the allegations by drag queens and transsexuals of supplying blow jobs in return for being let off soliciting charges in the late 1970's.

Beats were not the only source of sex partners, but saunas were not a favorite with Barney: "You'd get someone in a sauna—and this happened to me—I shoved it in a couple, come out, and next thing someone's down on me without [my] having a shower! And I thought: 'What are you going to catch down there?' " It is a beautiful moment of displacement. Yet it is not so foolish a thought, for Barney has had a variety of sexually transmissible diseases (STDs) in his time, including syphilis.

His varied sex life included visiting (male) prostitutes occasionally, and he liked them young. He reported that this use of prostitutes and the beats originated when P was on night shift for long periods of time and was too tired for sex, particularly Barney's favored "morning glory," that is, intercourse when one first wakes up. He talked of developing friendships with young rent boys, but it was clear that Barney was no pedophile. He regarded sex with a rent boy as a business deal. The terms were sex for money, and they were encounters that in general lacked that certain sociability he liked. Not surprising, given his own history, he registered something widely regarded as "true" about the sexual interests of boys: "You've only got to put your hand on their leg and [a gesture indicating an erection]. It's an old saying—a stiff prick has no conscience."

Barney reported that 10 percent of the men he has had sex with were not gay, and in referring to men's sexuality in general said: "Male sex. You've only, you know, got to look at someone, have a drink with someone in a pub or something and, er, get talking, go home and have sex. 'Cause that's what you went out for. Meet a woman and she doesn't want sex for six months later. . . . The right time and the right place, they'll [men] do anything. I don't care who it is." This kind of belief about male sexuality was very common among the men in this study, and certainly coincided with their experiences of sex as well as with the claims of gay liberation activists in the 1970's.

Although Barney enjoyed telling tales of derring-do in casual sexual encounters, the actual sex was not the purpose of the tale. It was not erotica like the Reverend Boyd McDonald's *Straight to Hell* books (for example, McDonald 1987); the purpose was in spinning yarns of risks taken, devilry engaged in, thrills pursued, narrow escapes. In this there was a language of sex, some of it general, some of it specifically gay, and some obviously a lingo related to his generation and class of homosexual man. Words used were "fondle," "suck," "stick his finger up me arse," "screwing . . . that [term] came from the Yanks," "go with," "pulling," "flip," "muck around," "go down on," "daisy chain," "morning glory." Unlike younger men, he rarely used the word "fuck"; "intercourse" and "screwing" were by far the most frequent words used for penetrative sex.

Barney mentioned "arses" a lot. He always preferred inserting to receiving in anal intercourse and by late adolescence he had become quite a fucker—there were more than just a few schoolboys during his college days who were on the receiving end. Yet his first experience of anal intercourse was not really pleasant. An army man at the same beach pavilion bathing shed shoved a finger up his bum—"Oh, no, get that out!" said Barney—and then the man fucked him. Barney did not like it. Yet he got used to it and started to like it as the next few years wore on. (Getting used to anal sex is an issue that was to come up more than once during this study.)

There was more than a hint in his account of his sex life that "real men" insert. This is not a crude idea of a strict "butch/femme" role allocation, but a good example of the finding on Australian gay men's sexual repertoire obtained in HIV/AIDS behavioral research: more men prefer to insert than to receive, but in general most men will reciprocate (Connell and Kippax 1990).

Barney preferred to be "butch." Part of the explanation for this is simple: "I just like screwing. I can remember going back when I was six, seven, eight, nine, ten, we had a pub in [country town] in '39 to '41. Saturday, Sunday morning, I'd lay in bed and flip meself ten or twelve times, and get the thrill not being able to ejaculate, you know. I've always been highly sexed." Further questions elicited more stories of how he contrived to make sure he got to do most of the inserting, as well as a number of other issues, such as the difference between sucking and fucking: some knew how to, others did not. As Barney put it, in sucking with "some: it's just like going into an empty bloody hole, with no one there." Those who knew how to be fucked were liked if they were "active" but not too much so: "I like him to be active a bit, but I'm always in control." He basically argued that anyone (including a bad sucker) could be fucked properly, that is, it essentially required one to take it as it is given, and any position would do: "face up, face down, saying their prayers on their knees"—again said with his wicked laughter.

These added up to what could be considered Barney's sexual ethic about insertive fucking, an ethic that placed sex for Barney in a single category—pleasure:

> I prefer to screw. You see, it used to come from the situations when I used to pick casual bits up years ago from Hyde Park, kind of thing. We'd go out and I'd want to screw them, kind of thing. I'd say: "As long as I can screw you." They say: "All right." [Then Barney would say] "But I'll go first." [We'd] be on our side or something because it would be out in the grass somewhere, you know. Couldn't take them home. And I'd always make certain I had a hold of them [their penises] and away I'd go. I'd know that they were about to blow their lot. And so would I, because when they blew their lot, they didn't want it [to fuck him]. So I was safe.

Condoms were a "bloody nuisance" but necessary. He had had no breakage problems, because he rubbed cream on his penis first so that the partner's anus gripped the condom and Barney's penis slid in and out of it. His lubricant was a vitamin E–based commercial skin conditioning preparation definitely *not* recommended in safe sex guidelines. Yet he went on to tell me that oil-based lubes were no good. If ever there was an example of experiential learning in action here it was.

Barney did not go in for *esoteric* sex[3] and saw this as being more related to drug use. He did not like "roseleafing" (oral-anal sex), or being tied up and whipped or belted. Much of his repertoire developed on beats and in casual sex; he was not a back-room fuck bar person and was not involved in the Oxford Street scene at the time when its (in)famous interest in esoteric sex developed. Sex for Barney had as much to do with *habit* as it did with *opportunity*: together these created his sexual history.

---

3 "Esoteric" sex here refers to sadomasochism, fist-fucking, watersports, scat (coprophilia), and bondage, including those activities which may or may not draw blood. This term was coined in early HIV/AIDS research in Australia as a category for these infrequent practices (Dowsett 1988).

The main impression gained from this account of Barney's sexuality is a strong sense of detachment. For Barney, sex is sex; it is in a class of its own. It is not the fulfillment of an identity, or an act of inclusion within a sexual culture, or the conscious exploration of the self. Sex is naughty, fun, an adventure, a gag; life does not depend on it. That is not to say it was peripheral. Barney spent a lot of his waking hours engaged in sexual activity of one sort or another. But he did not create himself through his sexual activity alone; nor did his sense of himself depend primarily on his sexuality. It was related as much to his trade, his interest in computers, his work with Neighbourhood Watch, his friendship networks, and, increasingly, his HIV infection.

He got close to something like a modern gay identity in his participation in parts of the emerging Oxford Street scene in the 1970's, that is, an identity formed through attachment to, and participation in, a gay community the likes of which have emerged in the last twenty years in cities in the West, such as San Francisco, Sydney, London, New York, Amsterdam, and Berlin. But Barney's identity did not gel into a modern gay identity. Why? Age perhaps. Maybe he just did not fit in. He was not of the Stonewall or post-Stonewall generation.[4] In this, he was strikingly similar to the two oldest men in Garry Wotherspoon's collection of Australian homosexual life histories, *Being Different* (1986). This begs questions about rapid generational changes in the formation of sexual identities: just how recently constructed is the idea of a sexual identity, what purpose does it now serve, and how long will it be of use?

Barney's personhood, his subjectivity, did not demand a central position for his sexual activity. Having sex with men required less of Barney in terms of his self-fulfillment than it does of those men of the post-Stonewall generation, those participants of the Gay and Lesbian Mardi Gras, those consumers of the modern gay merchandising dominating *Outrage* and *Campaign*, Australia's monthly gay magazines.

Barney did not experience the difference between the moments of recognition of homoerotic interests and "coming out," that moment of telling the world that one is "gay." For him there was neither a single moment of recognition of difference, nor a single instance when he started living a gay life. The whole process unfolded, it was an evolution, not a drama. When questioned, he registered the only differences between being homosexual and being heterosexual as, first, not having a family and, second,

---

[4] "Stonewall" is a shorthand term for a week of civil riots in New York City beginning on June 27, 1969, regarded as the birth of the modern gay liberation movement.

"not much at all any more," since the antidiscrimination laws (in relation to homosexuality) were enacted in New South Wales in 1982. This measured the extent of his gay awareness, and it is not to be sneezed at: how many gay men of his generation would be in Neighbourhood Watch, let alone tell the local police representative that he was gay?

There was a larrikin (a likable lout) in Barney. There is a phrase that also comes to mind in thinking about Barney's sexuality: *doing what you can get away with.* There was no existential concern with the sexual self and fulfillment through orgasm; but of a life lived in which there was also sex, and because his sexual interest was in men and because men are readily willing to engage in sex, he has simply had more sex than many men experience.

∽

(So what is happening with your sex life now?)

Just Mrs. Palmer and her five daughters.

By the second interview Barney's sex life was almost nonexistent. There was still a spark of interest in anybody cute and in the sometime boyfriend, M (who had become a thirty-four-year-old alcoholic with a proclivity for pills), with whom he occasionally still had sex. Sex with M conformed to Barney's usual wicked and "macho" mode:

(When you do have sex, what sort of sex do you have? What do you do, or what have you been doing over the last year or two?)

Not much at all, not much at all. But basically, well, with a friend I spoke about, um, he, basically, has always been 100 percent active, you know — ah, not active, sorry, passive. So I ride her. I told her — I said, if that asset of yours ever fails, I says, you're history. So don't lose it. Remarkably, he's seen a lot of traffic and he's still tight.

This was a glimpse of the old Barney, the wicked one, the same change of gender. He returned to a flicker of wickedness one more time when he unwittingly confirmed another of the consequences of gay body culture and age on an older gay man: "No, I wouldn't give you tuppence for a sauna. Although I must admit that saunas are good. You get into those dark corners and they don't know who you are, and you do get a bit of a feel."

For Barney, AIDS has added a considerable heaviness to the dilemmas he was already experiencing as an aging working-class gay man. As noted anthropologist Eric Michaels said in his remarkable biographical account of his fight with AIDS:

What a terrible psychic violence something like AIDS must wreak on most gays — and has perhaps done to me, although my analysis seems to offer a particular exemption for my case on this account, if only to rationalise and distance myself from the sad fact that I expect never again to engage in those caresses of the body which sustained and defined me for most of my adult life. (1990: 100–101)

Barney indicated that he still practiced anal intercourse without a condom with M, withdrawing before ejaculation, but there was some doubt about the success of this. The extraordinary thing is that this was probably how Barney became infected in the first place.

Barney had already made significant lifestyle changes by 1984 when AIDS became a big issue. He was still in the long-term relationship with P at that time. They decided to be monogamous and were so for a year. Then they broke up, and Barney pursued sex only with casual partners:

No, it wasn't "safe" sex during that time and, er, I asked down at the clinic and they said: "Oh, you know, if you give it, you haven't got much chance of catching it."

(You mean, if you're doing the fucking?)

Yeah. If you're butch, you haven't got much chance of catching it. So you don't know, do you? . . . Then you hear from [the clinic] that it's dangerous if you don't use a bloody condom, you know. So what do you do? And it's only speculation with the clinic.

(Do you reckon they're not certain?)

Well, they're not certain. If somebody gets screwed, kind of thing, they pull out, right, they don't [then] go and take a test.

By "clinic" he meant the main HIV testing site for gay men in Sydney at that time, and it would be an awful irony if they had indeed given him incorrect advice.

This quotation reveals something of the struggle Barney has had with HIV/AIDS. It may be that he did practice withdrawal and did not think of himself as being in danger in those days. He had tested HIV antibody seronegative a few times while having sex using withdrawal, and as a result of inappropriate, unclear, or misinterpreted information about that sex practice, it appears that he was infected. He was, in a way, retelling his own tale—an ongoing sense-making exercise for him, something that has been carried over into his understanding of his own state of health.

### AIDS and Being HIV Infected

Barney was HIV seronegative at the time of my first contact with him in a survey being undertaken as part of a large-scale HIV/AIDS research project, but had seroconverted by the time of the first interview. He was convinced that his was a case where seroconversion took place a couple of

years after infection, because he steadfastly maintained he had done nothing "unsafe" in the interim, and his partner was still seronegative. (It must
be pointed out that such a delayed seroconversion is extremely rare.)

Barney's knowledge of HIV/AIDS was fairly good on the whole, but
his language was revealing: he talked of having T-cells "going up" to 300
when he meant down, and of the main HIV testing clinic being a better
place to be tested because they did "all" the tests and a "thorough" test. Of
HIV he said: "I think it's more like a syphilis bug, you know, that will hide
in the body and then come out." There was a strong suggestion of imperfect knowledge, of a tendency to get things approximately right, or upside
down, or confused. This impression was confirmed at the second interview, which revealed that Barney did not have a clear understanding of his
deteriorating health.

At the first interview he claimed that being positive was having no great
effect on him. By the second things had changed. The death of his ex-lover/
housemate, P, in late 1991 had been quite a shock. P's state of health had
been a bit confusing for Barney, and with his characteristic approximation
he told me that P had "debenture" (dementia), and that it was P's "I don't
care" attitude that had led to the deterioration. Yet he also suspected a little
medical chicanery: "Ah no, no, I think something funny went on at [hos-
pice] you know, 'cause they give them these drugs and things and I think
it hurries the process along. So I don't know." Given Barney's precarious
health, the prospect of a premature death, the memory of conceivably inaccurate information concerning HIV transmission, and the possibility of
medical malpractice, one might think this would have induced in him a fair
degree of skepticism concerning the health professionals he dealt with, but
this was not the case.

The date of the second interview had been postponed because of the
house fire and because Barney had ended up in hospital with what he
simply called pneumonia:

(Do you know what kind of pneumonia it was? Did they tell you?)

Oh, yes, they did—don't ask me the name of it.

It was *pneumocystis carinii pneumonia* (PCP); this meant that Barney had
finally progressed to clinically defined AIDS. Aware of Barney's inaccurate
understanding of HIV transmission, I was curious to see how he understood
his deteriorating health. Was it also a case of approximate knowledge?

(Can I ask you a little bit about your health? Have you got a regular doctor
who is monitoring your health, 'cause you said, I think, in that questionnaire you'd been getting regular tests and things?)

Yeah, down at [the AIDS clinic], yeah, yeah.

(What sort of things are they checking for?)

Oh, just to see how you are and what you are and do you want anything, you know. Um [pause] what could I say, yeah, and if you've got any complaints or anything they'll look at it, you know, and if not they'll send you off to a specialist. See, I had this rash and they have got a dermatologist clinic down there now and I went to them, and they were excellent. When I went to the local doctor and he said, oh yeah, I think it's lice or something, you know.

(So you think they are much better down there?)

Yeah. And I went to a professor up at [a large public teaching hospital] and he gave me some ointment and that wasn't doing any good at all.

(Have you got a regular doctor at the clinic?)

Yeah, yeah, yeah.

(And how often do you go?)

Oh, I'm due to go again, and I'll just ring up and make an appointment. About once a month or so.

(So they've been looking after you for a while now, haven't they?)

Yeah, yeah, yeah. Well, the reason I went there in the first place back in '85, I think, I went to them originally, was because it was all the advertising and that was the place to go. They're the experts you know.

Barney is not an ignorant man, nor is he stupid. He is poorly educated and, like many working-class Australians of his generation who left school with few formal learning skills, experience has been his greatest teacher (Dowsett et al. 1981). Whatever he has been told by the clinic or doctors about his health and a disease that has a pattern of infection and progression only recently understood (and still disputed in some places) was mediated by an uncritical belief in modern medicine and by his usual way of making sense:

(Do you read up much about it or do you try to find out as much about it as you can?)

Oh no, no, you'd go mad if you started to read every bit, but you do hear bits and pieces, you know.

(Who is your own source of information, do you think, about that sort of stuff—friends?)

Oh, no, different people. Even the news coverage, you know.

(Right. Do you read the gay press: the *Sydney Star Observer* and— ?)

Yeah, when I get it.

(You don't always get it?)

Well, I haven't gone chasing it for a while.

The dilemma for HIV educators with reference to prevention interventions among men like Barney is to understand their learning and information-mediation processes, and recognize that it is unlike those of the educated professionals the educators work with and for. The dilemma is exacerbated in the case of HIV treatment information and its part in assisting better self- and medical management of the disease among those infected.

How do we begin to provide programs for Barney, a man given to approximations, exaggerations, tall tales, inattention to detail, and clichéd understandings? He is a working-class man. His life has been lived by "getting by"—in his work, his knowledge, his satisfaction. The models of safe sex exemplars—modern gay men and model PLWHAs—used in gay community agencies are so embedded in that milieu that they are of no use to him, and to create from his approximations a resource for his education and survival would be very difficult.

Another dimension of this problem was his uninformed criticism of the support services available to infected gay men:

Well, I don't know, I think there are too many of them. You pick up the *Sydney Star* [*Observer*] and there is a support group for this and a support group for that, and it would be better if it was all under one umbrella, much rather, than being scattered out, right. Um, just like any association, when they're scattered out you've got presidents, chairmen, and what for have you. And most people could be used if they were all under one umbrella. Instead of having a dozen, say, people in charge, you could have one person in charge, that gives you another eleven to do more . . .

(So you haven't been to any of those sorts of things?)

No, no.

(Nothing interested you about them?)

No, not really, not really. Oh I've read about them, support groups and what for have you. Oh yeah, just another meeting. 'Cause I've been involved in meetings and committees all my life, so why should I waste me bloody time listening to a bunch of fags that they don't know what they are talking about.

The resentment expressed in these comments has been building for a long time. The net consequence of this growing estrangement may be the risk that Barney will not obtain the best possible health care as he deteriorates. He used the words "AZT," "ddC," "ddI" (antiviral treatments for HIV infection), but knew only that AZT slows down the growth of the virus and that "Baclin" (his mispronunciation of "Bactrim," an important antibiotic in AIDS prevention), which he was taking sporadically, stops his "chest infection."

This represents the limit of Barney's knowledge of his HIV infection and its possible treatment options. He was quite uninformed compared with gay men working in HIV/AIDS agencies and organizations and those living within the gay community itself.

In terms of self-management of his health Barney was as resourceless as he was ignorant:

I've been looking at this, whether you do the right things or don't do the right things. Ah, and they talk about eating this and eating all the right nourishing things and everything, but, yet I've known people who have done all that and they've gone down the spouts quicker than I've gone down the spouts, you know, because sometimes I abuse the food. Sometimes I go without a meal or something you know. I try not to now. Um, a lot of these people go jogging, physical and lift all this stuff.

(You're not interested in that?)

Oh, I could show my energy in better places [meaning sex].

A few final questions about other gay HIV/AIDS services and organizations elicited more of the same detachment and resentment:

I've heard a little bit about the Quilt.

(What have you heard about it?)

Oh, I don't know, I've heard the name or something. Oh, yeah, yeah, yeah, of people making these things and designs to put on the Quilt.

(What do you think about that idea?)

Oh, I don't know, I don't know. It's definitely not me, you know. You get a thousand people who've got names on it and you know. How big is it going to end up and where is it going to go finally?

(What about something like ACT-UP? Have you heard of them?)

Ah, yes. I've heard of them but I don't know a great deal about them. I don't know. Actually, P got something sent to him about ACT-UP the other day something. I didn't take much notice of it. But evidently, they do fight to get drugs into the country, saying why can't we get AZT or ddC in or something. What's the bloody hold-up. I believe they're all right in that respect.

Barney's situation is similar to others in this study who had failed to develop the social relations that could sustain them in their fight with AIDS. Barney's increased exclusion from the emerging gay community from the late 1970's onward had finally come home to roost, not only in his bitter accusation that the gay community had failed to support him when he needed it, but also in the sad fact that he had not obtained the best possible care and support services available in Sydney.

⌒

Barney Sherman was still alive at the time of writing but may not be so for much longer. His tale is unremarkable in many ways, yet his life history and his fight with HIV reveal much that concerns this study. His life history raises questions about the historical formation of a homosexually active man and about the contribution of sexual experience to the creation of a sexuality. His sexual sense of self, his subjectivity, cannot be reduced to being someone who was "camp" in an increasingly "gay" world, but clearly reveals that the relationship of a man of his generation and class to the transformation of homoerotic desire produced during the 1970's and 1980's is problematic and far from satisfactory.

Barney offers, then, a starting point for the evaluation of the gay liberation project and in particular of its creation of a vibrant gay community. What is Barney's place in that history? What will be its place in his life now that HIV/AIDS is drawing a cordon around his social and sexual possibilities, and as his health, mental and physical, deteriorates in the context of his increasingly uncomprehended isolation? What can he teach us about the lacunae in the conceptualization of gay community that underlie the HIV/AIDS strategy in Australia (and elsewhere) and the effort to stop the epidemic?

Finally, is Barney just an exception? It is possible that his life story is simply about someone being born in the wrong time in history. Or are younger homosexually active men having the same dilemmas? Is Barney really a quite ordinary Australian gay man like many others after all?

# 2

# Finding Out

There was this blond at the gym—tall, slender, with broad shoulders and long, muscular legs. Dave always made sure that he was in the changing room when this guy had finished working out. And there he was, standing, taking off his sweat-wet T-shirt as Dave sat down on the bench opposite. Slowly, gracefully like a dancer, this hunk bent over to take off his sneakers, revealing thighs to die for. Dave was pretending not to notice, and trembling so much that he knotted the laces on his gym shoes and couldn't get the damn things untied. The blond slipped out of his tight cotton shorts and then slowly turned to face Dave, completely naked. Gorgeous! He threw a glance at Dave's swelling groin, and offered a slight smile as he leaned forward to grab a towel from the shelf behind Dave's head. As the smell of that body reached him, Dave felt the heat rise in his cheeks.

The guy headed for the showers, leaving Dave fumbling with a glued-on singlet and an embarrassing lump in his lycra as he raced to undress and follow. Dave pushed the door open to a darkened room filled with steam. He couldn't see as he edged his way toward the noise of the shower pole, its four nozzles streaming hot water. Just as Dave got wet all over, he felt a hand on his nipple. A face emerged from the steam and kissed him squarely on the mouth and then slowly turned him around. Dave felt one hand running lightly over his arse, its probing fingers sending shivers up and down his spine. Dave glanced over his shoulder to see a hand pump a pulsing cock as the blond inched closer. Dave reached around and gave him the soap.

At this point yours truly, the intrepid social researcher, reach for my trusty instrument and enter the shower:

Would you please fill out the following survey?
How often, now or at any time in the last six months, with either a regular or casual partner or partners, have you engaged in any of the following sexual practices? You may answer each question: "Never," "Sometimes," "Often," "No Response."
First one—oral-oral contact. Ah, no—I mean kissing.
"Often," good. Wet and deep? Or dry and light? Righto. Now, oral-anal contact.

Err, rimming—roseleafing—tonguing him out—licking his bottom! Aha. Insertive? Were you the insertive one? Did you stick your tongue in?

Right, you were the one with the bottom. Okay. Ah, no—I don't have a box for "it felt great"!

Next is "Anal intercourse"—right, you guessed it, the F word!

Okay. With or without a condom?

*Without* a condom, but no ejaculate? No, semen—spunk—did you cum inside him? You do know that you're not supposed to do that, don't you?

Mm. Promise?

Okay. Was this a regular or casual partner?

Regular, right. How often do you have unprotected anal intercourse with this boyfriend? He's not your boyfriend? I thought you said he was a regular partner. He is, but—I see—you meet with him regularly for sex, but he's not your boyfriend. He was once—for two weeks—about a year ago—mm.

Last question now. Do you use your HIV-antibody test result in negotiating sexual events with your reg—ah, your boyfriend, or—your—um—any person you have sex with regularly, or with any other casual partners?

You don't have casual partners. You always know their name. Really? How interesting!

No—"negotiate" means talk about what you're going to do in bed—whether you'll be "safe" or not. No—it doesn't have to be in bed, you're right there.

You don't talk—I see—you just writhe around and moan a lot and you—ah—poke it here or there—wherever it fits.

Many thanks for your time.

I am sure my research will be a successful contribution to HIV prevention: those two men will probably never have sex again!

Since the early 1980's, gay men through their organizations and personal efforts have been trying to ensure that men use condoms in such moments, and if they do not actually engage in anal intercourse then they follow the other safe sex guidelines. Researchers, determined to document the changes in sexual behavior that many knew were occurring, have doggedly pursued such men, asking them to recount their sex lives over the last month, half-year, year, or lifetime, on various scales and measures, and inventories.

But do we really understand sexual behavior change? More important, are researchers really in a position to assess it and advise those trying to produce such change, when there is an obvious difference between sexuality as it is experienced and sex research as it is done? This story points not just to the incongruity between method and setting, but to one between the conceptualization of sex and sexual desire in much social research and sex as it is actually experienced.

## The Dangers of Positivism

In recent years most research into homosexuality has been either historical or set within a psychosocial framework derived from classical sexology and psychology. Positivism dominates much of this work, irrespective of its often clear desire to be pro-homosexual, or at least be anti-homophobic.[1] There is also a particular way in which this kind of research has dominated the HIV/AIDS social research agenda. Elsewhere I have argued that in the Australian context the dominance of behavioral and positivistic research in medicine and public health has made it very difficult to pursue even empirical work not based on positivist assumptions (Dowsett 1988, 1990a). For the sake of argument, this kind of work could be deemed as belonging to *sexology* or *sex research* and its scientific traditions.

In contrast, there has been considerable research in cultural studies and humanities that offers other analyses of homosexuality, but which most often has been concerned with history and the development of social theory. Sometimes this is called *humanistic* research, and much of it has been pursued in what could be termed "gay and lesbian studies." Judith Allen (1992) would all but restrict the site of theory development on homosexuality to this category of research. Janice Irvine (1990) describes the contribution of (North American) sexology more generously, allowing the tension and conflict within the sexology project itself to emerge as a reminder of the historical construction of the frameworks researchers adopt and sometimes uncritically employ in research on sex and sexuality. This is not to detract from Allen's strong case that, along with feminism (and led by it to a certain degree), gay and lesbian studies have offered a substantive and significant critique of the so-called "scientific" project of investigating that phenomenon, "homosexuality," over the last 150 years.

This critique has called attention to some consequences of that kind of positivistic science—aversion therapy, chemical castration, the equation of homosexuality with mental illness, and so on—and to the connection between scientific discourses on sexuality and the political and sociolegal consequences for homosexually active people. Early gay liberation activists

---

[1] Positivism is a worldview that dominated the physical sciences of the nineteenth century. Positivistic social science regards social life as observable in much the same way as rocks, chemicals, and star constellations are. It presumes that testable scientific laws can be inferred from social phenomena. Its preoccupation with cause and effect, quantifiability, rationality, and objectivity has led it to be bypassed by social theorists and researchers concerned more with discourse, politics, motive, symbol, culture, history, interpretation, and understanding.

offered considerable insight into the oppressive consequences of the overall scientific project in its challenge to psychiatry (Bayer 1981) and advanced the approachable idea of *self-* or *internalized* oppression (Hodges and Hutter 1974) to register the operation of powerful ideas and forces in shaping people's often detrimental beliefs and understandings about themselves.

Much of the work done to gain for homosexually active people a sense of centeredness and social equality has emerged from what might be called the "international gay history project," a synergetic effort across language and culture, although it is largely confined to the industrialized world. Some of this work is based on recent findings in comparative anthropology that suggest that sexuality is a culturally specific phenomenon.

Although the empirical work of historians, anthropologists, sociologists, and cultural theorists has vastly increased our understanding of homosexually active people, this increase in knowledge and the certainty it brings about the existence in history of "gay persons"—to use John Boswell's (1989) term—has not grown without a corresponding increase in positivistic, so-called scientific research, which has continued to attempt to reduce homosexuality to a set of characteristics of deviancy and manifestations of psychic or biological damage to be somehow repaired or rendered inoperable and noncontagious.

Much of this type of work lays claim to a certain kind of scientific method, and I am not going to navigate its twists and turns here. Michael Ruse (1988) documents very adequately the scientific gaze on homosexuality; Kenneth Lewes (1988) has performed the same valuable service with reference to psychoanalysis. The research documented by these commentators represents a particular view of science; one not shared by all claiming the label (for example, Bhaskar 1989). Here I am not concerned with the debate about science, the challenge of Thomas Kuhn (1962), or the claims of Marxism. But I do want to register the *incommensurability* (as Judith Allen uses Kuhn's term) of a particular kind of "scientific" approach to homosexuality and the humanistic effort, and query the part played by gay researchers and intellectuals in the production of such work.

This incommensurability is never more evident than in social research on HIV/AIDS, with its psychologistic emphasis on behavior, and its method dominated by large-scale survey technique and correlative analyses of individual characteristics. The questionnaire parodied earlier—which came from my own research team's early work, I might add—reduces sexual interaction to a technical inventory, its sequence related more to researchers' fastidious minds that to the sex acts themselves. Why is it that "watersports," "scat," "fistfucking," and "sadomasochism" are always grouped in the same section of the inventory? Who decided the terms used? Try this one on for size: "brachioproctic eroticism" (Donovan, Tindall, and Cooper 1986), meaning "fistfucking"; or another, again from my first involvement with HIV/AIDS research (Kippax et al., *Sustaining Safe Sex*, 1993) — "Anal intercourse (fucking) without ejaculating (cumming), no condom."

When renowned gay science-fiction writer Samuel R. Delany in a article on HIV/AIDS delivered an impassioned plea for "street talk" rather than "straight talk" (1991: 22), he was advocating not lay speech over jargon, but subcultural language forms over those of established or hegemonic discourse. But the language and rhetoric of research is only one side of the issue. It is the actual configuration of the sexual in much research that should cause alarm.

A good example of this scientific distortion of sexual life is the positioning of *anality* in much positivistic research. The confusion between the sexual possibilities of the human body and the sexual orientation of desire —namely, the notion that sodomy equals homosexuality—has underlined almost all accounts of homosexuality for at least a century. This confusion has now been compounded by the ease with which anal intercourse facilitates the transmission of HIV. In much research, particularly in HIV/AIDS, a man's interest in sex with men (that is, *being* homosexual) seems to be seriously confused with the pleasurable experience of anal sex (namely, *doing* sodomy), which heterosexual sodomites, male and female, also enjoy.

Recognition of the historical collapse of sodomy into homosexuality and the transformation of the sodomite into the homosexual are cornerstones of recent theoretical insights into sexuality (Weeks 1990; Foucault 1978). Yet these insights seem to have been ignored by HIV/AIDS researchers, who instead collect huge data sets on sex practices with scant regard to sexual meanings or pleasures. Not only do some respondents seem genuinely perplexed at having to recall their sexual activity in the time frames offered (which are then debated in endless articles on research method), but many struggle to recognize in the sequential inventories the complex interactions and sensations they experience in sexual activity. How often are respondents ever asked what it felt like? I am convinced that the accuracy and time frame question, as just one problem in current sex research, is less related to memory and reliability issues than to the alienation of research inventories from respondents' sexual experiences.

It must be said of recent work that in the search for a nonoppressive politics of HIV/AIDS, many researchers participate in the development of a non-sexuality-specific notion of *high-risk practices* (flying in the face of the historical elaborations referred to earlier). One consequence has been the creation of categorical absurdities: stratifications such as gay community-identified men, gay men, bisexually identified men, behaviorally bisexual men, other men-who-have-sex-with-men, exclusively heterosexual men, and finally men who are periodically one or any of the above. (This is almost a new Kinsey's seven-point scale, but one focused on a very confused interpretation of the relation between sexual identity and practice.)

The net result is a new, hasty continuum of male sexuality; an analytical "camel" on which we merely count the humps, but which is completely devoid of logical structure other than sexual difference (that is, the logic is *gender*). The seductiveness of gender in progressive social science obscures the worrisome effects of its deployment in such research. The relations of power that suffuse sexuality are completely lost in the search for those ideologically sound categories of practice among those still at risk.

Phrases such as "men who have sex with men" transmute into "men who have sex with women," or "men who have sex with women and men," ultimately tying all men together. Homosexual transmission of HIV becomes a simple variation in a unitary domain of *male* sexuality. This, first, ignores the subordinate position of homosexuality and the struggle of gay men (and lesbians) to resist the structural relation between heterosexuality and homosexuality. Second, it obliterates from view the struggles of gay communities with the HIV epidemic and foolishly conceals the massive contribution of "gay identity" and "gay community" to their tremendous success at prevention.

In tandem, the inexorable process of mainstreaming HIV/AIDS programs and services in most Western countries (which seemed to perturb so few at the 1992 Amsterdam conference) is producing, as one consequence, the "de-gaying" (as distinct from de-homosexualization) of HIV/AIDS. There is a trap in this and it is one of the researchers' own making: in an attempt to defuse homophobic responses to HIV/AIDS, an insidious form of heterosexism has emerged to rid research of an analysis of sexuality as a multidimensional structure of power and praxis affecting all lives, as a product of iterative cultural production, an accumulation of experiences and meanings. Instead, it reduces sexuality to a washed-out, one-dimensional, sketchy differentiation of practices and interests — merely individual preferences in a unitary domain, a program of graded and categorized delights.

This should not be a surprise; there is a long history of this conceptualization of sex. No researchers are more renowned for this model of sex research than Masters and Johnson (1966, 1970), whose famous work reduced sexual behavior to sequence and technique to the ludicrous point of comparing anal intercourse between men with that between men and women. This complete excision of all beyond the immediately observable and measurable marks sexology at its worst, and the support they lent the "homosexuality can be cured" quest has earned them significant, well-deserved criticism (see Irvine 1990). Masters and Johnson's (and Kolodny's) unfortunate contribution to the HIV/AIDS debate (1988) brought them into significant disrepute, in particular through their claim that HIV can be transmitted through casual contact, for example, on toilet seats. Perhaps this augurs the end of that particular paradigm in sexology. One is ever hopeful.

The participation of gay researchers in similar reductionist accounts of sexuality is not without its compassionate motivations; nor is it without its benefits. Nor do I stand outside this critique. But its inability with reference to HIV/AIDS to explain—*beyond a retreat to voluntarism alone*—changes in sexual behavior, the continued homosexual transmission of HIV, the complexity of infection patterns within relationships and among the newly homosexual, or the accusations of sexual marginalization made by PLWHAs within gay communities should alert researchers to the dangers of this positivistic, undertheorized approach, its niceties and its neatness, its lack of sweat, bump, and grind.

It is this lack of the relational character of sexual activity, the inattention to sexual meanings and their creation, an ignorance of the social constituents and contexts of sexual activity, which deprives much research of the answers so urgently required. Men in this study consistently refer to the importance of intimacy in anal sex, to emotional qualities in HIV/AIDS educational images, and to their need for relationships. This is not the researcher's variable "relationship status," but a complex ideological and emotional response to desire, oppression, and the pursuit of a homosexual life.

There is a need, therefore, for better science, for research that can take developments in social theory about sexuality and pursue empirically its investigation without falling into the traps of positivistic approaches to science or retreating into a phenomenological languor. The dilemma for the researcher is to inquire deeply and rigorously into the operation of desire without abstracting it, on the one hand, or making it concrete, on the other. These research paradigms, the so-called scientific and its psychosocial derivatives, reify sexuality and only allow one view on the object of their gaze as valid.

The humanistic tradition, however, has its own problems. One of the striking aspects of the 1987 Amsterdam conference was the lack of empirical research being reported on homoeroticism, its lived experience and constructed meanings, its rituals and relations, its discords and dangers, its artifacts and fantasies.

The formidable international gay history project seemed singularly unimpressed with the challenge to its unifying and convergent analyzing by theorists pursuing the essentialist/social constructionist debate. The endless search for gay generals, artists, nuns and priests, court officials, aristocrats, ancient Greeks, and so on (see, for example, Gerard and Hekma 1989), has been at least as obsessive and blinkered as much of the psychosocial work. Elements of the debate about whether homosexuality is essential or socially constructed have been accommodated to a certain extent (see Duberman, Vicinus, and Chauncey 1989), yet convergent universalizing tendencies remain.

Both kinds of research appeared in the *Journal of Homosexuality* during the 1970's and 1980's. The psychosocial work was preoccupied with, for example, the "Klein Sexual Orientation Grid" (Klein, Sepekoff, and Wolf 1985), the five-stage "Proposed Model of Lesbian Identity Awareness" (Chapman and Brannock 1987), or administering the "GAL Q" (Gay and Lesbian Questionnaire) to youngsters (Savin-Williams 1989). Similar work identified the contribution of "attention to mother's fashion" and "cuddliness" to parenting in the development of "sissies" (Green 1987), a six-stage model for analyzing the gay male couple (McWhirter and Mattison 1984), or the more impressive work of the later Kinsey Institute researchers (Bell and Weinberg 1978).

There is value in this work. Its descriptive detail is useful raw material and its contribution to legitimation of studies of homosexuality outside homophobic frameworks must be recognized. Its clear intent to move on and construct an objective and, therefore, unoppressive analysis of homosexuality must also be lauded. Yet there is a terrible normalizing tendency in much of this work—almost a plea for respectability—within which the sexuality of gay men and lesbians is sanitized and redeemed. In contrast, again in the realm of gay *practice*, the late distinguished gay photographer Robert Mapplethorpe's famous shot of himself as subject, photographed in full leather gear with the handle of a bullwhip inserted into his anus, offers a far more disturbing counterpoint to the naturalizing and normalizing tendencies of such humanistic research.

The dilemma remains: How should a researcher conceptualize homoeroticism in order to pursue it in research, without losing sight of the object itself, particularly when the object is moving so swiftly?

## Gay Sex and the Endless Transformation of Desire

From the start, gay men working on the ground in HIV/AIDS prevention believed that gay sexual behavior could be changed to prevent the spread of the virus. This belief has proved generally accurate, and the documented changes in gay men's sexual behavior show that there is a profound difference in the structuration of sex practices and sexual preference. If sex practices can be changed, then sexual experience is adaptive. And so, sexual feelings and meanings also are malleable. Once it is agreed that actual sexual sensation, experience, feeling, and meaning are changeable, it must also be recognized that homosexuality is profoundly *social*, influenced by history, culture, and experience: it is something we ourselves make.

Beyond that, it must be remembered that gay sex is perverse; gay sex is different. The physical sensation of male-to-male sex is different from sex between women or between women and men. The combination of possibilities for sensation and pleasure in two male bodies is quite different from other combinations available. It is clear that the physical possibilities of human bodies play a definite part in what we call sexual pleasure; a prostate is a prostate and uniquely male. To deny this basic biological contribution would be foolish. But more than physical sensation is involved. Gay sex encompasses the interaction of sensation and meaning unlike any other kind of sex. Every man knows when he engages in anal intercourse with another man that he is engaging in something perverse. It is or was illegal. It is still often severely frowned upon, disdained, or persecuted.

Early Australian HIV/AIDS survey work on gay men indicated that, although most gay men had tried anal sex, only about half actually practiced it. Although anal intercourse was rated as extremely pleasurable, it was fellatio and mutual masturbation that were practiced almost universally (Connell and Kippax 1990). Nevertheless, almost all gay men consider anal sex the symbolic center of gay identity. It is central to the social definition of male homosexuality and, therefore, claims its erotic core. Beyond its unique physical pleasures, it is perhaps this symbolic stature of anal sex which acts as a crystallizing force on male homosexual desire.

Yet it is clear that homosexual sex is more than anal sex and mobilizes other sensual possibilities; it extends to contextual domains, historically constituted sexual events instantiated anew—all laced with multiple manifestations beyond the narrowly defined sex acts themselves.

The sexological tradition has proven mostly incapable of making the connection between, for example, a counting of orgasms and the concept of *sexuality* more likely to be used by more humanistic social science. There is a new task awaiting researchers: how to investigate homosexuality as a practice, a pleasure, a culture, an icon, a fantasy, a threat. Grappling with the motivation and operation of homoeroticism requires a keener sense of the "content" of sexuality as being far more diverse than the sex acts themselves, far more unsettled and seemingly contradictory than that captured within the binaries of homosexual/heterosexual, male/female, gay/straight, and as something capable of endless transformation, representation, and elaboration.

This is a task not peripheral to the HIV epidemic either, but central to the understanding of social process in sexual behavior and the ever-changing responses of homosexually active men to HIV/AIDS.

## HIV/AIDS and Research

The HIV epidemic has provided social science in Australia and elsewhere with a series of challenges and dilemmas. HIV infection and AIDS are not simply diseases; the epidemic has become an arena for significant debate about the formulation of knowledge about HIV/AIDS and the right to speak about it (Treichler 1988; Coxon 1988; Horton with Aggleton 1989; Weeks 1989). Too often issues within this debate go unnoticed by those who take for granted the privilege accorded academic and political discourse.

 Medical and quasi-medical discourse has achieved a hegemonic position in Western society not only in medical matters but also in many other fields of human endeavor: sexual activity, concepts of public health, ideas of human normality (to include mental well-being), and so on. Other, nonmedical disciplines have similar capacities for powerful consideration of human behavior, notably psychology, and to a lesser extent history and sociology. As the range of issues affected by HIV/AIDS has expanded, these nonmedical disciplines have been increasingly called on to offer assistance. However, these disciplines have often found it difficult to make inroads into the institutions and procedures that govern national AIDS programs, revealing an implicit hierarchy of knowledge and the relativities of power within which even the privileged academic disciplines exercise their influence in social life.

Others have analyzed the developments and contests that marked the political response to HIV/AIDS (in Australia—Reid 1988, Ballard 1989; in the United States—Altman 1986, Shilts 1988; in Great Britain—Watney 1987b, Strong and Berridge 1990). The axes of these debates have been: a public-health versus a narrow medical response to the epidemic; struggles within medicine itself between epidemiology, virology, venereology, immunology, and community health; conflict at times between health professionals, public servants, and politicians over political control of the national AIDS efforts; jousting over the participation and influence of the community sector, in Australia, particularly, its well-organized and politically skilled gay communities; a discernible absence of serious debate over the very obvious part played by the media (Watney 1988b; however, see Lupton 1994).

Few in Australia have analyzed the debate between medical and social science to determine the relative importance, nature, and amount of the contribution each can make to efforts to minimize the impact of the HIV epidemic. It is within this context that any social science research related to HIV/AIDS must operate and contest the definition of issues and the conceptual domain being mapped out.

The nongovernmental sector (often, but not only, the gay communities) has resisted political solutions to public-health issues that do not recognize concerns such as discrimination, homophobia, sexual politics, and community consultation and participation in decision-making. And the community sector has had considerable impact on some public-health procedures such as notification of HIV infection and AIDS, and contact-tracing and partner-notification practices. As possible treatments for HIV infection have become available there has been substantial debate about the drug companies and their economic interests.

PLWHAs have rejected the traditional (passive) role of the patient; other medically untrained people affected by the epidemic have mounted a collective challenge to standard medical procedures such as treatment, drug-trial, and drug-evaluation protocols (see Ariss 1990). These issues, long on the agenda of feminists, workers' health activists, and the community health movements, have been brought sharply into focus by the HIV epidemic (Ballard 1988; Altman and Humphery 1989; Hicks 1989; Lloyd 1990).

It is in this context that the contribution of social science research to the Australian HIV/AIDS effort should be examined. Justice Michael Kirby (1989), erstwhile member of the World Health Organization Global Commission on AIDS, has noted the apparent failure of social science to make a significant contribution to HIV/AIDS research. In mitigation, he comments on the small expenditures in most developed countries on social research and the failure of governments to encourage such contributions. Yet all the social sciences have a lot to offer. In particular, social science, as distinct from more narrowly defined *behavioral* sciences, which are customarily part of medical discourse, are able to offer a range of distinct bodies of theory and research methodologies less often used in the medical sciences, but which require different research structures to support them.

There is an informal but rather rigid division of labor between HIV/AIDS prevention and what might be termed *care/support* issues, paralleling the medical/social split. The prevention of HIV infection, called at one time the "education vaccine [*sic*]" by the Commonwealth Minister for Health most responsible for Australia's initial response to HIV/AIDS, Dr. Neal Blewett, was seen as having been a more appropriate issue for social research to investigate. As a result, social science has made very few inroads into care/support issues in the last few years. This disappointing level of activity is reflected in steadily more demanding calls from PLWHAs for research into their educational and social needs (Ariss 1991).

The social/medical science split influences the institutional arrangements of research as well (Ballard 1990; Dowsett 1990a), producing a failure to involve many disciplines that could offer broader perspectives — anthropology,[2] adult and community education, philosophy, politics, media studies, mass communications, and sexology — to name a few. One effect of this narrow conception of social research has been a dearth of new research on gay and homosexually active men.

⌇

Sociological research attempts to move beyond a conceptualization of the individual and his or her responses to the world to a collective and societal analysis. Personal activity and response are always based in social dynamics. This is more than a simplistic view of the person in context; it is a study of the mutual production of both persons and societies. A sociological focus attributes to individual action only part of the responsibility for the unfolding of a life. Sociology seeks to understand how individuals live their lives within highly complex, historically constituted, *social relations*. It recognizes that history and culture produce and shape the potentials and constraints within which individuals live their lives. It recognizes that and seeks to understand how human actions and relations are embedded in *social structures* that provide both the patterning of human action and the tools for understanding their meaning. All human action then is both constituted within, and in turn constitutes, these social structures.

The "sociological imagination" (Mills 1959) allows a breadth of concerns not dissimilar to those of anthropology and history. There is a focus on social process rather than individual development or progress; a moni-

---

2 This is not only an Australian problem; see Bolton 1989.

toring of collective effort; a utilization of theory that describes the operation of societies with concepts such as class, power, gender, the state; a reliance on historical analyses that recognize the contingent nature of present-day explanations and awareness about reality. There is also a perspective on understanding the role of knowledge itself and its production—that it is not static, absolute, or neutral, but challengeable, changeable, and provisional.

This is particularly important in HIV/AIDS, where issues such as sexuality need to be explained not as attributes of individual will but in terms that permit rapid intervention at a collective level to change sexual behavior. It is in the area of sexuality studies (in Australia in particular) that sociology has made most of its contribution to HIV/AIDS research with reference to the transmission of HIV. Such research has drawn on the work of modern gay liberation theorists and activists, and from second-wave feminism and revisited sexology. Less often utilized in Australia have been studies of the state, cultural studies, the sociology of deviance, and the sociology of knowledge.

A knowledge of the history and structure of human sexual activity is needed as a context for understanding what is happening in a world in which sexually transmissible diseases, such as HIV infection, have become so widespread. For many, sex seems a knowable, definable entity; its parameters are the sexual activities and the relations within which we pursue sex. Some people talk about their sex lives with ease. As a consequence researchers can readily obtain detailed sexual information. But what is often obtained is a description of activities, the frequency of practices, and a counting of partners, which offer only some guidance on the possible arena where problems such as HIV/AIDS are being played out.

Large-scale descriptive surveys of sexual behavior have been given a tremendous boost in the last ten years, so that governments might estimate the possible impact of the HIV epidemic. This kind of research assumes that sexuality is a readily knowable thing, accessible to cognitive process, capable of abstraction, intelligible in language, and describable. The meaning of sex is deemed irrelevant to an inventory of the practices themselves. Rarely are subjects asked about the circumstances, their emotional and relational context, the significance of the events, and the fantasies behind them. All of these have a profound effect on the *choreography* of sexual practice and are important in any understanding of sexual behavior.

Such research assumes a sharp difference between the observer and the object of research. It ignores a more *reflexive* approach where those being researched are part of the research team, and where learning is linked to action. Reflexive research recognizes that the research object is not static, a photograph that is once taken and forever captured. This is important in a situation where community action has been relied on to prevent the transmission of HIV.

Contemporary social theory offers a view of sexuality wherein sexual activity and meaning is seen as historically and culturally specific. For example, the word and concept "homosexuality" does not exist among those New Guinea societies where male-to-male sex is a compulsory part of all male adolescents' initiation (Herdt 1981). Western concepts of sex do not fit that culture. An understanding of sexuality is not found in the outward appearance of sex acts to be counted and documented. Sexuality has an internal structure, a history and a cultural production within which sexual experience takes place, is organized, and is understood. The concept, sexuality, is itself a modern invention, emerging in nineteenth-century European culture (Foucault 1978). "Sexuality" is not a fact but an artifact of life.

A sociological approach is concerned with this relationship between experience, understanding, and structure. It seeks to explain, not just what we do sexually, but why and how our choices of partners and practices are formed. This involves not just counting the frequency of the sex act but understanding the experience of sexual engagement. It seeks to explain the shaping or limiting of choice and action and the resistance to that constraint. For example, the resistance of gay communities to criticism of all homosexual acts regardless of their relation to HIV transmission represents another moment in a social dynamic of sexuality. This resistance was not only a political struggle by gay communities but a personal sexual response by gay men as they dealt with a growing awareness of the epidemic.

The actions of the individual are only intelligible in relation to a social analysis. Activity seen often as external background to the person and his or her response to society and culture becomes an integrated part of a social analysis; it is seen as the reality to be investigated and not just its context. This is what a focus on the social means, and this is why social science is different from behavioral science. It is this perspective that sociology can bring to sexuality and to HIV/AIDS.

A second feature of the sociological gaze is a focus on collectivities rather than individuals, which permits the development of strategies that utilize collective patterns of behavior and practice as the basis for conceptualizing action. Understanding the operation of collective action and its structure is crucial to HIV/AIDS prevention, because of the impact of the epidemic in Australia (and in many other countries) among identifiable subcultures, for example, gay communities and clusters of injecting drug users. Theory about the structuring of collective social and sexual practice enables us to comprehend the dynamics of what are sometimes simplistically called "norms," a term remarkably void of analytical thought.

A norm is simply a social "biopsy" performed at a given moment, which is then frozen for later examination, the body (politic) having moved on. It "represents" nothing more than the state of play at a second in history observed in its hegemony and/or its dominance, and must, as a result, ignore the contest in action. The norm is a concept that ignores the actuality of domains of contested power operating in the structuring of relations in any society. As a result, the notion of subcultural norms is an oxymoron.

The very findings from so many surveys of the changes in sexual behavior among gay men reveal a wonderful paradox: if sexuality were such a constraint, an individualized fetish, an Oedipally fixed concern, as conventional wisdom would have it, how could so many gay men change their sexual behavior, both practices and relations, so quickly? Further, if modern, postmodern, anti-homophobic, or other progressive theory could easily apprehend *abstractly* these sexual changes, why was such theory of so little use to the HIV/AIDS activists and workers dealing with the epidemic on the ground?

In order to address these epistemological and methodological issues with reference to homosexuality in social analysis, I chose a specific method of inquiry—the life-history method—to obtain the detail required to locate the analysis at a deeper level of comprehension. I was keen to inquire empirically into homoeroticism in the era of AIDS, to subject theory to a good dose of fact. But I was also keen to avoid the more positivistic and schematic approach to sex derived from the psychosocial tradition. This study was conceived as one that would rest on a large amount of detailed information from a small number of men, intensely scrutinized to glean from individual detail the social character of the process and experience of becoming homosexual and being homosexual within the HIV epidemic and AIDS.

## The Life-History Method

The life-history method is common nowadays in the social sciences, yet still causes controversy in research circles, especially those whose claim to science relies heavily on issues of quantifiability, generalizability, reliability, and validity. Researchers working in HIV/AIDS know only too well the ongoing debate between the disciplines about the scientific contributions to fighting the epidemic (see Horton with Aggleton 1989; Patton 1990). But we should not confuse a debate centered on objectivity and subjectivity with a debate about research method, that is, a debate about "quantitative" versus "qualitative" method. It must be conceded, however, that it is usually on this latter axis that the struggle acts itself out.

The clinical case history is a classic example of this confusion. Medical practitioners frequently publish reputable papers in refereed journals based on very small numbers of clinically observed cases. In 1990 Lifson et al. published a paper documenting HIV seroconversions in gay men, related, it seems, exclusively to receptive oral intercourse with swallowed ejaculate. Given the ongoing unresolved debate about the likelihood of HIV transmission through oral-genital sex, this was a sensational finding. The article, however, was based on two cases, and although the authors' conclusions were properly cautionary, the example demonstrates that the chief concern need not always be the sampling method and sample size. (Indeed, it has been said that Freud invented psychoanalysis essentially on only one case—himself!)

The case history is the primary mode of medical reasoning. Medical practitioners use a combination of experience, training, information, and knowledge of the patients and their quirks to make considered judgments about treatment. This is not scientific method as such, but a combination of training, experience, and professional reasoning. It could be argued that, beyond the clinical domain, most medical knowledge is actually generated in more rigorous procedures: clinical trials, behavioral surveys, epidemiological research, and so on. Yet it is important to acknowledge the intimate and productive relationship between these scientific *research* modes and the more intuitive, clinical *practice* of medical care. It is in this closely structured relationship that we find the genesis of progress in combating disease.

There are other difficulties and blind spots in the scientific model. A very clear example was the notion early in the HIV epidemic that homosexuality itself caused AIDS (see Altman 1986). Gay men the world over "smelled a rat" instantly. Their challenge to this notion and its implied call for sexual abstinence led to the development of safe sex (Patton 1989; Watney 1988a). PLWHAs have been vocal on this kind of issue, uncovering logical inconsistencies in scientific and medical procedure and pointing out at times the highly subjective nature of much scientific work. Their success in transforming the procedures for developing new therapies is a tribute to the capacity of lay persons to unravel the scientific gobbledegook that often clouds good common sense. Science is not above human frailty and the operation of culture and history. The point here is that all research work is shaped by various intellectual relativities, emotional caveats, cultural cul-de-sacs, and that strange thing called judgment.

In the humanities there is far more recognition of the worth of work that documents and analyzes an individual life. Social and feminist histories in particular have made great strides in moving beyond the "Great Man" theories to analyzing the lives of ordinary people. Some of this work is document-based, as is much of the work done in reclaiming gay history; other work is more strictly biographical in form.

Biography is rightly regarded as a legitimate form of recording and analyzing the living of a life. Historical and literary biography is a distinct, recognized form and can range in quality from the sensationalist to the highly analytical. Reviews of biography often reflect the concern with authenticity and accuracy; yet the biographical form is widely regarded as a valid and valuable mode of knowledge production. Seldom does the issue of authenticity and accuracy in biography emerge more clearly than in the issue of homosexuality, as in David Marr's (1991) biography of Nobel laureate and homosexual author Patrick White. White himself resisted the label "gay" and was quite estranged from the gay community in Sydney; yet he remains a gay hero among the gay intelligentsia (Hurley 1991). The question remains: Which interpretation of White is correct? Was he a gay writer or a social analyst in fiction who happened to sleep with men? This is not an idle question: much of the sense of liberation of gay people has come in the last twenty years from uncovering the lives of predecessors in such biographical research.

Other recent and highly regarded theoretical work on sexuality by writers in the humanities, the social sciences, and cultural and literary studies has alerted us to the contingent nature of homosexuality as category, culture, discourse, experience, and meaning. It has been exciting to read much more of this work recently in new journals such as the *Journal of the History of Sexuality* and *GLQ: A Journal of Lesbian and Gay Studies*. These theoretical advances are not merely interpretive tools, offering new ways to analyze the same old thing. They argue that there is no fundamental homosexuality, no ever-present truth we can regard as certain and immutable; (homo)sexuality is in constant movement—a social construction on a shifting cultural and historical terrain.

It could be said that this is all very well, but there are viruses, arses, and cocks, and the meeting of these three is a scientific "fact"; it does not really matter how this fact is interpreted. There are lots of so-called scientific facts around at present about gay brains and the genetic bases of homosexuality and the like, which should alert us to the tentative nature of fact. Fact retains its status only until it is disproved.

There is no issue, to my mind, less able to be bent to a rigid scientific model, to be awarded the status of fact, than human behavior. The reductive nature of positivistic research on the behavior of gay and homosexually active men renders it much less productive in comparison with close-focus research methodology in general and semistructured interviewing and life-history work in particular.

Let me give an example.

In the early days of the epidemic, many North American studies, unlike Australian ones, found little evidence of a relationship between gay communities and success in changing sexual behavior. It was soon clear that this was a conceptual difference, not a factual one. In the early North American studies there was a tendency to conceptualize gay community participation in terms of questions such as "Are you a member of the gay community?" "Do you identify with the gay community?" "Are you involved in a gay community?" as well as identity-related questions such as: "Do you see yourself as gay, bisexual, heterosexual?" and so on.

This contrasted sharply with the first major Australian study, the Social Aspects of the Prevention of AIDS (SAPA) Project (Kippax et al., *Sustaining Safe Sex*, 1993), and its formulation of gay community participation as related sets of interlocking social, sexual, and politico-cultural practices. The SAPA researchers had found that "gay community attachment" was the most significant variable in predicting the greatest sexual behavior change toward "safe" sex practices, pointing to the *collective* and *social* nature of sexual behavior change (see also Kippax et al., "Gay Community," 1992).

Yet these measures are not the be-all and end-all of gay community attachment. In fact, they barely scratch the surface when it comes to understanding extent of practice, variability over time, issues of meaning and importance, even in measuring the contribution of items left out. The SAPA measures are precis of gay community life, useful sketches that alert us to contributing factors. They neither fully explain these men's lives within gay communities, nor do they alert us to everything we can utilize to maximize the potential of gay community attachment to change sexual behavior.

This is something often forgotten about questionnaire schedules—the questions left out or not thought of, the conceptual decisions affecting analyses, the technical decisions to omit items to achieve reliability, the influence of the order and labeling of items on respondents' hunches about researchers' information requirements. This so scientific of instruments, the questionnaire, is actually a highly subjective measure. The process of knowledge production embedded in the technique itself is deemed largely irrelevant as figures and "fact" fuse to become scientific "truth."

Such techniques also reduce sexuality to a list of discrete practices, unrelated to one another, from which we merely choose. Such a representation of sex lacks color, movement, and sinewy action. Many men in this study talked of the intimacy and pleasure of anal intercourse. It is this relational character of sexuality and the vibrancy of participation in a homosexual community that can be explored in life-history work, as we seek to understand how gay and homosexually active men got to where they are today, how they understand that process and themselves, what contributes to the history of their lives and to that of the friendship circles, social networks, institutions, and organizations that frame the living of lives and the loving of men. In recognizing the limitations of surveys and moving on from their findings to explore these issues in depth, this study seeks to contextualize (homo)sexual activity in a more historicized and sociological framework.

The information gained from life histories is not fact per se, but it is possible to verify some of the information obtained across subjects and in reference to other material at hand—local histories, related studies, similar material gleaned elsewhere, and other empirical work that has sharpened a theoretically informed vantage point. Facticity may not always be the major concern: the discursive framework used and the persona or subjectivity constructed in the interview itself will be revealing. Yet the issue of validity remains for a study based on life histories retrieved from interviews with "real" gay and homosexually active men. Martyn Hammersley (1992: 67ff.) argues for two criteria on which such work can be judged: validity and relevance. To this a third could be added: purpose.

Two claims to *validity* are offered here: first, case material is presented at some length to ensure that the reader through familiarity with detail can judge the conclusions drawn from and across individual cases; second, at times, the interview material is linked to data available from survey research (utilizing quantitative methodology) to establish any generalizability of findings.

*Relevance* can be judged from how well this study examines the empirical evidence relevant to the essentialist/social constructionist debate, whether it expands the methodology available to gay and lesbian studies and offers new ways to relate conceptual work to daily life, and what conclusions it draws about living a homoerotically focused life in the era of HIV/AIDS. The immediate impact of this study on such day-to-day responses to HIV/AIDS as activism, advocacy, and gay community AIDS service organizations may be scant at first, but I hope that it will offer, ultimately, some corrective to the mutual failure of theory and practice that has plagued gay and lesbian studies.

This study is a theoretically driven concern. I am not attempting here to explicate yet more gay history, investigate the lives of, for example, working-class gay men, or examine the plight of gay men infected with HIV, living with AIDS, or affected by either of these. I am concerned with the everyday construction of gay men's lives, with the ever-changing character of gay social and sexual relations and the reiteration and reinvention of homoerotic pleasure in sex and the manufacture of responses to these things by men, individually and collectively. My purpose here is to theorize beyond the individual to the emergent collectivity called "the gay community" and thereby offer a useful commentary on homoerotic desire in the era of AIDS.

A major resource in any study is the researcher him- or herself. If the issue of the social production of knowledge is to be recognized fully, then the fact that I am a gay man in early middle age with a long history of gay activism and, until recently, a full-time researcher working on HIV/AIDS social research of course has an impact on what information I seek and on shaping the starting point for analysis. My long familiarity with gay and, to a lesser extent, lesbian and feminist theory certainly colors my view of the world and the place of sexual politics within it. But my almost equally extensive history as a teacher in, and a researcher of, Australian education at many different levels offers another vantage point; one that conceptualizes HIV prevention, for example, in terms different from those, say, a health educator with a nursing background might employ.

Nineteen years of research using face-to-face interviews with a life-history focus as raw material for the study of social process develops skills in information retrieval, analysis, and interpretation and offers a dexterity in "reading" the texts generated by this method. This is not a simple claim to accuracy or veracity; it is a presentation of the intangible contribution of familiarity, no different from that provided by a statistician skilled at multiple regression analysis.

Ken Plummer's *Documents of Life* is the best guide to, and explanation of, life-history work, its purposes in humanistic research, its relation to other qualitative research techniques, and its value in the area of sexuality in particular. However, I do not develop the methodology used in this study from textbooks, but from experience. A brief history of the development of my approach to life-history interviewing should explain my fascination with it.

My first exposure to semistructured interviewing and life-history work came with reading a book by Richard Sennett and Jonathan Cobb, *The Hidden Injuries of Class* (1972), in which the effects of class inequality and conflict in the United States unfold through the authors' accounts of the internal struggles of men and women in their daily lives. It was a challenging account that maintained its focus on the object of its analysis—how an unequal society works—without reducing the people in it to ciphers or victims.

Inspired by this, in 1977, as part of the team of four people working in two different cities, I began interviewing fifteen-year-old high-school students, their parents, and their teachers in twelve of the richest (private) and poorest (public) schools in Australia. My colleagues and I were researching the effects of class and gender inequality and the involvement of the education system in the production of unequal educational outcomes (Connell, Ashenden, Kessler, and Dowsett 1982; Connell 1985). It was a moving and bruising experience. We met, or rather encountered, arrogant corporate bosses; aggressive, anti-gay factory workers; raving, "neurotic" parents; and idiosyncratic school principals. The major source of exasperation—and hope—was, however, the often wicked resilience of the kids. Although sexuality was not a top priority in that inquiry, it could not be ignored. One teacher asked a colleague for a date; one father felt up my leg during the preliminary interview; the woman on the team was sometimes subjected to sexism; and I, the only gay person in the team, investigated more nuclear families than I ever want to see again and sat often helplessly distanced from the obviously gay young men and women I met in every school. The strength of face-to-face interviewing in that study was reinforced by an early use of classroom surveys (replicating a previous study); the greater complexity and wealth of information obtained through the interview established its superiority to the classroom survey in no uncertain terms.

Since then I have interviewed teachers of English-as-a-second-language around Australia; subscribers to mainstream arts programs such as *Musica Viva*, *The Australian Opera*, and the *Sydney Film Festival*; artists employed by trade unions; and for the past ten years gay and bisexual men about their lives, their sexuality, their actual sexual activity, and their response to HIV and AIDS. Often the purpose of these interviews was not to obtain life histories per se; for example, there is no immediately clear and direct connection between life histories and teaching English to adult migrants. However, in all these various projects, some perspective on the lives of the subjects and how they got to be where they are has proven central to understanding the issue at hand.

There are other examples of interviewing I found inspirational: Studs Terkel's *Working: People Talk About What They Do All Day and How They Feel About What They Do* (1972); Rhonda Wilson's *Good Talk: The Extraordinary Lives of Ten Ordinary Australian Women* (1984). Good examples of more weighty theoretical work done using similar methods are Mike Donaldson's *Time of Our Lives: Labour and Love in the Working Class* (1991) and Rosemary Pringle's *Secretaries Talk: Sexuality, Power and Work* (1988). Pringle questions, inter alia, the explanatory power of "class," so often thought of as determining the position of men in the relations of production, but clearly inappropriate as a tool for examining that very large section of the workforce—secretaries. Pringle actually proposes that sexuality is more useful than gender and investigates the sexual *structuring* of work rather than the simplistic sexual (or gendered) division of labor. Using semistructured interviews with secretaries and their bosses, Pringle goes on to argue that work is much more sexually suffused than is taken into account in many social analyses of the workplace. (Were that analysis applied to a gay bar—one interviewee in this study worked in a gay bar— a picture of the barmen as "sex workers" might emerge.)

In "Live Fast and Die Young: The Construction of Masculinity Among Young Working-Class Men on the Fringes of the Labour Market" (1991) R. W. Connell used life-history work to investigate how gender processes work in the lives of marginalized working-class heterosexual men. This investigation also recruited a few men who had had sex with other men yet inhabited a largely heterosexual domain. The study proposed some quite radical ways of thinking about what are normally regarded in Australian parlance as "yobbos"—or, more formally, as delinquents—and reinforced Connell's (1987) work on gender as a social structure and the part played by sexuality within that structure.

This capacity of life-history interviewing to uncover more than is immediately obvious in the individual life makes it useful for investigating social processes. To quote Connell: "[The] life-history method is particularly relevant because of its capacity to reveal social structures, collectivities, and institutional change at the same time as personal life . . . [and] the interplay between structural fact and personal experience. . . . Where the research is based on a theory of social process we may speak of the *theorised life history* as a specific method" (1991: 143). This is not a process of theorization by generalization, but a systematic method of investigating the operation of social processes through the recounted experiences of individual lives.

### Research Themes

Some of the recurring themes or issues that guided this investigation emerged from HIV/AIDS research undertaken in Australia and elsewhere from 1985 onward. Other issues arose directly from my own involvement as a volunteer and as a researcher working with gay community-based AIDS service organizations. Yet a third group of issues were derived from the theoretical work on sexuality and from gay liberation theory and politics. Finally, a fourth set were part of the intellectual "capital" I carry with me as a result of many years working as a social researcher. Some of these themes changed as the study proceeded, but a number remained constantly useful and important.

*Identity* is a dominant concept in sexual politics and current sexuality theory, but it is a worryingly inadequate one. Identity is often thought of as a very personal or individualistic construct and, like "personality," has become dangerously reified in the second half of the twentieth century— one "has" a sexual identity. Yet work on arts audiences undertaken with colleagues (Kippax, Koenig, and Dowsett 1986) indicated, in contrast, that identity formation is a continuous and profoundly social process in which the self is defined and redefined in relation to *collective* practices and discourses. It is at one and the same time: (1) a process of belonging to, and being recognized as belonging to, certain collectivities; (2) a statement about oneself and one's capacities and skills in relation to others; and (3) a way of distinguishing oneself from others. One only has to listen to a bevy of opera "buffs" during the second interval at a performance of Puccini's *Tosca* to recognize exactly how these distinctions operate! In this study the concept of identity, in particular sexual identity, is regarded more as a box of tools with which to demolish and then rebuild the sexual self.

*Sexual initiation* is an important story in many gay men's lives, and it becomes important to capture memories of earliest homosexual experiences in order to analyze a number of issues. There is ongoing contention surrounding Freud's functionalist account of passivity and anality in homosexuals, particularly in the hands of conservative, North American, neo-Freudian psychoanalysis (see Lewes 1988). Yet the more social aspects of Freud's work beckon any investigator of homosexuality. The "passivity" of many working-class men in this study (Freud originally intended the term to reflect a lack of assertiveness and a tendency to masochism) in dealing with the social world seemed to have as much to do with the effects of class inequality as with sexual orientation. And anyway, a number of these socially "passive" men were distinctly oriented to doing the inserting in gay sex. Actively pursuing passivity became a major theme for this study.

In life-history work, it is important to investigate sexual histories and current sex lives at the level of meaning and experience, through the telling of tall tales, the boasting of dirty deeds, and the frank recounting of failure, fears and doubts about anal sex, and so on. The purpose is not, for example, to generalize about the centrality of anal sex in formative sexual experience; rather, it is to theorize the relation of homosexuality to anality through the relations of gay men to their anuses and anal penetration. The focus of the analysis is on the positioning of experience within a collective and symbolic order.

One interviewee claimed to have been fistfucked for four days on two occasions, the first time at age twelve. The issue here is not the truth of the claim, but its meaning and its significance in the relations of the interview itself and within the broader relations of that man's life. This story was a claim to sexual precocity and sophistication and to membership in a relatively exclusive sexual club, as well as a representation of this man's relation to gayness and to gay identity. What such a claim raises for this analysis is the question of *sexual motive*: Is sexual practice more about joining in, of belonging, than it is about satiating a deeper, unknowable need? Is sex simply fashion?

Much work on sexuality is fixated on sexual *object choice* understood as the binary determined by gender, so that other defining aspects of desire are neglected. There are a number of axes to explore here. How does desire change? Is it something that occurs over time, as an artifact of generational and maturational processes? Does it occur in relation to collective practices of sex-object redefinition, such as backroom fantasy and fuck bars, or does it occur in pornography and the explosion of gay male art photography? How fixed is fetish? How is it explored? How does it become fixed and unfixed? (One of the subjects in this study was a heavy S/M leatherman who simply decided to give it up one day.) How influenced are sexual needs, desires, and pursuits by the effects of a hegemonic, North American, minority-style gay politics and culture?

There are further themes concerning the *cultural production* of modern gay life and modern (homo)sexual practice. Is it possible, for example, to comprehend the development of the HIV identity, community, and career mentioned earlier as (following Altman 1982) the "Americanization" of the PLWHA? And to come back to the findings from the SAPA project: How does gay community attachment operate? Could it be a process of exclusion as much as one of inclusion? And are these processes random or structural? Is there a legitimation of some subcultural expressions of homosexual desire and the delegitimation of others? Are gay communities really the distillate of a contingent and brittle process of enculturation and appropriation, rather than the aggregation of men's discovery of their true selves? What more than a homosexual orientation is required in order to become "gay"? This list of questions grew as the analysis grew, and the material was revisited a number of times to investigate the evolving focus of the study.

Semistructured Interviewing

The technique used to obtain life histories can be called *semistructured interviewing*. The definition used here is not that of, for example, psychology, where "*semi*structured" indicates a loosening of an interview schedule from the strictures of forced-choice questions, allowing some flexibility to use open-ended questions and some alteration in the actual wording of questions to suit the circumstances of the interview and the respondent.

In this study the method approached a state that some researchers might consider *unstructured* interviewing. This term refers to a method of interviewing that allows maximum flexibility for both interviewer and interviewee to follow any path they choose and yet always maintain the focus on the research question the researcher has chosen. The interview is guided minimally by the interviewer, and it is even claimed at times that in this form of interviewing the respondent and the researcher are more or less equally able to influence the research process and agenda.

However, this term "unstructured" is misleading, because no researcher enters an interview without ideas, issues, interests, experiences—indeed, research questions or topics—which inevitably structure the interaction. The interviewing in this study did have a definite set of issues to explore and the process, while very flexible, was ultimately managed and controlled by the interviewer. This type of interview can be also called *nonstandardized* or *focused* (Fielding 1993), but I prefer the term "semistructured" in order to clarify that this is not inductively pursued research; there is definite theoretical and methodological logic guiding an ongoing process of induction and deduction, which deeply structures the investigation.

In this form of interviewing there is usually a list of themes to be explored rather than a set inventory of standard questions. The sequence, timing, and depth of that exploration depends on the interview itself. These can be somewhat formal, or more conversational and interactive; the capacity of the interviewer to generate a comfortable rapport is important (Dowsett 1986). The structure of the interviews for this study became less and less obvious and formal as the fieldwork progressed, which allowed the respondents to shape the interviews as much as possible and to lay out for the interviewer what constituted for them the categories of desire, sex, love, work, family, and so on, rather than having these determined a priori.

The patterning of the interview depended on its dynamics and its purpose. Most often the interviews occur singly, but I have interviewed couples together (one couple in this study) and groups (in other research). Sometimes respondents were asked for second interviews (four subjects in this study) to resolve ambiguities and clarify issues found puzzling in the analysis of the first interview, or to complete a life history too long for a single session. The interviews were always audio-recorded, which allows the interviewer to concentrate on the interaction and the content by reducing technical aspects of the interview to a minimum. These interviews were transcribed on a word processor, allowing for easy correction and textual interrogation. After correcting and "cleaning" the transcript (using previously agreed-upon confidentiality stipulations), the transcripts were indexed automatically by computer and printed. Other material used in the analysis included field notes, post-interview commentary recorded on tape immediately after the interview, and in the case of nine men in this study who had participated in earlier surveys undertaken by colleagues and myself, their questionnaires.

Confidentiality was a key issue, in particular because of the intimate sexual detail obtained on individual lives. Part of this was handled mechanically: changed names, details and places, split or partial characterizations at times to ensure extra protection, and sometimes amalgamated or reassigned characterization to prevent identification. This was done without distorting the processes under investigation. Informed consent, though a standard practice in such research, was obtained in almost all cases verbally rather than in writing because at the time it was unclear how the new public-health laws on HIV/AIDS enacted in New South Wales were to be administered.

## Analysis

The initial analysis occurred during the writing of a case study. The case studies varied in length from three to ten thousand words, depending on the information obtained and the position of the interview in the analysis—later interviews often generated much shorter case studies than the earlier ones. The case studies took the form of brief biographies, followed by explorations of both the themes that had originally informed the study theoretically and those new issues and ideas which had arisen from the interviews as they proceeded. One of the major benefits of this method is the possibility of reworking the interview schedule as the interviews progress, and where the analysis is simply being confirmed each time and little new or contrary information is emerging. The second level of analysis involved thematic interrogation of the case material in order to pursue the theoretical and inductively derived issues.

The use of case study technique is explored in various ways in this study: in a single story, for example, Barney; in sets of three sequential stories; through thematic interrogations of three stories; and in integrated theorizing across stories. This employment of different analytical possibilities permits the reader to evaluate the methodology and to witness the emergence of the theory directly from the analysis.

The key to the theorized life-history method is its intent, the explication of social process, not biography. It is important to make no special effort to avoid paradox, contradiction, or inconsistency. There should be no "papering over the cracks," but an embracing of discontinuity and ambiguity within a subject's life. One should look for inconsistency in the telling of the tale, and one needs a keen ear for the revelatory slip of tongue, the disclaimer, the prioritizing of events, and the subjective importance of avowal. These apparent paradoxes, these inexplicable moments, these inconsistencies, eventually fall into place as part of larger, more social processes and patterns.

## Sampling

Sampling is an issue for many researchers used to more quantitative methods. It is less important than one might expect. If I were studying the experience of sexual oppression suffered by gay men and lesbians in homophobic societies, would I really need to know how much oppression goes on? For some purposes it might be important to know, for instance, that there were, say, five gay bashings a week in inner Sydney in 1993. For other purposes it may be more important to investigate the one case, say, where a gay man was gang-raped by the youths who bashed him. That latter investigation might reveal more about the construction of homophobia and its relation to heterosexual masculinity-forming practices and rituals than a quantified procedure ever could. Sampling, then, is directly related to the research question being investigated; not all issues are reducible to sizes and numbers.

Plummer (1983) talks about sampling eloquently, and Anselm Strauss and Juliet Corbin (1990) argue the value of *theoretical sampling*, which they define as "sampling on the basis of concepts that have proven theoretical relevance to the evolving theory" (p. 176). The theoretical issues and the information gathered progressively through the interviewing and analysis interact and inform the development of the sample, until "theoretical saturation . . . is reached. . . . This means, until: (1) no new or relevant data seem to emerge regarding a category; (2) the category development is dense, insofar as all of the paradigm elements are accounted for, along with variation and process; (3) the relationships between categories are well established and validated" (p. 188). The material collected in the course of this study met and exceeded my demands for theoretical saturation. Indeed, there was more material obtained in the interviews than presented here, mostly pertaining to specific issues of HIV prevention (see Davis et al. 1993).

The interview themes covered in each interview (though rarely in this order) were current broad circumstances, living situation, housing, social milieu; family origins and background, family members, schooling, friendships, current family ties; early sexual experiences and sexual relationships history; working life, training, work history; current sex life, regular and/or casual partner(s), sex practices and fantasies, sexual interests and preferences; sexual identity and gay community definition and participation; HIV/AIDS issues in general and personally, including HIV-infection status and health, safe sex knowledge, and "safe" and "unsafe" sexual behavior; and finally, reasons for participating in the study. As the fieldwork progressed various themes rose to prominence or sank into the background, depending on the interviewee's capacity to contribute on these issues and on their progress in the saturation of categories process.

The men selected for this study were chosen partly on the basis of the issues that arose from the findings of the early Australian surveys on HIV/AIDS (see Chapter 3). A second consideration was the set of issues emerging from the theoretical debates about essentialism and social constructionism and my decision to investigate these empirically. A third consideration was an attempt to explore evenly the three different sites on which this study is based: the inner-Sydney gay community centered on Oxford Street, and the epicenter of the HIV epidemic in Australia; western Sydney, a vast conurbation of over one million people stretching from Parramatta to the Blue Mountains, which has developed since World War II, and is considered largely a working-class area, heavy in industry, light on services; and Nullangardie, a provincial town in New South Wales with a history of trade unionism and industrial militancy, a predominantly Anglo-Australian population, a local gay community, and an HIV epidemic of its own. Some chosen for this study were also asked to recruit friends, mates or sex partners, members of gay organizations, or participants in HIV/AIDS programs with whom they were familiar.

Twenty men in all form the basis of this study. All were interviewed by the author. Their ages range from twenty to sixty. There are one or two quite well off, a few professionals, some tradesmen, some unskilled workers, a number quite vulnerable in the job market, and two on social security benefits. A few are in long-standing relationships, some in newly established ones, and others have spent their adult lives as singles. Most of the men were interviewed in their homes; however, four were interviewed in local gay community organization offices. The first interview took place in late 1987, the last in late 1990.

The material is presented in two forms. Eleven of the men provided the basis for the core of the analysis. I will present their life histories in some detail, as I have already done with that of Barney Sherman. The other nine will be referred to when their contribution illustrates or adds to the analysis of particular issues. All the men have been given pseudonyms and certain details of their lives have been changed to protect their identities. For example, occupations have been altered—one trade ticket substituted for another—and towns and cities have new or different names. Third persons have been renamed and similarly altered.

In order to assist the reader in differentiating these twenty men clearly, I have prepared the following capsule biographies:

*Barney Sherman*, approaching sixty, lives in inner Sydney. Formerly a tradesman, Barney is now on the Invalid Pension as a result of AIDS. His partner of many years, though estranged of late, died recently of an AIDS-related condition. Barney has a sometime lover but is facing increasing isolation as his health deteriorates.

*Peter Standard*, in his late thirties, is a teacher who had spent many years abroad before returning to Sydney to live in the Oxford Street area just as the HIV epidemic was becoming very serious. A volunteer in various gay agencies, Peter still has difficulties with coming to grips with safe sex and its impact on his sexual and emotional life.

*Harry Wight*, early forties, a large affable man, on the pension as a result of an injury, lives in Nullangardie with a lover of many years standing. Once married, Harry sees his children often and they know he is gay. Harry spends much of his spare time having sex and working as a volunteer for local gay and HIV/AIDS agencies.

*Ralph Coles* was in his late forties, lived in Sydney, and was professionally employed. He was a gay activist and later an HIV/AIDS activist and educator. Ralph was in his third significant relationship, with *Dennis Partridge*, Sydney born, thirty, a community worker and an ex-prostitute. Dennis is now in the process of rebuilding his life after Ralph's recent death, and is facing his own uncertain future as a gay man living with HIV infection.

*Neil Davidson*, mid-fifties, was born in Nullangardie but now lives in Sydney. An educator, Neil was married for many years and finally left his family to live a gay life. He lives with his first-ever gay lover, and they work hard to negotiate workable relations with Neil's wife, children, and other family.

*Huey Brown*, late thirties, is better known as "Harriet" by everyone he knows. A tireless worker for HIV/AIDS fundraising in Nullangardie, Harriet has been variously a bar attendant, drag performer, stripper, and transsexual prostitute. Harriet now makes sandwiches in a café.

*Ren Pinch* has an independent income and lives in Sydney. He is in his early forties, an active member of the Sydney gay community for many years, and very active within that community sexually. He reckons that he has had over ten thousand sex partners in his lifetime.

*Richard Cochrane* lived in Nullangardie for many years, then joined the Sydney gay community to have the time of his life. Richard returned to Nullangardie to be looked after by his family as his HIV infection progressed to AIDS. He died not long after I interviewed him. He was in his early thirties.

*Robert Cusack* is fifty and though not HIV infected, his once active sexual and social life in Sydney's gay leather set has almost been devastated by AIDS. Robert seeks an early retirement from a white-collar job that never turned into a career. He is virtually celibate.

*Phillip Gibbs* is twenty-five and lives in western Sydney. Phillip is poorly educated, and at a bit of a loss after ten years of sex, a stint in a reformatory, a few black-economy jobs, unemployment, retraining and more unemployment, and a little prostitution. Phillip is HIV negative, but he has been the victim of anti-gay violence on two occasions and is unwell as a result of that. He has what could well shape up to be a problem with drugs.

*Simon Little* is twenty, cute, and not completely happy to find himself a gay man. He finds living in a gay part of inner Sydney a mixed blessing, but it is far better than being in western Sydney with his family. Still lacking a firm sense of direction in his working life, Simon seeks security in his primary emotional-sexual relationships, all of which have been short term and unstable, in Madonna memorabilia, and in dancing as the "boy" in drag shows at a western Sydney gay social group.

*Pip Bowles* is in his early twenties, extremely sexually active and very popular with his friends. His form of gayness is more European than West Coast American. Although Pip has a university degree, he has had trouble settling into a career as yet, preferring parties, recreational drugs, and sex to meetings, memos, and management issues.

*Dan Berger* is in his late forties and HIV infected, and still resents the recent breakup of his partnership of nearly twenty years. Well-educated and erudite, Dan has enjoyed the homosexual subcultures of a number of places, preferring nowadays a more sedate pace but with no less enthusiasm for the occasional "hot" time.

*Geoff Harris* is a country-bred, gentle young man, now dealing with an unexpected HIV infection that was diagnosed just as he began to embark on his chosen career as a performer. He is anxious about developing AIDS without a much-desired partner to help. Although Geoff resists a gay self-definition, he sees his reliance on gay community HIV/AIDS organizations growing as his health deteriorates.

*Jack Sayers* is retired and lives in western Sydney. He spent his whole working life refusing advancement beyond a minor supervisory level and in seeking sex with young workmates and occasional hitchhikers. At fifty-five he has just buried a young lover who died from AIDS, after nursing him for a number of years.

*Morrie Layton* is bisexual, married, and has AIDS. A classic working-class bloke, Morrie has had good times in the saunas and beats of Sydney. Though now living in western Sydney, he had until recently put the CB radio to good use seeking sex partners, male and/or female, for himself and his wife. Morrie is now cared for by his wife, who remains HIV negative despite their active sex lives. Morrie found out his HIV serostatus when an interviewer in an HIV/AIDS research study encouraged him to get tested. The result came as quite a shock.

*Martin Ridgeway* is twenty, in love, and has settled in a gay "marriage" with an older man, complete with sheepdogs, bungalow, and a pool, in western Sydney. Gay sex all started in the local public toilets at age twelve in his western Sydney housing commission estate. Gay community has little meaning for him as he pursues a white-collar career and escapes the cultural poverty of his upbringing through his relationship.

*Alan Cunningham* is a welder in his late twenties, retraining himself for community work in Nullangardie. Bright, chirpy, sexually active, he lives with a considerably older lover of a number of years standing. Alan pursues an openly gay lifestyle and is "out" to his family and workmates at the factory.

*Alex Lawes* is married, bisexually active, and somewhat unclear about the risk at which his sexual activities place his wife. Alex finds his sex partners in local pubs, and through "swingers" newspapers and magazines. A car salesman, his economic situation is often unstable, relying as he does on commission. Now in his mid-forties, Alex's favorite sexual encounter is with a heterosexual couple, but they must be older than him so that his "youthful" appeal still contributes to the occasion.

These are the men who contributed their lives to this study. They will appear in passing or in detail as the themes of the study unfold and are explored. And to them go my grateful thanks.

# 3

# AIDS: A Fact of Life

AIDS has touched all the men in this study—all live with AIDS in one way or another. There are one or two who seem to have escaped the tragedy of the epidemic; yet even among these men the Australian experience of HIV/ AIDS performs as mise-en-scène, either at the level of framing their own sexual practices or as a discourse suffusing gay culture in Sydney.

In 1995 there were very few Australians unaware of HIV/AIDS. Extensive public education programs, although controversial at times, such as the infamous "Grim Reaper" television advertisements of 1987, have argued that HIV/AIDS is a problem for everyone. Yet it is clear that many non-gay Australians still regard the epidemic as a gay problem and that persuading non-gay Australians to give up behavior deemed to be of "high risk" for transmitting HIV has been difficult (e.g., see Crawford, Turtle, and Kippax 1990; Kippax et al., "Establishing Safe Sex Norms," 1990; Kippax, Crawford, and Waldby 1990; Rosenthal, Moore, and Brumen 1990; Gifford et al. 1994; Rosenthal and Reichler 1994).

For gay and homosexually active men the possibility of HIV infection has been an urgent, difficult, and terrifying threat for over a decade now. Because the HIV virus is most easily transmitted during anal intercourse, gay and homosexually active men who practice anal intercourse are at far greater risk than those who do not, and than those who do not venture into sexual milieus that already have high HIV rates. Even though sodomy is almost universally associated with male homosexuality in the key academic, professional, and popular conceptions of gay sex, in practice the picture is far more complex. Each gay or homosexually active man's relation to the epidemic needs to be assessed in the light of more than a simplistic categorization as "gay."

For each man in this study HIV/AIDS issues have had an ongoing impact since the early 1980's, and each has dealt with his particular experience of the epidemic in his own way. Whatever the nexus between sexual practice, sexual identity, and the discursive reordering of both as a result of HIV/ AIDS for gay and homosexually active men, it is necessary to register the *fact* of the epidemic clearly. In order to gauge this impact on these men's lives, it is important, first, to recognize the specificity of the Australian HIV epidemic and, second, to understand the responses of the Australian gay communities to that specificity, for this constitutes an often crucial mediation of each man's experience of HIV.

## The HIV Epidemic in Australia

The first case of AIDS was diagnosed in Australia in 1982 (Penny et al. 1983). The HIV epidemic, as it came to be known, had begun here. Health professionals, however, were only one of the "expert" social groups that contributed to the national response to the epidemic. By the time the mass media began to inform the Australians of this new public-health threat, the gay communities were already well aware of what was coming: they had been discussing the illnesses appearing among gay men in North America in their local gay newspapers (e.g., *Sydney Star Observer*, June 7, 1981) and had been reading the overseas gay press.

By 1984 it was clear that Australia was facing a significant epidemic, and government public-health machinery, after a faltering start in 1983, moved into top gear, establishing the institutional arrangements and policies that have guided the country since. It is important to recognize that from the start the national response to the epidemic in Australia has involved three groups: the Commonwealth and State governments, and their public-health officials; the nongovernmental sector, initially and predominantly the gay communities' HIV/AIDS organizations; and health professionals and research academics.

### AIDS

By June 30, 1995, 6,035 cases of AIDS had been recorded in Australia, 71 percent of whom have died (National Centre in HIV Epidemiology and Clinical Research [hereafter NCHECR] 1995). Men account for 96 percent of AIDS cases. The rate of increase in new AIDS diagnoses in Australia has slowed dramatically—from 40 percent in 1988 to 19 percent in 1991—and even began to decrease by nearly 3 percent in 1992. However, 827 new cases of AIDS were diagnosed in 1994, an increase of just over 4 percent (NCHECR 1995).

TABLE I

*AIDS Cases by Sex and Exposure Category to June 30, 1995*

| Exposure category | Male | Female | Total | Percent |
|---|---|---|---|---|
| Male-to-male sexual contact | 4,978 | — | 4,978 | 82.5 |
| Male-to-male sex and IDU | 239 | — | 239 | 4.0 |
| IDU (heterosexual) | 93 | 55 | 148 | 2.5 |
| Heterosexual contact | 153 | 95 | 248 | 4.1 |
| Hemophilia/coagulation disorder | 84 | 1 | 85 | 1.4 |
| Blood components/tissue recipients | 89 | 55 | 144 | 2.3 |
| Mother with HIV | 9 | 9 | 18 | 0.3 |
| Other/undetermined | 144 | 11 | 175[a] | 2.9 |
| TOTAL | 5,789 | 226 | 6,035[a] | 100.0 |

SOURCE: from NCHECR 1995

[a] Persons whose sex was reported as transsexual included here.

Table I shows a patterning of HIV transmission that would place Australia among "pattern I" countries like the United States and Great Britain. However, this taxonomy of patterns (which divided the world into three types of epidemic by dominant HIV transmission mode and a timetable for the global epidemic) has come under considerable criticism (Patton 1990).

In "pattern I" countries HIV began to spread in the late 1970's and early 1980's, largely through male-to-male sexual contact. The blood supply was usually protected early in "pattern I" countries resulting in minimized blood product–related infections, but early heterosexual HIV transmission was noted, related often to injecting drug use, but feared more as a result of "bisexual" activity by men. A consequent "heterosexual" epidemic was expected in many "pattern I" countries, and certainly in the United States and Great Britain significant heterosexual transmission has occurred.

The Australian epidemic is still spreading mostly through sexual contact, predominantly male-to-male sexual contact at that; other transmission categories have grown in significance only slightly over time (see Table 2). This marks one of the basic differences between the epidemics in other "pattern I" countries and in Australia, and therefore its "pattern I" designation is somewhat misleading.

Yet to speak of an Australian epidemic is misleading. Sydney, the capital of New South Wales and the largest city in Australia (population 3.5 million), accounts for over 58 percent of the national AIDS total (New South Wales Health Department [hereafter AIDS Bureau] 1990). But to speak of

TABLE 2

AIDS Cases by Exposure Category, 1982–1994

(in percentage)

| Exposure category | 1982 | 1983 | 1984 | 1985 | 1986 | 1987 | 1988 | 1989 | 1990 | 1991 | 1992 | 1993 | 1994 |
|---|---|---|---|---|---|---|---|---|---|---|---|---|---|
| Male-to-male sexual contact | 100 | 66.7 | 71.7 | 80.8 | 87.2 | 86.9 | 88.8 | 87.2 | 86.1 | 83.4 | 84.4 | 83.3 | 82.6 |
| Male-to-male sexual contact and IDU | 0 | 33.3 | 2.2 | 0.8 | 4.8 | 2.1 | 3.0 | 2.6 | 1.6 | 3.1 | 3.0 | 3.5 | 4.0 |
| IDU (heterosexual) | 0 | 0 | 0 | 0 | 0.9 | 0.5 | 2.1 | 2.2 | 1.8 | 3.4 | 2.0 | 2.0 | 2.3 |
| Heterosexual contact | 0 | 0 | 0 | 0.8 | 0 | 1.6 | 1.5 | 1.4 | 3.0 | 3.8 | 3.0 | 3.6 | 3.9 |
| Hemophilia/coagulation disorder | 0 | 0 | 4.3 | 0.8 | 0.9 | 1.6 | 1.3 | 1.7 | 1.9 | 1.0 | 1.6 | 1.5 | 1.5 |
| Blood/tissue recipient | 0 | 0 | 21.7 | 13.6 | 5.3 | 5.3 | 1.3 | 1.7 | 1.8 | 1.7 | 2.8 | 3.2 | 2.5 |
| Mother with HIV | 0 | 0 | 0 | 0.8 | 0 | 0 | 0.2 | 0.2 | 0.5 | 0.3 | 0.3 | 0.2 | 0.2 |
| Other/undetermined | 0 | 0 | 0 | 2.4 | 0.9 | 1.9 | 1.7 | 2.9 | 3.4 | 3.3 | 2.8 | 2.6 | 3.0 |

SOURCE: NCHECR 1992, 1993, 1994 and 1995.

a Sydney epidemic is also misleading: three inner-Sydney health districts, the Eastern, Central, and Northern Sydney Area Health Services, together account for 48 percent of national AIDS total (AIDS Bureau 1990). Two of these inner-Sydney health districts take in the Oxford Street precinct.

### HIV Infection

The overall level of HIV infection in Australia is harder to gauge. By June 30, 1995, 19,087 diagnoses of HIV infection had been recorded, 84 percent of them in men (NCHECR 1995). It has been estimated, however, that between 20,000 and 25,000 Australians could be infected (Solomon et al. 1991), and as time goes on this estimate looks as if it will be reasonably accurate. New South Wales has an HIV case rate of 203.6 per hundred thousand people (nearly three times higher than the next hardest-hit State, Victoria, with a case rate of 77.3 per hundred thousand), and accounts for 65 percent of the national HIV infection total (NCHECR 1995).

*Newly diagnosed* HIV infections increased by 897 cases during the twelve months from July 1, 1994, to June 30, 1995, a 5 percent increase in the overall numbers of infected Australians (NCHECR 1995). By exposure category, the pattern of reported HIV infections remains stable and was substantially ascribed to male-to-male sexual contact (81 percent). Again, this marks an important difference between Australia and many other "pattern 1" countries. Other transmission categories accounted for the following: male-to-male sexual contact and injecting drug use (3 percent); injecting drug use among heterosexuals (5 percent); heterosexual contact (7.5 percent); hemophilia and coagulation disorder (2 percent); blood or tissue recipients (1.5 percent); mother with HIV (0.4 percent); and healthcare setting (0.1 percent) (NCHECR 1995).

Research that monitors *newly acquired* HIV infections (as distinct from newly diagnosed infections) recorded 231 cases between July 1, 1994, and June 30, 1995, 186 (81 percent) of which were related to male-to-male sexual contact, with a further ten cases (4 percent) related to male-to-male sexual contact and injecting drug use.

### Gay and Homosexually Active Men and HIV/AIDS

To date, the Australian HIV epidemic has been one overwhelmingly related to male-to-male sexual transmission of the virus, and the great majority of such infections occur among men in the identifiable gay communities. The earliest prospective study of HIV/AIDS among men recruited in inner Sydney who identified with a gay community found that 39 percent of these men were infected in 1985; this had risen to 49 percent by 1987, but the rate of new infection had dropped from 8 percent per year to less than 0.5 percent per year (Burcham et al. 1989). Research comparing data from this prospective study, an anonymous HIV-antibody testing site in inner Sydney, and the blood-donor screening program has confirmed these substantial decreases in the HIV-seroconversion rate among gay and homosexually active men (Kaldor et al. 1991).

The earliest behavioral study of gay and homosexually active men in Sydney and parts of New South Wales, the SAPA project, found in its first cross-sectional survey in 1986–87 that 68 percent of respondents had been HIV-antibody tested and of those 25 percent were infected. Of those infected, 76 percent lived in inner Sydney (Dowsett, Davis, and Connell 1992a).

These are not definitive figures for HIV seroprevalence in the gay communities in Sydney, but do indicate the intensity of the epidemic there. Estimated infection rates in gay communities in some other Australian cities, based on early cross-sectional surveys, can only be regarded as a rough guide: 16 percent in Melbourne (Campbell et al. 1988); 7 percent in Brisbane (Frazer et al. 1988); 5 percent in Canberra (Kippax et al. 1989). The more recent national cross-sectional survey of gay and homosexually active men, Project Male-Call, found that 6.7 percent of the whole sample (and 9 percent of those tested) were HIV seropositive, and the figures for each State were lower in this study than in earlier ones (Kippax et al. 1994).

Although not all those infected through homosexual transmission are part of organized and recognizable gay communities in Australia, it is clear that gay communities—the inner-Sydney gay community in particular—are the most affected social groups in the country. Project Male-Call reported that 11 percent of all men tested in New South Wales were HIV seropositive and of the men living in "gay Sydney" 14 percent were infected (Kippax et al. 1994). This is probably the closest to accurate figure so far available.

## Australia's Response to HIV/AIDS

Even though the expected increase in HIV infections among heterosexuals and injecting drug users has not occurred in Australia, a watchful eye is still kept by public-health officials on these transmission categories. It seems increasingly clear, however, that infection rates via these transmission modes will not reach a "take-off" point, and Australian public-health officials have finally resolved that the epidemic among gay and homosexually active men is the main game (Feachem 1995).

From 1984 onward the Australian government pursued a policy of cooperation and consultation with the affected communities, national medical bodies, and other State and Commonwealth institutions, in order to create a unified national response. This policy was necessitated partly by Australia's federal system of government—the States are wholly responsible for the delivery of health services—and by an initial recognition that the first affected communities, the gay communities, were already mobilized and informed about the problem and had taken their own steps to deal with it.

Relations between the groups involved in HIV/AIDS work were patchy until late 1984 when the first fully fleshed out national policies emerged (see Ballard 1989). As government funds began to flow to the already active gay community AIDS service organizations and other nongovernmental bodies, more systematic preventive education strategies and programs of care and support were developed. The activist and volunteer-based gay community AIDS Action Committees, established in each State in 1983 to lobby and provide the first education and care/support efforts in the gay communities, became AIDS Councils in 1985 and soon federated into the Australian Federation of AIDS Organisations.[1]

A division of labor in preventive education was soon established: the Commonwealth Government was to retain responsibility for overall policy guidance and funding, and for the national mass-media (largely) education programs; the States would be mainly responsible for health service delivery and some State-specific prevention activity, for example, schools programs and coordinating the nongovernmental sector response in their States; the nongovernmental organizations would undertake the task of educating their affected communities. Similar specialization was to occur in care/support programs, for example, the national health scheme, Medicare, assumes most hospital costs associated with HIV infection in Australia, but the gay community care/support organizations provide much of the volunteer home care for those infected with HIV or living with AIDS. Research, however, was to be funded separately through a special Commonwealth AIDS Research Grants Committee (now part of the National Health and Medical Research Council).

These arrangements mean considerable direct government funding of gay community agencies and programs, of injecting drug user groups, of

---

1 The Australian Federation of AIDS Organisations (AFAO) is the peak HIV/AIDS organization for nongovernmental and community-based AIDS service organizations. Through AFAO the Commonwealth Government deals with the whole community sector input into the national AIDS program. AFAO now also contains many other non-gay community organizations, such as prostitutes' collectives and injecting drug users' self-help groups.

sex worker collectives, of hemophilia organizations, and so on. Although some of these funds are delivered directly to the nongovernmental organizations by the Commonwealth, most are dispersed via the State health departments' HIV/AIDS units/bureaus in relationships marked in the main by a high degree of cooperation and mutual respect.

From 1984 until 1989 this policy evolved, redistributing the tasks as needed, guided by various national advisory bodies, which were eventually combined to form the Australian National Council on AIDS. Gay communities have had spokespersons on all these bodies, as have other interested groups. Considerable increases in funding accompanied these policy developments until the early 1990's. The national HIV/AIDS program and its mechanisms for consultation and decision-making were definitively outlined in a series of strategy documents (Commonwealth of Australia 1989, 1993) designed to guide the country through successive three-year cycles. The third such national strategy is to be in place by mid-1996. (See Timewell, Minichiello, and Plummer 1992 for an overview of the Australian experience of the HIV epidemic.)

The cooperative political and institutional arrangements for the Australian response to the epidemic are important to keep in mind when assessing the programs of prevention undertaken among gay and homosexually active men. While the relations between governments, health professionals, and the community sector have often been difficult, even abrasive, and have led to direct political action on the part of gay communities at times, these arrangements allow for considerable flexibility in program management and delivery. The gay community AIDS service organizations have been given significant funding and considerable liberty to undertake their programs of prevention. As important is the overall sense of a nation *not* at war with its gay communities in this epidemic. Indeed, three States have legalized homosexual practices between men since 1985. Only one State, Tasmania, has yet to do so, and its anti-gay laws were overridden in 1994 by Commonwealth legislation guaranteeing a right to sexual privacy, passed after a successful submission to the United Nations Human Rights Committee by Tasmanian gay activists. The international repercussions of this United Nations ruling are yet to be fully assessed. Several States have anti-discrimination legislation related to sexual preference, and some have also included HIV infection and AIDS as grounds for legal complaints about discrimination.

These political and institutional arrangements, in part, structure the epidemic experienced by gay and homosexually active men in Australia and by the men in this study. Some of these men are intimately involved with and understand clearly these structural issues. For others, like Barney, HIV/AIDS is a personal issue only. However, none is unaware of the consequences of the consistency and predominance of male-to-male sexual transmission of HIV in this country, and the ambiguity it generates in the national political arena and in the media about the "gayness" of AIDS. The homophobia that has burdened HIV/AIDS work elsewhere (Altman 1986; Treichler 1988; Watney 1988a, 1988b; Weeks 1988; Bronski 1989; Davenport-Hines 1990) has not been absent from this country either, with its deeply anti-homosexual history (Hughes 1987; Altman 1992; the epilogue in Wotherspoon 1991).

This epidemiological pattern and the structuring of HIV/AIDS at the political and social/cultural level have a powerful counterpoint in the responses of gay communities to the epidemic. The gay communities have been deeply involved in the formulation of Commonwealth and State policies and are major program deliverers. More important, the representations of the epidemic exhibited at the affected-community level are mostly products of gay community efforts and thereby provide authoritative signifiers for gay and homosexually active men to appropriate for themselves and with which to comprehend what is happening to them. The men in this study are deeply affected by the organized gay community, in Sydney in particular, and it is useful at this point to describe the communities' responses briefly.

### Preventive Education in and Beyond Gay Communities

In the early 1980's the gay communities of Australia rapidly developed their own early analysis of the looming HIV epidemic, its political setting, and the emerging discursive positions of the actors and embarked on a remarkably astute response.

Australian gay community–based educators of gay and homosexually active men have developed significant expertise in the last thirteen years in devising and delivering educational programs on HIV/AIDS. Their AIDS organizations did not come to HIV/AIDS work cold: many of their workers and volunteers had long histories of gay activism, and some work in gay health had been occurring in the early 1980's. There had been more than a decade of National Homosexual Conferences from 1975 onward, creating a more unified national gay liberation movement than had existed in many other Western countries. The earliest news stories of the diseases that became AIDS were carried almost exclusively by the gay press in Australia until 1983–84, when patchy and often sensational coverage began in the mainstream media. The gay press has remained the most important site for community debate about prevention, policy, treatments, and so on, ever since.

Almost all preventive education directed at gay and other homosexually active men in Australia has been developed and delivered by nongovernmental gay community–based agencies.[2] These preventive education strategies involve much that is familiar in health promotion on other issues: information distribution through pamphlets and posters; community newspaper advertisements; information and support activities, usually involving group processes such as seminars, conferences, and discussion nights; promotional activities geared to special events. Gay community groups were able to rely on an existing culture of considerable open discussion of sex among gay men. This facilitated an approach to education messages in image, style, language, and meaning that could be sure of direct effect, particularly on gay-identifying men. Many of these interventions are shaped by the culture of the existing gay communities themselves. The institutions, organizations, and commercial venues that constitute the infrastructure of the gay communities have been utilized as distribution and reinforcement points in education.

A prominent example is the work done at politico-cultural events such as the annual Sydney Gay and Lesbian Mardi Gras, particularly its street parade watched in 1994 by over 500,000 spectators and followed by an all-night dance party attended by over 21,000 gay men (mainly) and lesbians. During each month-long Mardi Gras festival there are special safe sex campaigns, featuring posters and pamphlets, sometimes disco songs or video clips in gay community venues, and thousands of condoms are distributed in special flip-top packages, called Safe Packs. Floats in the Mardi Gras parade, costumes, and street theater activities by groups such as the "Safe Sex Sluts"—a group of educators in "radical drag"—exhort gay men to practice safe sex to protect themselves and their community. Community leaders, entertainers, and gay media are all involved. Other moments in Sydney's gay calendar—the Sleaze Ball, the Pride Party—receive similar educational attention. The Mid-Summa Festival in Melbourne and comparable events in other cities focus on taking the message about HIV and safe sex to gay men wherever they are, whatever they are doing.

These community events become moments for educational campaigns

---

2 No national preventive education campaigns by government public health services were directed specifically to gay and homosexually active men until 1991, nine years after the first AIDS case.

that attempt to link gay men to a *safe sex culture*, invoking the notion of a community acting to protect itself. These *community intervention strategies* (Dowsett 1990b) rely on inserting safe sex information and other educational materials into the existing framework of gay community life. They utilize existing cultural forms, institutions, and practices as the vehicles for the transformation of sexual behavior. These are important because they create a continuity between existing gay culture and "safe" sexual practice. They acknowledge, but also reduce, the dislocation caused by the epidemic in the lives of gay men. Such interventions also directly address those aspects of gay community life which were implicated in creating the environment for the homosexual spread of HIV, such as sex-on-premises venues, events with considerable sexual activity and partner acquisition, beats, and so on. They modify a culture of sexual recreation and exploration to ensure it is conducted safely.

This notion of safe sex culture is not about describing a majoritarian behavioral response to the epidemic; rather, a safe sex culture creates an overarching discursive "hum" that attracts gay men by situating safe sex within collectively defined and recognized activities and meanings. Keeping the momentum of that "hum" going; renewing and re-presenting its message; amplifying its inclusivity: this has become the ongoing work of gay community–based prevention interventions. The insinuation of HIV/AIDS in more formally recognized aspects of gay cultural life, particularly its creative, artistic, and representational activity, underscores the centrality of HIV/AIDS within gay communities in Australia today (see Gott 1994). These formal and informal cultural efforts intersect in the safe sex culture constructed by gay communities.

These community intervention strategies have changed as the epidemic itself changed. During the early years, the various print materials produced concentrated on the symptoms of HIV infection and a growing list of judgments about the safety of, or risk associated with, certain sex practices. In the hands of the gay community AIDS organizations these print materials were a far cry from dry clinical lists of do's and don'ts of the sort typical, for a time, of government-produced materials. Increasingly, images and iconography from the gay communities themselves have shaped the form, tone, and delivery of their educational materials and programs.

These more subculturally specific configurations of homoeroticism were (and are) controversial, and at times have angered more conservative Australians and worried supporters within government and the public-health bureaucracies. Debates continue over the use of homoerotic imagery, explicit language, and the access of the "general public," especially youth, to such information and its representations of homosexuality. At times government funding has been, and occasionally still is, withdrawn from specific materials, revealing something of the underlying tension in the response to HIV/AIDS between Australian society and its conspicuous homosexual communities.

Stuart Marshall (1990) argues that these pro-gay configurations are the only countervailing imagery available to gay men in the face of the mass media's distinction between "innocent" and "guilty" and media photos of those ravaged by this "killer" disease. As such, these pro-gay representations constitute another significant method of attaching gay community-identified men to a collective project of stopping the epidemic.

The content of much of the education campaign material actually encodes and discloses a history of previous tumult and debate within gay communities about the epidemic and its likely transmission routes. Australia had its parallels to the *How to Have Sex in an Epidemic* booklet (Callen 1983) and the debates about anal sex and gay saunas in the United States (Shilts 1988). These early collective debates and actions produced considerable change in behavior as a result—change already available to be capitalized on by gay communities as HIV/AIDS became more serious (Dowsett 1989). In much of this work Australia's efforts have been informed by, and have in turn informed, activity among other established gay communities in the Western world. The international character of gay culture has been a significant factor in the largely successful containment of the epidemic in these gay communities. (See, for example, Mantell 1989, Pollak 1989, Tielman 1989, and Weatherburn 1989.)

The level of activity involved in this work by Australian gay community-based AIDS service organizations has been enormous, and some of the men in this study have been directly involved in the process. They exercise a strong sense of ownership and commitment to the ins and outs of gay community politics about HIV/AIDS and share common understandings of the disease and its implications for gay communities and the men who identify with them. For others, the gay communities are part of their very difficulties in dealing with HIV/AIDS.

The research programs funded to monitor the gay communities soon revealed the beginnings of a differentiation in response. This research confirmed that measures of knowledge of HIV transmission and responses to other HIV/AIDS issues were related to geographic proximity to an established and observable gay community, in addition to a significant degree of participation in it, the details of which are explored below. Subsequent research among working-class homosexual men indicated difficulties related to gay community participation and in response to educational materials produced by gay community programs (Dowsett, Davis, and Connell 1992b). The reach of the gay community prevention programs had a definite limit.

This posed problems for community educators: how to devise strategies for preventive education that relied less on print (and therefore, literacy) and "gay" iconography, and reached those homosexually active men distanced or detached from gay communities? To reach these "hard-to-reach" men, the gay community educators were by 1988 developing *community attachment strategies* (Dowsett 1990b). These take the form of peer education programs, which differ markedly from State to State, but which in essence offer opportunities for men linked by age, sexual interests, or region to participate in programs of education about HIV and its transmission and to sustain safe sex (Davis 1990; Parnell 1989). These are particularly important for men seeking to join gay communities. One of the men in this study was recruited through just such a peer education program. Similar programs for men of Asian heritage and from other non-English-speaking backgrounds, for the hearing impaired, and for bisexually active men have been established. In addition, education programs for HIV-infected men are developing, as yet with less than adequate government funding, since many policymakers consider those infected only in need of medical help and fail to recognize the health enhancement support and assistance HIV-infected people need in adapting their lives to the infection. Barney Sherman clearly exemplifies this need.

A second form of attachment program is the outreach project, such as telephone hotlines, local or regional programs supplying educational materials and condoms to suburban social networks and groups, and developing programs especially designed to educate men who use beats. Teams of educators regularly monitor the activities of men at these places, distributing condoms, handing out pamphlets, and referring men to other programs and agencies if necessary. This beats program started in Sydney (van Reyk 1990), but similar projects operate throughout Australia (Dowsett and Davis 1992). Although each takes a slightly different form, most projects recognize that for many men their lives do not allow them to leave family, region, background, job, and personal history to move to inner-city gay communities. Some of these men are gay-identifying; others find it easier to handle homosexual interests in clandestine and casual encounters than in the glitter of gay bars and discos. Often these programs are developed by paid staff with volunteer workers, and the range of these programs has increased considerably over the past six years. Increasingly, in these programs a patterning of homosexual interests by the effects of social class has become evident (O'Reilly 1991; Dowsett, Davis, and Connell 1992a, 1992b; Connell, Davis, and Dowsett 1993).

These outreach programs target men like many in this study. Beats emerged as a vital component of the sexual practice of these men and became one of the focuses of the investigation. Concurrent research done in collaboration with outreach educators began to reveal a "beat culture" (Davis, Klemmer, and Dowsett 1991) and sexual milieus significantly different from that of the Sydney gay community, and this reinforced this study's concerns about "gay communi*ties*" and the problematic notion of "membership" therein.

This successful response to the HIV epidemic by gay communities is not without its problems. Indeed, a key stimulus for this study was the particular shape and character of these community efforts and the images, representations, and language they use to conceptualize the epidemic, gayness (whatever that is), gay community, and most important, homosexual sex itself. It became obvious that a massive collective effort without parallel was under way to transform the historical and discursive link between gay sex and anal intercourse, the sex act that had always signified homosexuality. If sodomy is as central to the psychic makeup of homosexual men as our societies have been led to believe, then the outcome sought by these prevention efforts should be well-nigh impossible. Surely, after years of fighting for the civil right to engage in anal intercourse (and other sex acts), gay men cannot simply transform, omit, defer, "re-code," the central symbolic and sensate core of their sexuality. Or can they? Can some of them? Which ones? And how? The framework being utilized in HIV/AIDS politics and public-health patois was of a simplistic modification in "behavior," akin to giving up nicotine, alcohol, or chocolate. There has been little research on the psychic and social cost of pursuing changes in sexual behavior among gay men. It is important, therefore, to find out how men are handling the deep disturbance that sexual behavior change was and is.

## Australian Social Research on Gay and Homosexually Active Men

A considerable amount of social research into HIV/AIDS has occurred in Australia, almost all of it funded by government. There are a number of Australian data sets pertinent to gay and homosexually active men, most of which concentrate on men attached to gay communities in the various capital cities.[3] In a sense these studies form a de facto baseline for current knowledge of the behavioral responses to the epidemic in this population. The SAPA study (noted earlier) is the single most influential Australian study, forming the basis of two follow-up studies: the Sustaining Safe Sex (Triple S) study undertaken in New South Wales and Tasmania in 1991 and Project Male-Call, undertaken Australia-wide in 1992. This latter, a national study of gay and homosexually active men, was undertaken by the National Centre for HIV Social Research (Macquarie University Unit) in 1992 and relies heavily on the questionnaire and many of the analyses from the original SAPA project, but offers truly national baseline data for the first time (Kippax et al. 1994).

There are many other smaller behavioral studies done in various parts of Australia, but the conceptual strengths of the original SAPA study place it among the five or six major data sets on gay men in the English-speaking world. Although the data from the original SAPA study are now ten years old, it is these conceptual strengths that make it worth returning to for guidance on current HIV/AIDS prevention issues. Moreover, the findings of the SAPA study, later confirmed nationally by Project Male-Call, raised many questions that went beyond the scope of their classically quantitative methodologies. These questions stimulated the current study and offered many starting points for the close-focus investigation reported here.

Barney Sherman's extensive sexual experience seems to indicate considerable lability in the sex lives of Australian men, an issue to which this study will return later. Even with all these behavioral studies on gay and homosexually active men, however, we can make only an educated guess at the extent and social dynamics of homosexual activity among men in Australia. General population studies of sexuality are rare in Australia and much needed, not just to ground HIV/AIDS research but also for sexual health policy and planning in general. Those small studies which have been done offer little assistance in estimating the size of the population of homosexually active men. Three AIDS-related studies of Australian sexual

---

[3] For Sydney, see Connell et al. 1988, 1989, and 1990; Connell and Kippax 1990; Kippax et al., "Question of Accuracy," 1990; Kippax et al., "Gay Community," 1992; and Crawford, Kippax, and Dowsett 1990. For Brisbane, see Frazer et al. 1988. For Melbourne, see Campbell et al. 1988; Burgess et al. 1990 and 1992; and Sinnott and Todd 1988. For Adelaide, see Ross, Freedman, and Brew 1989. For Canberra, see Kippax et al. 1989; for Western Australia, see Waddell 1992 and 1993, and Waddell and Buchbinder 1992. For regional New South Wales, see Dowsett et al. 1989; and for working-class gay men, see Connell et al. 1991, and Dowsett, Davis, and Connell 1992b.

behavior can be scrutinized for some information concerning the extent to which, in such surveys, men will admit to being homosexually active.

The Australian Market Research Company was commissioned by the Commonwealth Government to survey the Australian population in 1986 in preparation for the launch of the first mass media AIDS education campaigns. That survey found that 6 percent of adult males reported sex with another man at some time in their lives and 3 percent reported having done so in the previous twelve months. For those between sixteen and twenty-four the figures were 6 percent and 2 percent (Australian Market Research, unpublished). Unfortunately, just what the "sex" was, in terms of sex practices, is unclear. M. W. Ross (1988) found that 11 percent of his sample had male-to-male sex at some stage and that 6 percent had done so in the previous twelve months, that is, twice the Australian Market Research figures. There were sampling difficulties in this second study, but the doubling of the figures should alert us to the relationship between a research method and its findings. Various studies report small percentages of homosexual behavior among university students: 2.2 percent at Macquarie University, 2.4 percent at the University of Sydney (Crawford, Turtle, and Kippax 1990). Similar student studies report degrees of anal intercourse of between 10 percent and 25 percent, mostly without specifying the partner's sex; much of this may be with a female partner (Rosenthal, Moore, and Brumen 1990; Turtle et al. 1989).

There is little comfort to be had from these figures. These small general population studies have problems of sample and method. The student studies focus on university students, a middle-class sample, and one noted for having less sexual experience than their nonstudent contemporaries (Kippax and Crawford 1991). That said, others would argue that homosexual sex is and has always been a significant part of Australian life, from the male initiation rituals of Australian Aborigines, about which little is generally known, to the sodomitical origins of the institution of Australian mateship (Hughes 1987). The sexual habits of Australians from non-English-speaking backgrounds have received much attention, most of it, however, only speculative (see Rosenthal, Moore, and Brumen 1990 on young Greek-Australian males; Australian Market Research, unpublished, on anal intercourse among adult, non-English-speaking men; and more recent, Gifford et al. 1994).

It is probably not possible to know the extent of homosexual behavior among men. What is clear from the research findings is that an incalculable number of Australian men can and do have sex with other men, some frequently, some occasionally, in the right circumstances or at certain times in their lives, in certain sites or in certain institutional settings, with certain cultural overlays, or all the above. The interviews in the current study, in investigating this particular issue, revealed a considerable diversity of contexts in which men pursue sex with other men.

Many of the standard survey techniques may never obtain sufficiently accurate accounts of the extent of such activity. This is particularly true when such sexual matters are deemed unreportable for moral or legal reasons. Despite the legalization of gay sex in Australia, certain discriminatory restrictions still apply in many States, such as different ages of consent, restrictions on public sexual expression, control of permissible images in film and media representations of homosexuality, in differential standards in pornography, and so on. These political/cultural dynamics will always confound attempts to uncover just how sexually active—whether "deviant" or conformist—Australians are.

The search for a definitive answer on the extent to which men have had and will have sex with other men is not going to offer a clue to the likely extent of this form of possible HIV transmission and its geographical location. There is considerable doubt whether it is necessary to know the extent of homosexual practice among men in any country in order to develop public-health policy and to implement HIV and STD prevention strategies. More important is the consideration that no statistic on the extent of male-to-male sex, even of anal intercourse, should affect policy and budgetary decisions concerning prevention. This is so because it is not the *extent* of male homosexual behavior that needs to be addressed but the *diversity of the contexts* in which it is practiced.

These *sexual contexts* determine, to a large extent, the nature and cost of effective health promotion among gay and homosexually active men. For example, the chances of an eighteen-year-old youth contracting HIV from having receptive unprotected anal intercourse with a schoolmate in a small town in far-western New South Wales are slim; if he pursues the same activity with a passing truck driver on the way from Sydney to Adelaide via Broken Hill, the chances increase dramatically. A married man who does the beats each week in inner Melbourne, but only engages in mutual masturbation, runs no risk of contracting HIV, no matter how many partners he has. A homosexually active but heterosexually identified man who goes to a gay sauna in Sydney once a year and engages in receptive unprotected anal intercourse, maybe with one or two partners, runs a high risk. Prevention needs to address the diversity of these sexual contexts and the meanings they generate, irrespective of the frequency of homosexual events.

So although surveys are conducted the world over to inform public-health initiatives about the sexual behavior of gay and other homosexually active men, counting the condoms used, the number of partners coupled with, and sometimes even the memory of motivations surrounding sexual events, they cannot capture the complexity of sexuality or its meaning, intention, desire, and contextual contingency. Different research is needed to explore the desire for, and the sexual contexts in which men seek, sex with other men.

Yet behavioral surveys have revealed a remarkable transformation of the homosexual repertoire since the onset of the HIV epidemic. The SAPA study (Kippax et al., *Sustaining Safe Sex,* 1993) revealed that considerable changes in men's sexual behavior had already occurred by 1986, and those documented changes threw light on some very interesting aspects of gay community life. Therefore, a brief summary of the SAPA project's findings is warranted.

## The SAPA Study

Over the southern-hemisphere summer of 1986–87, a team of twenty-five field-workers surveyed "men who have sex with men" in Sydney; the nearby commuter cities of Wollongong, Newcastle, and the Blue Mountains; two country areas—the Orange-Bathurst area in central New South Wales and the Northern Rivers district of New South Wales; and Canberra, the national capital. These largely gay, mostly male, field-workers administered, face-to-face, a lengthy structured interview to 535 men, yielding up to 1000 items of information per subject. The questions covered topics such as social descriptors, background and personal circumstances; gay identity and participation in gay community life; sexual experience and practice with regular and casual male partners, female partners, and prostitutes; knowledge of HIV/AIDS issues, safe sex practices, and awareness of local HIV/AIDS educational initiatives and programs; and health status, history of STD infection, contact with PLWHAs, and HIV test status and result. A full account of this survey method and the sample achieved is discussed in Connell et al. 1988.

Findings from the project embrace a range of issues: knowledge of HIV transmission and attitudes to HIV/AIDS; behavior change in terms of sex practices, sexual relations, health care, and drug use; the continuance by some men of unprotected anal intercourse; regional differences in men's responses to the epidemic; the behavior of men who have sex with both men and women; the impact of HIV-antibody testing; the effects of close contact with the epidemic; and the importance of gay community attachment to HIV prevention.

The SAPA study confirmed the success of the gay communities' education and prevention strategies to date. Gay community sources of information about what is "unsafe" and, in particular, what is "safe" in homosexual sex were the most cited in achieving the widespread awareness found among the respondents (Kippax et al., "Question of Accuracy," 1990). These sources include the gay press, gay organizations, and friends. This overall level of knowledge of HIV and AIDS was widespread through the sample, but accuracy of that knowledge was patterned. Knowledge of what is "safe" was related to men's awareness of AIDS pamphlets and membership in gay organizations, pointing to *attachment* to an organized gay community, whether in an urban or rural area, and its education strategies as an important contributor to successful health promotion.

Further findings indicated that assessment of the safety of sex practices is related to experience. For many practices, the least experienced underestimate the safety, and possibly restrict the range, of sexual activity available to them; the most experienced underestimate the risk of practices they are used to. Again, a link to area of residence pointed to a social patterning of knowledge acquisition and mediation, indicating that the immediate context—social networks, support systems, a secure place to be gay—were important for accurate assessment of risks associated with sexual activity.

Knowledge does not necessarily produce the changes in behavior that are needed to prevent the sexual transmission of HIV; and the process of mediation involved in absorbing information proved to be more complex for Barney Sherman and for Peter Standard, the first man actually interviewed for this study and who, though a volunteer in a gay community AIDS service organization, was having great difficulty in dealing with safe sex, in particular, the uncertainty concerning the safety of oral-genital sex and of getting semen on the skin during mutual masturbation. It was Peter Standard who first alerted me in 1987 to the ongoing nature of gay men's struggles to sustain safe sexual behavior over time.

The SAPA study revealed that change in sexual behavior was also related to the context in which men deal with HIV/AIDS. There are different ways to react to the threat of a sexually transmissible virus: some men might stop having sex altogether, or cut down on the amount of sex; some might become monogamous, or at least more nearly so. None of these strategies replaces abstaining from those sexual practices which transmit HIV. Unfortunately, mixed messages were broadcast during the early days of the epidemic calling for partner reduction or monogamy, which grew from a mistranslation of epidemiological correlations between partner numbers and HIV infection, and from a desire to stop gay sex entirely. Such a request has never been made of heterosexual men and women anywhere in the world.

Safe sex was, at one and the same time, a demand by gay communities for sexual rights in the face of anti-gay forces and an intelligent reading of gay sexual activity and the necessary modifications that would make it "safe." There is still resistance to safe sex, whether heterosexual or homosexual, from those who will not accept any departure from their particular interpretation of the purposes of sex. Notwithstanding, health programs on AIDS around the world quickly adopted the term "safe sex"[4] in one form or another, in a realistic response to the growing awareness that sexuality encompasses such cultural and social diversity that uniform strategies of prohibition and regulation will not work. In this, the international gay community led the world.

One legacy of the confusion about the transmission of HIV and the political arguments about sex is that some men adopt incomplete strategies or incorrect ones in the belief that they may be doing enough. For example, monogamy without the benefit of HIV-antibody testing is not a protection against HIV infection. Neither is a reduction of partner numbers in and of itself. Only the adoption of "safe" sex practices (or celibacy) prevents the transmission of the virus. The SAPA project recognized this pattern of response and assessed changes made in both the relations of sexual activity— whom you have sex with—and in the practices of sex itself.

The SAPA study reported that a change in behavior in male-to-male sex occurs most among men who have friends practicing safe sex, who have seen the pamphlets produced by community health organizations and know what is "safe" and "unsafe," and who are more immediately in contact with the epidemic. Less effective behavior change occurs among men who are economically and sexually less secure and who are in circumstances where an interest in male-to-male sex is difficult to explore or reveal (Connell et al. 1989). These men were likely to try changing their sexual relations, which, without a change in practices, is not adequate in reducing their chances of HIV infection. Interpersonal relationships and social networks, we may infer, are important in producing changes in sexual behavior, pointing toward group or collective educational strategies rather than those focused on individuals. The significance of this *relational* aspect in homoeroticism became an important issue for the current study.

Attachment to an organized gay community and its safe sex education programs was significantly related to successful behavior change among gay-identified men (Kippax et al., "Gay Community," 1992). The different

---

4 Some countries use "safer," as the term to describe risk reduction strategies with reference to HIV transmission, and the same arguments are used for and against either term. It is Australian policy to use "safe," and this study, therefore, uses this term.

patterns of participation in gay community life and their differential impact on behavior change were as pertinent for the rural and provincial gay communities as for the large inner-Sydney gay community. These findings reinforced the need to investigate in more detail the enactment and meaning of "gay community" (see Chapter 6).

Together these findings pointed to the need for *informed social support*, not just as a context for understanding the seriousness of HIV/AIDS and for producing behavior change, but as a vital ingredient in a *collective* response to the epidemic. This collective response appeared to work on two levels. The gay community AIDS organizations have worked hard in their education strategies to create a safe sex culture. There is also an interpersonal dimension to this collective effort, where men with differing patterns of attachment to gay community life are providing information, support, and encouragement to one another. Similar findings on the significance of this collective or communitarian aspect of successful behavior change later emerged in studies in other gay communities in the Western world (summarized in Dowsett 1993b).

The effectiveness of these interventions is confirmed by data that indicate a significant drop in rectal gonorrhea and other sexually transmitted diseases among gay men (Donovan 1988; Australian Gonococcal Surveillance Program 1988); a substantial drop in rates of new HIV infection (Burcham et al. 1989); and significant and sustained sexual behavior change (Connell et al. 1989; Kippax et al., "Longitudinal Study," 1993; Kippax et al. 1994).

The SAPA project asked some detailed questions about sex practices in order to assess major suppositions about homosexual sex. The research pointed to a definite patterning of the sexual repertoire among gay men (Connell and Kippax 1990). Although anal intercourse was regarded as the most "physically satisfying" and among the most "emotionally satisfying," it was practiced by only about half of the men in the sample. Oral sex, on the other hand, was rated very highly in terms of physical satisfaction and somewhat less highly in terms of emotional satisfaction and was practiced almost universally, along with mutual masturbation, kissing, and massage—all "safe" practices. It was possible to identify three repertoires differentially practiced by men. The first is the *oral/tactile* group consisting of largely "safe" practices, including oral sex and practiced by almost all gay men. The second group focuses on *anal* sex in various forms, excluding fisting, and these were variously engaged in by about half of the men. The third group is called *esoteric* practices and includes fisting, sadomasochism, and watersports, and these were practiced by less than 10 percent of men. It appeared that men who are economically and socially more secure had a wider and more varied sexual practice.

Although there was a decided preference among some gay men in their assessment of sexual "enjoyment" for the insertive or the receptive *mode* in anal intercourse, in practice such activity is commonly reciprocal, men moving from insertive to receptive modes at will. This focus on anal intercourse (and oral-genital sex) seemed to confirm a *genital primacy* in homosexuality, but the SAPA researchers also noted a *communicative primacy*, again reinforcing the relational character of homosexual sex (Connell and Kippax 1990: 180–81). There is also a conscious element in gay sex: men choosing to forgo pleasurable activity in order to pleasure others and in order to remain safe from HIV infection.

Given the significance of anal intercourse to the definition of male homosexuality, this analysis was provocative: it tends to play down the centrality of sodomy to gayness. Yet I would argue that, irrespective of the frequency of anal intercourse revealed in the SAPA study, anality *is* central to gay men but perhaps in different ways than previously conceived. As a consequence, I added the range of experiences of, and meanings attached to, sodomy to the growing list of issues for this study.

Despite this remarkable level of change among gay men in their sex practices, various studies noted significant pockets of continued unprotected anal intercourse among men (Morlet and Guinan 1989; Connell et al. 1990; Kippax et al. 1991; Kippax et al., "Longitudinal Study," 1993). These findings confirmed growing concern in many gay communities in Australia (and abroad) that some men persist in engaging in unprotected anal intercourse for reasons that are none too clear. (For an international summation of this issue, see Stall et al. 1992.) Much of this concern centered on the concept of *relapse*, and much research has pursued the men who still engage in, or who have reverted to, such practices (for example, Stall and Ekstrand 1989, and Lynn et al. 1989).

The term "relapse" does not adequately describe the dilemma for gay men at all. "Relapse" is a health promotion term more appropriate to issues of alcohol and drug use. Like the equally unfortunate term used in criminology, *recidivism*, it purports to describe a return to unfortunate or dangerous behavior. But for gay men the sexual activity now called "unsafe" was not an unfortunate or dangerous behavior; it was ordinary sexual behavior, validated historically by homosexual communities, their cultures, and political struggles for the decriminalization of that specific sex act. It just so happened that a virus got in the way.

A higher frequency of unprotected anal intercourse with regular partners in the SAPA study indicated decisions being made about safe sex in the context of intimacy, with a judgment about the quality of the relationship being a basis for assessing risk. This may prove a correct judgment in some cases: in Canberra, for example, well-educated gay men were involved in a quite sophisticated decision-making process, drawing finer distinctions between insertive and receptive anal intercourse and oral sex involving ejaculate (Kippax et al. 1989).

In Melbourne, Gold et al. (1991), pursuing cognition and its relationship to sexual behavior, noted that 69 percent of "unsafe" sexual incidents happened in private homes, with only 18 percent occurring in sex-on-premises venues. This finding gestured toward some effect in the interpersonal negotiation of sexual encounters. The data also reflected the continued prevalence of "unsafe" sex within regular relationships, although more than half the incidences occurred with a casual partner.[5]

The SAPA project also noted that such decisions about "safe" sex are less well taken by some men: men in the "high danger" group (defined as those who reported having unprotected anal intercourse with a regular or casual partner sometime in the previous six months) showed higher use of sex-on-premises venues. The differences between "high-danger" men and "low-danger" men occurred in "settings where the making of casual sexual contacts is informally but definitely institutionalised" (Connell et al. 1990: 202–3).

These findings would seem to indicate that the social structuring of sexual events themselves is important in understanding events of unprotected sex. Overall, they point to the contexts in which men who are interested in sex with other men live their sexual and social lives. When the findings, reported earlier, on which men had more effectively changed their behavior are also taken into account, the idea of social constraint seems very applicable here; men with fewer personal resources and skills in situations where homosexuality is difficult to explore do less well in coping with adopting and sustaining safe sex. The circumstances that led to Barney's infection come to mind immediately here. In contrast, it is in an alternate pattern and structure of immediate relationships, social networks, and at-

---

[5] This finding on casual partners does not agree with those of the SAPA study and the Victorian Gay and Bisexual Men's Health Survey (Campbell et al. 1988). These two studies found less "unsafe" sex in casual encounters. The Gold et al. sample was recruited from gay venues and the men surveyed were younger than in the other studies: this may explain higher levels of sexual activity with casual partners overall. Moreover, the men sampled in the study were *only* men who had experienced "unsafe" sex on some occasion(s), making it impossible to generalize about the patterning of "unsafe" sexual events in populations of gay and homosexually active men.

tachment *to* gay community practices, institutions, and infrastructure that the generation of successful responses to the epidemic are to be found.

The SAPA analysis stands in stark contrast to that which seeks to isolate the characteristics of persons who, for example, practice "unsafe" sex, and points to the contextual nature of a decision to adopt "safe" sex. Such decisions are contingent on circumstances—intimacy, settings that encourage a slip "just this once," restricted access to accurate information, group support—and must be reaffirmed at each challenge. The ongoing prevention of HIV infection among gay and homosexually active men requires a different account from that focused on the correlates of individual behavior change—an account that generates a range of educational opportunities at the collective level, and thus avoids focusing on what is wrong with the individual. This concern with the "problem individual," which continues to emerge in much HIV/AIDS research leads, on one hand, to a pathological account of gay men and, on the other, restricts the health promotion response to therapy (Roffmann et al. 1990). This reduction of focus merely offers a prevention strategy that no country can afford.

What is beginning to emerge is an account of men grappling *collectively* with this epidemic and its consequences. More important, the ingredients for developing and sustaining a response to HIV/AIDS that prevents infection, I would argue, are to be found not so much inside individuals as in their social relations, in the collectivities in which they live. This analysis contains important challenges for health promotion and HIV prevention, which if it relies on traditional health education models of knowledge and behavior, tends to focus only on individual behavior change. Although a focus on the person with problems is often helpful, the construction of the "problem person" is one consequence. Rather, successful strategies for education and prevention lie not so much in remediating the individual as in providing the collective strategies and support programs for groups of men in which to deal with the constant task of sustaining "safe" sex.

### Working-Class Men Who Have Sex with Men

Some of the SAPA project team launched a second study in 1989, which focused on working-class men who had sex with men—the Class, Homosexuality, and AIDS Prevention (CHAP) study. Using measures of "income," "education level," and "labour market situation," the original SAPA survey data were reexamined for more detail on the subtle class effects that had emerged in the original analysis. The responses of men with lowest incomes, least education, and greatest vulnerability in the job market indicated that their sexuality was less separated out from the heterosexual social matrix as a distinct and acknowledged cultural form. There were slight differences in sexual histories: earlier initiation, more often by older partners; overall smaller numbers of partners and suggestions of more reactive sexuality; a sense that solutions to AIDS will be found "out there"; less involvement in softer, "safe" sex; less condom use, and a greater likelihood of unprotected anal intercourse with casual partners; less HIV-antibody testing; and various indications of less accurate knowledge of safe sex (Connell et al. 1991).

Many of the men in this current study were recruited through the CHAP project when it became clearer that class and the effects of social inequality were deeply implicated in their responses to the epidemic (Ariss, Carrigan, and Dowsett 1992; Dowsett, Davis, and Connell 1992a; Connell, Davis, and Dowsett 1993). There are present-day concerns about utilizing class as a theoretical tool, but it is important to state here that whatever the criticism of structural concepts such as class in social theory today, the attempt made in the CHAP study has shone a light on issues concerning AIDS, HIV prevention, homosexuality, and gay community that had not emerged before.

The CHAP research pointed to a dissonance between working-class gay men's lives and gay community–inspired representations of safe sex (Davis et al. 1993; Dowsett 1994a). The unity of homosexual desire and of "gay" started to dissolve as these men talked of their sexual experience in different terms. This dissolution is explored in detail in Chapters 6 and 7.

### Other Studies

The Triple S (Sustaining Safe Sex) survey, undertaken in 1991, followed up a subsample of the original SAPA study four years later via a shorter telephone interview—in essence a successful trial run for the methodology later used in Project Male-Call. The Triple S results (Kippax et al. 1991; Kippax et al., "Relapse," 1992; Kippax et al., "Longitudinal Study," 1993) revealed little evidence of relapse. There was also a firming of accuracy in knowledge levels, particularly on the issue of oral-genital sex. A significantly larger percentage of men had been HIV-antibody tested (88 percent in 1991 compared with 68 percent in 1986/87), but HIV-antibody test result was still unrelated to successful behavior change. However, it was clear that in regular relationships, gay men with concordant HIV serostatus, namely, both seropositive or both seronegative, were negotiating unprotected anal intercourse using their test results as one factor. This was termed by the researchers as *negotiated safety* and is the subject of considerable controversy (Ekstrand et al. 1993; Davies 1993).

It is important to note that such negotiation about unprotected anal intercourse using HIV-antibody test status was occurring in a highly informed population that had already achieved a high degree of compliance with safe sex regimes. It was also a population that had been encouraged to test and which had almost reached testing saturation. More recent, close-focus research has revealed less successful employment of the negotiated safety strategy among younger men and those less supported by an attachment to gay community (Chapple, Dowsett, and Smith 1994). The Triple S findings also confirmed Vadasz and Lipp's (1990) earlier report on gay couples and the negotiation of condom use. The strategy of negotiated safety is another example of the need to understand the contexts of sexual activity, in that it illustrates both the interpersonal and social structuring of sexual expression within relationships.

Triple S holds one other important piece of information about gay and homosexually active men. Previous SAPA work (Crawford, Kippax, and Dowsett 1990) indicated that, among men who engage in few or no practices of gay community attachment, personal experience of the epidemic was important in changing sexual behavior. In the Triple S study many more men reported personal experience of the epidemic. This far wider personal experience of the effects of the epidemic than evidenced in 1987 indicates that the level of pain and loss throughout the gay communities of Sydney had deepened and widened significantly. This collective experience of pain has not ever been addressed in any Australian educational or support program for the gay community funded since the epidemic began.

Project Male-Call pursued many of the measures developed in the SAPA and Triple S studies and applied them nationally for the first time to a population of 2,583 gay and homosexually active men (Kippax et al. 1994). Measures used included scales such as those describing sexual repertoire (three scales adapted from the SAPA study), HIV avoidance strategies (four scales), and a set of ten indicators that assessed knowledge and eight that assessed practice.

Project Male-Call confirmed the high degree of compliance to safe sex regimes nationally among gay-identifying men. The patterning of that safe sex compliance was analyzed through five central factors: age, region, education level, gay community attachment,[6] and sex of partners. It is the rela-

_____

[6] It is important to avoid confusion here between the Project Male-Call discussion of "gay community attachment" and the more complex analysis of intersecting practices described in the original SAPA study. The Project Male-Call analysis uses the same term to refer to a single measure of involvement in gay communities' *social* activities. For that reason, and so as not to confuse the later discussion of attachment to gay community (see Chapter 6), the Project Male-Call findings will be referred to as "social attachment."

tion between these factors, especially the intersection and overlap between the last three factors, that is highly suggestive of a particular social structuring of sexual contexts.

Among the Project Male-Call sample in general, accurate knowledge about HIV transmission and AIDS was widespread among gay and homosexually active men. Less accurate general knowledge and knowledge about specific "unsafe" sexual practices were found among men not living in "gay Sydney" and "gay Melbourne," men with low levels of education, men with low levels of social attachment to gay community, and men not tested for HIV antibody. Among those less socially attached to gay community, mainstream media were an important source of information. This finding would seem to have two implications: (1) mainstream media would appear to be an important component of any future prevention activities directed to homosexually active men less attached to the gay community; (2) its lack of use in Australia (and in most Western countries) to date in attempting to send a clear message to this particular population about the specific dangers of unprotected anal intercourse between men has been an unfortunate loss of opportunity.

Interestingly, men who had sex with men only were more knowledgeable than those having sex with both men and women about the risks associated with unprotected penetrative sex with women. It may be that gay men have a sense of "ownership" of HIV/AIDS information. Men who do not identify with a gay community, irrespective of their sexual activities, may not take as much notice of the available HIV/AIDS information.

It is important to note, however, that 31 percent of the Project Male-Call sample had *never* practiced anal intercourse with other men, only 8 to 12 percent had practiced unprotected anal intercourse with casual partners, and a small 5 percent had practiced unprotected intercourse with both men and women partners. Most unprotected intercourse took place within regular relationships, confirming the possibility of negotiation of sexual activity and reinforcing the importance of regular relationships as a major sexual context for risk-taking, an issue this study pursues.

In relation to avoidance strategies measured by the Project Male-Call analysis, a wide variety of strategies had been adopted. Younger men were more likely to use condoms, but older men were more likely to avoid anal intercourse. Differences related to regional distance, low education levels, less social attachment to gay community, and having male and female sex partners were associated with less effective behavioral responses to the possibility of HIV infection. The three factors, education level, social attachment to gay community, and sex of sex partners, are very closely related.

These factors do not measure the same subsample of the Project Male-Call respondents, but all three are remarkable in predicting similar less-effective responses to the epidemic.

This raises the question about the interrelation between these factors. The less well educated were also significantly more likely to have sex with both men and women, as were those less socially attached to the gay community. And the less well educated were also less socially attached to the gay community. Of interest is the region factor, where, on many Project Male-Call indicators, men not living in "gay Sydney," "gay Melbourne," or Canberra were responding less well. Similar associations were found with lower levels of education, less social attachment to gay community, and more likelihood of male and female sexual partners.

The size of the Project Male-Call sample allows some generalization with confidence beyond its immediate findings. The intersection of factors is too strong to go untheorized and the start of such theorization must be the relation of the sexual to the structural in social life. These key factors in the Project Male-Call analysis are measures of the experience of social inequality and difference. Inequality does not simply mean having more or less of some social good: less education is also a product of unequal access, inequitable provision, and cultural marginalization; geographic distance poses real limits to opportunities; social isolation can lead to constraints of sexual expression. Social difference is also not simply about distinction between equals, but about hierarchies of validation and prospect. The relation between factors that sketch or approximate the experience of social inequality and homosexually active men is too strong to ignore.

When the overall amount of sexual activity reported in Project Male-Call by homosexually active men (as distinct from gay community–identifying men) was assessed (even if it might be more unsafe than among gay men), there was less sexual activity in all going on and with fewer partners of either sex. It would seem that a sexual boundary of some sort between gay men and other men undertaking homosexual activity is in place. Just what that boundary is and how it functions led this study to explore the complex structuring of sex between men outside of "gay" as it was comfortably regarded at the Amsterdam conferences discussed in Chapter 1.

## Conclusions on Prevention and Behavior Change

It is clear from the interrelatedness of aspects of behavior change, monitored by such measures as the SAPA project developed, and Project Male-Call generalized, that the behavior change process is a dynamic one—one where the political and bureaucratic arrangements for the development and deployment of preventive education among gay and homosexually active men mesh with the historical emergence of the gay communities' responses to the epidemic. This convergence not only facilitated, but also structured, the nature of the educational interventions directed to gay and homosexually active men. The uniquely gay character of educational approaches and representations, the utilization of the cultural, social, and sexual aspects of gay communities in the community intervention strategies, combined with direct, knowledge-focused attempts to secure an informed collective movement toward adopting safe sex, has worked well. For men attached to gay communities this dynamic process of change has achieved its goals. The evidence of significant behavior change, large reductions in STD rates, and a greatly reduced incidence in new HIV infections among gay men is clear.

For homosexually active men not attached to a gay community, a complex interaction of geographic and social distance and the inequities of social class has hindered the appropriation of gay community–identified messages, largely through a lack of informed social support. This finding emphasized the social character of behavior change, the dynamic interaction between the overall national prevention effort, that of affected communities through their institutions and practices, and individual lives. This largely successful response was tightly woven within the fabric of the gay communities themselves, but somewhat frayed at the margins where men's attachment to gay life was less established or pursued.

The statistical data also provided indisputable evidence of a different "positioning" of anal intercourse in many gay men's lives than might have been imagined by, on one hand, the homophobic, and on the other, by those with psychoanalytic analyses of desire. Also, the exhibited capacity for sexual behavior change could not go untheorized. The patterning of the findings of the SAPA project offered another possibility: that of postulating a more *social* motive in sexual activity, something less *un*conscious, something more collective or relational, more experiential and embodied; indeed, the findings indicated a possibility of investigating a dramatic moment in the social construction of sexuality.

Barney's story took on a different shape against the backdrop of the SAPA findings, but gestured toward a more complex picture. At each point of the fieldwork for this study, pressing questions were raised by the behavioral research findings. Could failures to sustain "safe" sex be explained in part by, for example, Barney's approximation learning strategy? Does the unfolding of Barney's exclusion from gay community life suggest how a process of gay community attachment operates? Further, are there lessons to be learnt from Barney's unraveling life about the meaning of gay community? More important, are there limits to "gay community" itself? What is the relation between gayness and the recurring theme of less-educated, lower-paid, working-class men handling less well not only HIV/AIDS, but also a wide range of issues to do with homoeroticism and gayness?

It is this behavioral research—which in a way raised more questions than it answered—that this study took as a starting point, embarking from its overall pattern to proceed with some confidence to begin close-focus work. With Barney Sherman's life history as a model, the study interrogated further interview material for the possibility of addressing these pressing issues of HIV prevention as well as those concerns arising from the international conferences outlined in Chapter 1. My fairly confident approach was, however, soon blown out of the water by my first meeting with Harriet.

# 4

# Gender Bender

My birthday in 1991 was my fortieth, and I received a homemade card of an attractive, nearly naked woman (something I am rarely sent by my almost uniformly nonsexist friends). The snapshot was a full-length color portrait of a slightly chubby, very bleached blonde, wearing naught but a shocking-pink strapless brassiere supporting a prodigious cleavage, a pair of similarly pink garters holding up a pair of black stockings. The model, perched on black stilettos, stretched somewhat pudgy arms upward, fingers extending outward at right angles, in a pose of defiant allure. The legs were pinched together at the knees, framing a carefully shaped pubic region of deeply black hair. The face, heavily made up, offered an enticing smile full of sparkling teeth. This was Harriet's birthday present to me.

Who is Harriet? Actually, *he* is Huey Brown, late thirties, sandwich maker of Nullangardie. Harriet became one of my favorite people interviewed in this study. He was one of the most straightforward and candid men I met. We talked first in one full-length interview, then in a number of group discussions and during a few meals together with other men. I encountered a thoughtful, amusing, and reflective man, courageous in a way not often ascribed to either homosexual men or drag queens. The interview, for all its wonderfully camp, self-deprecating humor and tales of glorious adventure, revealed a quietly determined person in charge of his life as he saw it. It also revealed a life operating within a particular set of social limitations.

Huey/Harriet problematizes the usefulness of making gender the central organizing concept for analyzing sexuality. He cannot be understood in terms of gender binaries, and forces us to question the almost automatic link conventionally drawn between gender and sexuality. He also allows the investigation of the process of the construction of a sexuality through practice; and in this his life history questions the usefulness of the idea of a gender identity and a sexual identity. Finally Huey/Harriet demands a broader concept of a *sexual subjectivity* within a larger *sexual order* as a better way to understand the structure and practice of desire.

## Harriet Rules, OK!

Huey Brown was born in Nullangardie to a truck driver and his wife. His parents knew he was gay and accepted his sexuality immediately. Huey attended local primary and junior boys high schools. Boys schools are notoriously difficult places for "different" kids, and he was "poofter-bashed" more than once. Although Huey mentioned knowing other kids in school to be gay at that time and later met some of his teachers on the beats, school was an isolating and painful place and he left at fourteen. In those days of full employment in Australia (even for youth), Huey found a job immediately at a local supermarket as a "cash-register girl," a job he held until age twenty-one.

Since then Huey's work history has been dominated by two themes: first, friends helped him get most of his jobs, almost always in the food and hotel services industry; second, he entered into pub work as, variously, a housemaid, a bar worker, and, eventually, a drag performer—a "show girl" as he termed it. These jobs were always concurrent: whatever else he did in the entertainment industry, Huey always kept a steady day job as a sandwich maker on shift work for the same café. The contrast could not appear greater.

The future is of a life running more or less along the same lines until he retires on the aged pension. It is important to note that working-class men like Huey live on meager incomes, often have unstable employment, and have skills of limited value in an ever-changing labor market. Lives such as his also include limited opportunity to explore that middle-class notion "choices." There is sometimes real poverty and restricted access to wider cultural resources.

Huey is always called "Harriet," which is not just a drag name, his showgirl character, or simply a "girlie" name. Everyone calls him "Harriet," and he calls himself that. I got the impression that if I called him Huey, I would be disapproving of him in some way—that I would be insulting him and his community.

Sexuality

Harriet's sexual history started early:

> I remember I was getting off with my next door neighbor R. This was when I was six, seven, and eight. There were the two brothers down the road. There was the boy S down the road. There was the boy B and his brother about two streets over from our place. This is in between a three-year period, right? And then I was having my first cousin and his brother down at my grandma's place. . . . They were rooting me or playing with each other or pulling each other off.

It did not take long for the neighborhood to get the gist of what was happening and for young Huey to get a few more serious offers: "An old man that used to be down the street used to, sort of, befriend me and play with me little wee wee and I used to let him. And anyway one day he offered me a shilling—[both laughing] don't laugh, it was fuckin' hysterical—to stick his cock up my bum." By early adolescence he was also touring the beats on his bicycle with a mate on Sunday afternoons, having sex with older men and youths. From this point, he eventually entered a few local homosexual friendship circles and social networks.

The bathing sheds at Nullangardie's beaches also provided a favorable venue for sex with men (cf. Barney's tales of the beach pavilion), and Huey's growing familiarity with beat sex was part of the collective knowledge among his peers and the men of Nullangardie:

> We used to have to go from our school, which was at the top of the hill, and walk down past the best known bog [toilet] in and out, which was Nullangardie Common, and it had about six or seven cubicles in it . . . and me and him would head for the biggest cubicle. While three or four of the other queens knew what we were going on to and they used to try to perve [steal a peek] through holes in the door. So we used to have to block it up. So we could get it off together. Never knew what happened to him, I always wondered. . . . God, he was a big boy.

By the time Huey left school, he was well and truly versed in the sodomitical delights of Nullangardie, and beat sex was to form a major aspect of his sex life from this time onward. Such sexual activity was widely practiced and commonly acknowledged by almost all the men interviewed in that city. This was the first indicator that the sexual order in Nullangardie was a little different from its public personation.

By his late teens Huey had met the local drag queens of Nullangardie and become Harriet. This already very sexually experienced Harriet was then ready for love. Harriet's first love was damaging. He was badly beaten a number of times because he would occasionally have a "bit on the side," describing himself at that time as a "slut." This looks very much like a modeling on heterosexual relationships, but it also looks like the brutal end of working-class life, where men use violence to maintain their control over others—men, women, or drag queens.

A brickies laborer called Jim was the second big love. This relationship lasted nine years: "Like brothers, like lovers, like friends. It was great." (Note: Harriet does not say: "like sisters.") This relationship was quite well accepted by parts of Jim's family, and Harriet and Jim even baby-sat Jim's nieces and nephews. Harriet said: "They thought I was the best thing that ever happened to him because I quietened him down a lot." It all looks a bit like a soap opera; even sex with Jim was a touch role-oriented:

Basically he did me. And he was excellent. He was that straight that he just didn't like a cock near his bum. A couple of times I did and he just . . . you know. But I always said to him, you know, after a few years, I said: "Look, you know, either you let me or I'm going to look for it somewhere else." So I was getting off with other guys behind his back. But he sort of knew but accepted it that way, because he knew that I was butch as well and couldn't get what I wanted off him. So he played around occasionally but I did it sort of mostly all the time. But he knew. It was a husband and wife team sort of thing. I looked after him and he looked after me. But it was okay.

After nine years, Jim left Harriet for a sixteen-year-old girl of whom Jim said: "She's everything that you are except she's a girl"; an extraordinary insult to Harriet, who by now had "tits" and was vaguely considering a "cut 'n tuck." One more hurtful relationship (this time with a preoperative transsexual drag artist) and Harriet called it quits. He has not had a close emotional-sexual relationship since.

Harriet was, by this time, clearly playing on the edge of transsexuality, transforming his body with breast implants, contemplating (but never going so far as to have) the "op."[1] But what are we to make of Jim? Working-class job and family; fearful of anal penetration in a "backs to the

---

[1] In Australia the term "transvestite" is reserved for men, usually heterosexual, who obtain sexual pleasure in cross-dressing. "Transsexual" (or "trannies") is the more widely used term to describe the varied experience of transsexual culture and activity and associated issues of sexual identity. The narrow psychosocial or clinical definition of "transsexual," related only to gender dysphoria or reassignment surgery, their issues and effects, is explicitly rejected by Australian transsexuals (see Collyer 1994) for a broader, more encompassing cultural definition.

wall, guys!" way; settled in a classic domestic relationship with a partner; baby-sitting siblings' children: it sounds like an ordinary suburban life, except his partner is a drag queen with breast implants and a penchant for insertive anal intercourse with casual partners on the odd occasion! Jim illustrates another instability in conceptions of working-class masculinity and male sexual interests and propensities. Whatever Jim was or is, he certainly cannot be called "gay," and when Harriet says: "He [Jim] was that straight!" he means a sexually conventional male, not a heterosexually identified one. This is not simply an example of the dissociation between sexual identity and sexual practice; it calls into question the salience of sexual identity itself.

Harriet explained how a gay boy finds his feet in Nullangardie: "Um, just probably hanging around toilets, I suppose, or will get the inkling that some of their friends have done somethin' in the toilet and been interested and sort of had a look." The beats were central to Harriet's sexual practice and to his public image. He was well known as a "beat queen" and would call into a number of beats on the way to and from work, friends' homes, or whenever he felt like it. If someone turned up, Harriet most often would suck him off, always using a condom (part of a rigorous "safe" sex practice Harriet sustained).

Almost any public toilet and bathing shed in Nullangardie offers the possibility of sex between men, and between youths and men. All men interviewed in Nullangardie knew about these possibilities and almost all utilized them. The history of these beats seems to be as long as living memory at least, and they were implicated in the sexual induction and initiation of most of the men interviewed. No man—gay or otherwise—could be unaware of the Nullangardie beats: the large number, their well-known locations, the clear markings on walls, and the frequency of their use must ensure they are part of the sexual possibilities available to the men and boys of that town. Just how many use them is anybody's guess. It is worth noting however, that although gay men in Nullangardie come in for some harassment and some homophobia, there is no history of serious bashing, even in the beats.

But is there another scene?

Shit yeah. (Made up of people like barristers and lawyers?) And hairdressers and all that sort of shit.

(And where do they hang out?)

I have no idea. I know that there are, but they just have private parties and all that sort of stuff. And doctors and dentists and hairdressers and a couple of lawyers or clerks.

This is an upper-crust homosexual social network, whose existence is quite widely known by Nullangardians from various scandals in the past and from their common link through a local church. There is certainly a class divide in Nullangardie, but Harriet's knowledge of the others and how privilege operates is sketchy.

The gay community for Harriet consists of a group of long-standing friends (some HIV-infected), other drag queens he has lived and worked with for years, ex-prostitutes, and old tricks. For years Harriet has been a part of the group of men organizing the annual Nullangardie Gay Fiesta. He organizes the entertainment, usually a classic revue with glamorous frocks, pretty boys, drag queens singing cover versions of recent hits and torch songs, raffles and prize-giving, and a good deal of unself-conscious humor and ribaldry. These are earnestly produced shows meant to entertain and to help raise money for various gay-related projects. The Fiesta is an important moment in community-building, and Harriet is central to that process.

Nullangardie's gay community does not have a definable precinct, although friends tend to congregate in the inner suburbs. There are some key institutions: a couple of AIDS service organizations; a fund-raising charity; a disco; some regular key events. But the heart of this community is formed from a set of overlapping, long-standing social networks of men in early middle age, with younger, newer acolytes who find their way into this unnamed and unnamable network, learning the ropes, and adding their youth, beauty, sexual interests, and a more modern "gay" sensibility to the configuration.

In this sense it is a historically formed "sexual community" (D'Emilio 1983), but it is also an older homosexual subculture with its camp elements being slowly overtaken by a newer "gay" community. As a result, Harriet was having his contribution to this community limited: younger "gay" men now want muscular male strippers at the Fiesta instead of the drag routines in which Harriet specializes.

### Sexual Identity

There are a number of facets to Harriet's sex life: the gay man, the "dragon," the prostitute, and the slut. Together these form components of what might be called a *sexual identity*, a concept greatly utilized in gay and lesbian theory on sexuality and increasingly generalized to encompass heterosexually active people as well. The term has assumed an existential function representing a psychic state, or a resolution of an individuated coming to the self. As such its effectiveness is increasingly questionable. Harriet's story reveals something of the "coming to," but also reveals the inadequacy of *sexual identity* to capture fully the process of self-formation that occurs.

(So you knew you were gay at school?)

Yeah, when I was five or six.

(How could you tell? What was the thing that convinced you?)

I didn't like girls and I used to play with dolls. I've always known about my sexuality, always. I got forced onto girls a couple of times by my parents and that, but never had an erection over them, never been interested at all.

Harriet is very definitely effeminate. His style is classically camp, replete with gender inversions. It seems very old-fashioned, even anachronistic in modern gay community terms, with a definite residue from the drag scene he had entered as a youth. That scene no longer exists in Nullangardie in anywhere near the same elaboration. Harriet also presents a blend of gayness and campness. He uses the term "gay," but just as a new word for "camp"; for Harriet "gay" is simply the fashionable term. He does not like "homosexual" and strongly dislikes "fag" or "faggot." This banter of terms pointed to the fact that gay liberation ideas had made only partial inroads into Harriet's life, in that some personal elements only have been appropriated.

Harriet regards liberation, though, as something he has known about for far longer than anyone else:

I've been liberated for years, forget it. If they can't be satisfied with living the way they are—I don't mind it, right, but I've always been the way I am and I've been liberated since I was a kid. I am the way I am because I am, and that's the way I present myself. And if you don't like it, well, tough shit to you. This is to anybody, right, and I'll say this to anybody. Um. If you don't like me for how I am, well, you're the one who's missing out, sweetheart, not me. Because I can be just as friendly and just as nice and just as much of a cunt as any straight person can be. And if that's the way you are gonna look at it, well, tough luck on your part, because I can be just as wonderful as anybody else. That's right, that's the way I live, you know . . . if I'm not liberated, nobody is. And I don't need to say that I am liberated because I am the way I am.

Harriet is rarely so serious and impassioned. Yet his language does not draw on a gay liberation rhetoric. It is not simply a liberal statement either, though it is cast in individualistic terms. There was certainly a moment when one hears a misquoted and all-too-familiar song title in the declaration. "Liberation" is equated with self-acceptance first and then a defensive distancing of the external world's response as *their* problem, *their* loss. The statement also reflects pain and hurt and the results of considerable mistreatment at the hands of others.

There was never a clearer, more purposive use for the "essentialist" notion of identity. Harriet's indignant determination in the face of oppression is something that cannot be understood fully by its relegation to one side or the other in some essentialist/social-constructionist binary. For Harriet, being gay is a personal resolution, not a political manifesto. No member of the gay intelligentsia, Harriet offers incontrovertible evidence of the performative basis of identity; he gains ground *in practice* against the effects of hegemonic heterosexuality. Harriet utilizes his sexual identity to deal with living as "gay" in a "straight" world each day. The dangers of a discursive deconstruction of the sexual identity "homosexual" (and the more insistent "gay") are clear: they would leave Harriet stranded like a beached whale.

Yet Harriet's manifesto only goes so far. He is aware that the cost of oppression to others like him is too high, but he simply remonstrates at their lack of strength or purpose. If there is political peril in essentialist identities, it lies in their limitation to individualized understandings and their validation of voluntarism. "Gay" for Harriet has yet to become a *collective* endeavor, one denoting immersion in a declared politics and culture.

There is a further significant element in Harriet's identity as gay, and that is a strong sense of distance and difference from the modern gay communities of inner Sydney: "Oh, I just don't feel adequate. . . . I don't feel comfortable amongst a group of gay men." In spite of this reservation and unease, Harriet has been very supportive of the burgeoning Nullangardie gay community. He has also hopped on a float in drag at the Sydney Gay and Lesbian Mardi Gras and talked of its parade as hard work with friends, thereby pointing out the group effort that constituted the "community" for Harriet. The larger political and cultural construct, The Gay Community, does not correspond to his idea of gay community. His alienation—and that is what it amounted to—is from, among other things, the commercial scene, where masculine beauty, muscles, the "SM bars" (he means "same models"), recreational drug-taking, and the high sexual and fashion stakes exclude him. Despite his centrality to his own vibrant local gay community, Harriet feels invalidated by the modern gayness of Sydney, instantly recognizable as similar to gay life in New York, London, Amsterdam, Berlin, and San Francisco.

Harriet might be "gay," but only in his own terms. It may be that "being gay" needs to be rethought; it may not be simply a psychic state, a resolution of desire in a singular manner. Rather, being gay may entail the negotiation of multiple possibilities, a declaration of belonging to different places, a daily performance rather than some sort of static achievement. It may represent a distancing from, as much as a proximity to, other collective resolutions of homosexual desire.

At age seventeen or eighteen Huey, physically, became Harriet. He had been hanging out with drag queens in a city that has quite a significant drag history of its own. Harriet's is not a transsexual story; he does *not* regard himself as a woman trapped in a man's body: "I like my dick." These networks of drag queens formed the first major social circle Harriet developed and with them he learnt his trade as a "dragon."

As a young drag queen, Harriet was lithe, pretty, and had a body good enough to be a stripper when he had "tits" and used a "fanny," that is, a *merkin* (a genital wig). He is now approaching forty, somewhat overweight and full-faced. The only common feature Harriet and Huey still shared was a brilliant smile. Dressed as Harriet, the "girl," he still glistens, gleams, and "vibrates" (his term) in his own way. But he is the same person or character frocked or unfrocked. The vocabulary, the intonation, the conversation are from one person only. Huey/Harriet is Huey-Harriet, one identity, person and character, namely Harriet; the difference is merely which "frock" he wears that day. Harriet is no *impersonation*.

Drag is a practice as much as an identity, and there is something about the construction of images of femininity that Harriet and other drag queens share. The common contention is that these drag queens derive their imagery and style from women, from heterosexual femininity in particular, and from an anxious identification with women. These accounts of the imitation of women and women's bodies in particular fail to recognize something more complex going on.

There is a very fine line somewhere between femininity and camp. Consider Joan Collins and her endless parade of new frocks in *Dynasty*, or Dolly Parton's exaggerated figure extending the female body into a realm of the improbable, or Bette Midler's conscious appropriation of camp in her early career as a performer in the gay bathhouses of New York. It is hard to tell whether these women are any less in drag than Harriet in his expertly executed, if homemade, creations.

For example, in *The Rose*, Bette Midler's Janis Joplin, now a famous singer, visits an old haunt, a drag revue bar, only to find herself included in its parade of impersonations of the famous. Called up on stage in recognition of her fame and her past association with the bar, Midler faces "herself" on stage, and the audience in the bar and of the film is forced to ask which is the more authentic construction: Midler's character, the impersonator, or even Midler herself?

There is another consideration. What might Joan Collins, Dolly Parton, and Bette Midler borrow from Harriet and his forerunners? The idea of authenticity is questioned here. Which came first: femininity or cross-dressing? Are they mutually constitutive? If femininity is to be considered socially constructed rather than "essential"—and there seems to be no doubt that drag, cross-dressing, and transsexuality (Connell's "daughters of the knife") are constructions—then what might the latter contribute in a femininity/drag binary not just to exaggerations such as Parton et al., but also to what Connell called "emphasised" femininity among ordinary folk (1987: 183ff.)?

The fixation of drag queens with representations of glamour is always tinged with parody, and the long tradition of drag as a representational and performing artistic practice and "character" might not only contribute to the construction of Harriet and his fellow dragons, but also inform emphasized and/or exaggerated femininity. It is doubtful that drag queens simply or only ape, copy, or want to be women. Nor do they merely elaborate a directly feminine image; there is an articulation and a refraction.

There is an authenticity in drag that comes from its long history in theater, in particular the pantomime and its "Dame," and in vaudeville and music hall. Its association with, in particular, British and Australian pubs and clubs illustrates a long-standing drag tradition (in the sense of collective practice rather than an elaborated and vaunted canon), which Harriet inherited at the hands of the Nullangardie dragons.

The motivations of each man who practices drag may be different. Some are transsexuals, pre- and postoperative. Others are transvestites whose sexual kick comes from cross-dressing. A third group live mainly as men but with alternate selves to perform on occasion. Still others are like Harriet—one person, one personality, two wardrobes. For all these different motivations and satisfactions, in a town as small as Nullangardie they all collapse into the single category "dragon."

For Harriet, being a dragon is not just about being beautiful; it is also about getting sex. It seems that drag has never been just about image and style. The eighteenth-century molly houses of London were clearly venues in which cross-dressing embellished and "dramatized" male-to-male *sexual* possibilities (Bray 1988). Harriet certainly has a sexual agenda in drag:

(But you wouldn't for instance go off to [the local night club] on Saturday night and try to pick up somebody to take home?)

As a boy or as a girl? (A boy.) Um, no one is really that interested. (As a girl then?) I'd manage quite well. Not for a queen, not for a gay guy. I could get a fuck any day goin' in drag. You know, that goes without saying.

(But that doesn't happen for you out of drag?)

No. I've never been that appealing.

This sexual success of Harriet, the girl, is an important part of his sense of self. The "tits" are an important part of this image and its success, so much so that he had them done twice after the first lot of silicone went hard:

I used to work at the [hotel] with a little tit top cut down to there, just to the top of the nipples and little scallops . . . so when you were pouring a beer you put your hands like that and [shows a gesture] behind the glass, the boys used to love it. I used to get all the surfies over my side and all the seamen would be over the other side [laughing]. It was fabulous. And all the bikies would be down the front, so I'd be serving. It was great. See-through tops with just me nipples comin' through a lamé top I used to wear, it was all floral. They used to love it.

Harriet came close to being a professional or as close as he could get in Nullangardie. At times in his career he was performing weekly in clubs and at the local seaside resort. He performed guest spots at famous clubs in Sydney and in other drag venues. He was often a stripper, using a good deal of tape and a merkin to produce with the right lighting the illusion of being a real female. Those years meant a considerable accumulation of experience and skill.

The songs are an important part of being a drag queen. They must "fit" the persona as a performer. Harriet bought records and if the songs "have guts," if "you can perform it" and "the feeling is there," this made the song appropriate for him. The performance might involve lip-synching, but the connection with the song is not merely imitative; Harriet does not pretend to *be* Shirley Bassey.

The dragon in performance may be a characterization to an extent, but in Harriet's case even performing is continuous with a single self. Harriet with "slap" on, gowned to the top of the very wig he is fond of, sells far more raffle tickets at HIV/AIDS fundraisers than Harriet the boy ever could. Drag is not a private act; it is a public statement. It receives its meaning from the collective witnessing of its enactment. This is not just a recognition by the boys at the bar of Harriet's pub, but also by a collective, historically formed "clutch" of dragons through their cultural processes, including various rites of passage (first outing, first performance, first sexual success). Drag is a product of the accumulated skill and dragon lore of Nullangardie.

Life as a dragon is not all glamour and glitter. There are always difficulties with the law. Bar work and drag shows do not pay well, and the "market" was small in Nullangardie. Those, like Harriet, seeking other work in the shrinking unskilled job market have problems enough in a postindustrial society like Australia, where work in manufacturing is decreasing rapidly. The service industry can absorb only so many. Add a penchant for wearing frocks and "tits" to the package they offer, and it is no wonder many transsexuals supplement their incomes by turning to prostitution. Harriet, living among the dragons in Nullangardie, was no stranger to their sexual activities. It is not at all surprising that he eventually tried his hand at a little prostitution.

In one sense, Harriet started earning money from sex earlier than most:

I think I went home one day with too much money and put it in my money box . . . and mum wanted to know where I got the money from. I think I told her. It was hysterical. . . . [The police] took me into a room and they had someone look up my bum with a torch. I don't think it was a doctor. I think it was all just to frighten me.

The three major aspects of prostitution—sex, money, and the law—were present in preadolescence.

Harriet got into prostitution accidentally. He had often been walking up and down the streets in drag on the way to work at the pub or in a show, and he finally accepted an offer. He was in his late twenties at the time:

And then when I discovered I could make money out of this, I thought, oh that's not too bad. And it's just like getting off in a bog with someone, you know, except you get paid for it. So I thought I don't mind this. So I worked on my corner for about two and a half or three years and made heaps. . . . They'd be waitin' for me, three or four cars lined up. I was good!

Harriet in his private sex life reported having sex a number of times each day, usually in beats. Harriet came to sex work at the same age Dennis Partridge stopped (see Chapter 7). It earned Harriet extra money beyond his very basic wage. A brothel also allowed him to do a shift now and then to earn money. He did not get involved in the drug use that often surrounds sex work. While this is somewhat similar to the freelance rent boys in Sydney, it is a far cry from tales of girls locked into sexual slavery by madams, brothel owners, pimps, and drugs that we hear so much about, and reveals an important stratification in the sex industry. The organization of sex work in Nullangardie enabled sex workers like Harriet to stay in control. Dragons, unlike girls, ran their own businesses.

The level of sexual skill involved in being a prostitute is an issue here, too. Harriet was not at all coy about sex, and handled his trade with dedication, wit, and humor:

> They want what you've got. That's why you can limit your services and they still get satisfaction out of the limit, you know. Like the end result will be that they'll still blow. That's what they want. . . . And as I said, if you are good business they'll come back, and I was having repeat business after repeat.

He commented on clients whom he found unattractive and I asked if he used his own sexual fantasies to help:

> Not necessarily. When you've got this big blob layin' in front of ya—I used to have to stick it up him—oooh, it was hideous—or he'd stick it up me and I'd just close me bum, because he was so fat he sort of didn't have a big dick and you could just tighten your bum and he'd think it was in ya [laughing].

Skill is obviously more important than fantasy. But sex work is work, similar to a trade in this case, and there also needs to be some kind of respect for the client:

> In particular there was one old guy—big, fat, hideous, warts, fat, and smelly bum and dick. Oooh, it was hideous. But like with anybody, I can find—if you're as ugly as shit, right, I can find something in anybody that can appeal to me or can be nice. And this fat hideous man was a nice man and I didn't mind pleasing this nice man. . . . I can still get an erection over it and he was hideous. But he was the nicest man, you know. He'd come back and ask for me specifically.

Harriet has played around with esoteric sex a little, mainly sadomasochism with a few customers, and the occasional moment of piddling on a lover or client. He expressed some disdain for coprophilia and fisting. He always insists on a condom and negotiates from a position of "condom or nothing." Harriet has remained HIV-uninfected even as a very active sex worker in a town with its own significant homosexually transmitted HIV epidemic. He was as skilled and careful in receptive intercourse as in everything else he does.

Harriet's skill in sex work, using beats, and in safe sex negotiation would seem to make him excellent material for an HIV/AIDS education outreach worker in his area. No wonder so few sex workers are infected in Australia, if he is anything to judge by. Yet the local gay community AIDS service organization refused to hire this "known homosexual." Even his gay community credentials and solid volunteer work are insufficient to guarantee him a place in the new-style professionalized gay community-based AIDS service organizations.

Harriet recognizes that there are dangers other than HIV in sex work (or in the beats, having been bashed once), but he puts his successful management of risk down to his "women's intuition," that sixth sense of what the punter is like. In this passage he revealed some of the danger and intelligence involved in successful sex work: "But you know, you can sense vibrations, like you're walking in a park at night and it's dark and you know you've got to be careful, you know you've got to be wary. . . . You're alert, yeah, always. Always conscious if you are sucking a guy off in a car where his other hand is, always."

Harriet proffered the following categories for prostitutes: queens, dragons, transsexuals, male prostitutes, boys, and girls. These are the different sex objects available in that sexual economy; they can also be taken as fine differentiations in categories of desire:

(So they wanted some men in drag at [male brothel in Sydney] as well . . . ?)

Oh yes. There were transsexuals working there, and dragons. Some very popular names in Sydney work out of the parlors [laughing] . . .

([The brothel] actually advertise themselves in the gay magazines, mainly using men's bodies. They don't in fact use drags at all.)

But that's it. They have another transsexual business name they use in most of the [non-gay] men's magazines. You don't advertise dragons in a gay magazine because gay men don't want dragons. So you advertise in straight magazines where a straight man would be interested. You don't think about that, do you?

This supersedes any simplistic, gender-defined reading that might interpret this differentiation as variations of the male/female binary. And there is also a clearly defined set of practices on which the sexual economy operates. Harriet, for example, offered only oral and anal sex.

Being a prostitute encompasses a number of facets, then. Harriet was one of an assembly of sex workers in Nullangardie who worked certain sites, offering a range of complementary practices; they recognized each

other and each other's speciality. Being a prostitute requires having a repertoire of skills and techniques for negotiating the relations of sex. It is also a
public identity. Even though Harriet was somewhat affectionately known
as a prostitute among his friends, it had serious consequences for his contribution to HIV/AIDS. Being a prostitute is a complicated state of affairs
reaching far beyond the name now often used for it—sex worker. Although
the term "sex work" emphasizes the industrial aspects of the job, Harriet
illustrates a clash of desires, skills, relations, and motivations more complex than the notion of work offers. Harriet must invoke his own desire in
order to undertake some sexual encounters; his body is intimately brought
into play, "greased" or otherwise, his erection must penetrate, his desirability as a "girl," such an important part of his own sexual self, must be
employed to gain customers. Harriet, the prostitute, *engages* sexual desire,
rather than *servicing* it.

Prostitution is not without its costs to those engaged in it. Dennis Partridge, who worked for ten years as a prostitute, reported that his private
sex life suffered as a result of being involved in sex work. There would
appear to have been far less damage to Harriet's private sexuality (Nullangardie may be less harrowing than Sydney). Harriet retained a strong sense
of self in the practice of his sexuality, even though it was Harriet the girl
who was most often desired.

Finally after being arrested twice for sex work, Harriet called it a day.
He had spent the money he had made on frocks, a few possessions, and a
trip or two. He'd never made big money, just a few hundred a week extra.
He retained one or two old clients and contented himself, sexually, with
daily visits to the beats.

Harriet has always liked sex. His apparent popularity with local boys,
one neighborhood father, other men later in the beats, and eventually on
the streets and in the hotels and clubs of Nullangardie drew heavily on
Harriet's own sheer enjoyment of and easiness in sex. As we walked the
length of Nullangardie's main street one afternoon, Harriet, dressed as a
"boy," brazenly pointed out each man he had had sex with: some rushed
past with downcast gaze; the Coke delivery man scurried into a shop; a few
queens shrieked "G'day"; and the number of furtive glances was astonishing. Either Harriet the "girl" was clearly recognized in Harriet the "boy"
by some of his trade, or an awful lot of men do the beats of Nullangardie.
And on his own or as a prostitute, Harriet had had them all.

Harriet certainly pursued everything with energy and will: "I just
pleased myself. If I wanted to go out in drag I did. If I wanted to put on
makeup I did. If I wanted to go out as a boy I still did. It didn't bother me."

But this willfulness was also about sexual success; Harriet the girl was far more successful than Harriet the boy. The boy did the beats, daily, offering blow jobs through glory holes to unseeing peers. Harriet liked sex a lot and saw nothing wrong with that, and he went on to make a distinction between being sexually loose and morally a prude, that is, one could have high moral standards but still enjoy sex.

Harriet the prostitute was no passive victim of the sex industry. His accounts of his explorations of drag and sex work are full of purpose and determination:

I think there were about six or seven guys—truckies, right. I had them lined up. . . . I think there was one, two, three, four, five, six, seven trucks. I mean those big semis, right. And they were all on the corner talkin' and I fronted 'em and had each one, one after the other. And then they went back and talked to each other. And I had every one of them. It was a joke, one after the other.

Harriet clearly likes sex and lots of it: "I'm a slut. I don't mind, I admit it. I'm the first to admit it. I'm good at it." Again, Harriet offers a personal statement of being a slut, both as a state of affairs so far achieved and as a promised continuation. It was also a comparative statement invoked as a defense against and in a recognition of others' ambivalent interest in his promiscuity. It is also a social identity: Harriet the slut is proudly ashamed and shamefully proud of his sex life, and this paradox is a significant aspect of his sexual self-assessment.

## Toward a Sexual Subjectivity

These four aspects of Harriet—the gay man, the dragon, the prostitute, and the slut—put in question the taken for granted categories of *sexual identity* and *gender identity*. The concept of identity is now increasingly narrowly defined as a distinction between sexual orientations—heterosexual/homosexual, gay/straight, and, maybe somewhere, bisexual; and between the sexes—male/female and, somewhere, transsexual. These binaries are useful; they do offer a grip on experienced inequalities and discursive distinctions increasingly deployed as definitions and defenses. They have a performative value: after all, even heterosexuals need a sexual identity, particularly when a homosexual walks into a room.

Sexual identity is generally seen as a psychic dimension. This might be regarded as its ontological function: one *is* homosexual; one's homosexuality is an internally experienced desire for one's own sex. But this psychic dimension seeks to elaborate and explicate little of the practices and relations of this mode of being, this homosexuality, this desire, or of its intentions and meanings.

The elements in Harriet's life that might constitute his sexual identity cannot be confined to the issue of his homosexuality. First, Harriet's sexual identity does not simply specify his sexual interest in men in response to a discursive definition as homosexual. It developed locally in the beats and among the homosexually active men and dragons of Nullangardie. Nor does "gay" offer him much; "camp" sufficed in this regard. This newer gay identity recalls elements of the countervailing discourses of gay liberation and gay community, but was developing under pressure from something that while renovating the homosexual subculture in Nullangardie, was also threatening elements of Harriet's identity and practice. It is important to recognize this relation between this essentialist function and its evolution.

But Harriet came to his gay identity through *practice*: years of sexual activity found a resolution in camp, later gay, and the shaping of his sexual identity by the experiences of sex itself is a major constitutive element of his being. Harriet's sexuality is a tested, experienced, and embodied capacity for pleasure. It could be argued that this is sexuality as *praxis*. The idea of sexual identity as psychic resolution barely captures this complexity.

Second, Harriet is also a boy-girl, and the girl is not an overlay on the boy. Harriet's is an integrated personality. He has played with what might be termed *gender identities* through the employment of the subcultural tradition of drag and all its historical baggage. Harriet the dragon is as much a product of Nullangardie's long history of drag as he is of the success he made of it in the eyes of others: other dragons, venue owners who hired him, patrons who liked the stripper, beautiful boys who admired the "tits," his lovers, the other men he had sex with. Harriet the dragon is a complex mix that goes well beyond drag, camp, mimicry, or, for that matter, sexual and gender identities.

The notion of gender identity as a concept, residing in and centered on male/female, man/woman, masculine/feminine binary oppositions, is not useful here. Harriet is Harriet, a dragon with "tits" and a "dick," both comfortably in and having their place. Harriet also confounds any attempt to seek some sort of "natural" definition of gender by appealing to the body as a source of definitive judgment. Harriet demonstrates that what is called gender might actually be raw material for a *sexual construction of the self*. What can Harriet's body be other than what Harriet makes of it?

Harriet's time as a sex worker adds a third dimension. Sex workers personify sex; they *are* desire. And they are not passive in this; prostitutes are "phallic Others" (Tyler 1991: 62), that is, they are constituted as eroti-cally powerful, sexually active, desiring (not just desired), whether they be women, men, or pre- or postoperative transsexuals. Harriet employed all but the last of these enactments as a sex worker at times, recognizing the value in each and in the mixing of them. He knew in practice not to mis-take the penis for the phallus and manipulated these unstable categories used only by theorists to produce pleasure for himself and others:

> If they thought you were a girl, well, naturally, they'd assume you'd have a fanny and they'd go for the tits first. But if they knew you were a boy and you had tits right—they could see that—the first thing they'd try to find out whether you had a cock. In some cases. And most cases they like the dick. . . . I guarantee—take a percentage—80 percent of the men that I had, right, were basically straight you may as well say, that liked to dabble with boys. Say, out of 100 percent, I rooted about 70 to 80 percent of them. And [they] loved it.

Fourth, this transgressive field of sexual pleasuring among men is the sexual world Harriet recognizes and inhabits, defining himself in the per-formance of sex itself. Harriet's body has been an ever-changing canvas for sexual expression, at one and the same time, a symbol of desire and its practice exercised exuberantly at the hands and bodies of other men. Harriet's *body* itself offers capacities and experiences that go beyond any-thing satisfactorily described by sexual identity or gender identity.

Last, one must ask the question looking at the sexually active and sexu-ally saturated life of Harriet: Where is all the urgency in sex, the getting carried away, the loss of the self, sex as the *le petit mort*, the disintegration of being? What of the "deep" murky side of sex that preoccupies psycho-analytically derived theory and commentary such as in contemporary film theory or scads of postmodern, meaning-driven accounts of sex? Barney's very conscious wicked fun in sex and Harriet's clearly consciously pursued, pleasured, and pleasuring sexual activity suggest a lighter enactment of desire. This is different from the heavily interpreted, multilayered, motive-prone, and deeply fractured reading of sex to which contemporary theo-retical discourse is prone. A discourse that from its progenitors (Freud in the main) to the present, may itself be as much a construction (and a bour-geois one at that) as Harriet in his frocks. But Harriet has few doubts about what his frocks signify. In order to take Harriet's sexuality seriously we must question discursive frameworks that render Harriet or Barney merely as "users" for whom the "operating system" is "transparent."

Harriet exemplifies the active construction of the self within a discursive framing of a homosexual desire. Yet the frame is very pliable and without its contents it threatens to collapse. To some extent being gay, that is, clarifying a sexual identity, is a discursive practice providing sufficient direction to enable men to cluster with like others; it is a collective resolution of individual desire. It becomes the vantage point from which the rest are assessed. But Harriet's example calls for a different conceptualization of sexual identity. To stretch the concept to include a preoperative transsexual prostitute, a dragon, a gay man with a sluttish sexual appetite, these experiences of transgressive male sexual interests, renders the term unwieldy. The term "sexual subjectivity" offers a larger conceptual space to encompass the ingredients Harriet illustrated.

## A Sexual (Dis)order

The considerable evidence of the collective (homo)sexual explorations of the youth and men of Nullangardie outlined by Harriet and other men in this study reveal a process whereby homosexual sex might not only be limited to a classifiable sexual orientation fixated on a same-sexed object, but might be a more general *experience*. Many of these boys and men later marry; others retain an interest in sex—with dragons, with prostitutes of dubious sex/gender, and with each other. These men explore their sexual interests largely tangentially to a definable gay community or its more discreet homosexual social networks. The evidence points to a larger, blurrier pattern and expression of homoerotic desire, which operates contextually and is related historically to the sex lives of working-class men in Nullangardie.

There is a multilayered sexual community of interest here: the dragons exist; the straight boys hanging on the corner for Harriet probably have girlfriends and even wives; the gay men live alongside the older queens; the bourgeois gays remain separate from the working-class ones, but meet each other on equal terms in the beats; younger gay men bring challenges from a newer gay order. The context is larger than the obviously gay, camp, or homosexual; there is a strong link with masculine sexuality and with a distinctly male sexual perversity.

Is this a counterhegemonic practice? It does fly in the face of the sexual order with its dominating male heterosexuality, denial of childhood sexuality, the insistence on private sexual expression, and so on. Nullangardie's men are certainly "sexual outlaws," yet they lack John Rechy's (1977) conscious and political pursuit of homosex. They do not present a gay liberationist determination to flout the sexual order. It is a group of working-class men and boys pursuing a tradition of sexual activity among themselves, reproducing the framework for the sex lives of generations of men in Nullangardie.

Robert Hughes (1987) may be right in his revelatory account of the Australian colonies' sodomitical past. The legacy of that almost obligatory fellowship of desiring male bodies might affect Australia's present in very deep structural ways, providing "mateship" with more "mating" in its meaning than we might like to acknowledge. Has a (homo)sexual order been constructed and preserved in Nullangardie through endless generations of first convicts and then working-class men pursuing their orgasms with/on/in each other? Harriet "worked" the local football clubhouse, doing blow jobs on "basically straight men" in the club toilets when short of money. Harriet's clients during his sex-worker days were young men wanting to get their rocks off and married men coming home from the local factories:

(What did most men want?)

Well, at that stage I'd give them what they wanted. They couldn't have straight sex. Like I wasn't a dragon, I was a girl, right [i.e., he pretended to be female, but with a restricted repertoire]. So as a girl I couldn't do straight sex, I could only do anal or, or I'd blow 'em. Some guys sort of knew the score and want to blow you. Want you to fuck them, you know. Whatever they wanted they got. . . . Anybody that wanted to, who could afford it. (Young boys?) Yeah, I've had one young boy pick me up in his car, drive me back to his place, raid his piggy bank and come out with, I mean, $40 worth of change. He made me wait in the car so he could count it out so he could have me. They come straight from the garages which are locked up in the night and have the rolled change, four lots of rolled 20¢ pieces—$20, joke! You go home with a pocket full of change! Then you get young boys pestering you—well, like when I was working on the street—young boys pestering you on their push bikes. . . . Sixteen or seventeen. We used to get a group of them. Ah, beautiful!

There is a strong parallel here with Harriet's lover, Jim—"He was that straight!"—in the fractured identities, the willful perversity of desire and the ambiguity in its enactment.

This local sexual economy ventures beyond Harriet's taxonomy of sexual partners to a flouting of these categorical sensibilities. Harriet's masquerade itself is central only for a time:

This customer that I said I have all the time, the only one I've got now, right. He fucked me for years before he found out. And then it didn't bother him. He never sort of thought about it . . . and then he sort of discovered my dick and, you know, I used to root him senseless. I still get paid for it.

With other clients eventually, even the masquerade is no longer relevant:

I started doing them in drag and then, sort of: "I'm as a boy at the moment. Do you still want to come over?" And they say okay, so I still have them out of drag.

This dissolution of categories cannot simply be explained away as a minority or the deviant few. Harriet's experience as a prostitute had him well placed within a working-class masculine sexuality that can swing any way, and which seems still to be somewhat beyond the deployment of sexuality.

There is a *discursive silence* that facilitates considerable sexual adventuring among men. By this I mean that the major discourses defining and elaborating sexuality are not in massive evidence. Their determinative power is limited and remarkably partial. More local narratives may be involved, but these must not be seen as derivative of, or simplistic responses to, a larger structural imperative. Harriet and his sex partners are not struggling with definitional issues of sexual identity through discourse, but are exploring a profound sexual ambiguity through daily practice. This discursive silence also registers homoeroticism as much closer to the consciousness of men and frustrates a conceptualization of such sexual activity as resistance to the sexual order as whole. Rather, the order itself begins to look increasingly shaky.

The structural tension between gay and heterosexual men is not that of polarities, but of interwoven destabilizing possibilities. Joseph Bristow argues that "we [homosexual men] are—to the heterosexual world—walking definitions of sex. We *mean* sex. Our lifestyle is defined as a sexual lifestyle, a lifestyle that says *fuck.* . . . The fascination of sex is endless. Gay men provide a convenient target for the displacement and projection of widespread social confusion about heterosexuality on to a small 'perverse' group" (1989: 74). Partly right. Gay men most clearly represent something disturbing for straight men: a pleasure foregone, a possibility, a representation of the unspeakable within. But the men in Harriet's sex life are not simply registering an unconscious confusion, a displacement, a straining at the "compulsory heterosexuality" bit and its problems of practice. Many of these men have *experienced* perversion itself.

It may be that gay men are not the "other" at all. Jonathan Dollimore's use (1991) of the term "proximate" rather than "other" in his analysis of anti-homophobic discourse captures a closeness, a nearby ever-present possibility and danger in the easy access to homosex available among gay men, but offered more widely by the likes of Harriet. Such proximity may explain homophobia as less an unconscious or abstract desire displaced sometimes into violence (in Australia generally at the hands of gangs of working-class youths) and more as a memory of experience, fantastic or material, invoking the "crisis tendencies" of masculinity (Connell 1983: see chapter 3). It adds weight to Eve Kosovsky Sedgwick's argument (1990) that homosexuality should be seen not as the sexual preference of a minority, but in universalizing terms as central to the social structuring of all sexual expression and the "pedal point" in the social relations between men.

It would be a mistake to place this sexual ambiguity into some kind of benign continuum of male sexuality: the "men-who-have-sex-with-men" group used so frequently by HIV/AIDS researchers, policymakers, and educators. For there is quite clearly danger in these exploits. Such desire is not free-floating. This *sexual (dis)order* is not some Rousseau-ian fantasy. Harriet, as a prostitute, has been hassled by police (who continue, literally, to police his desire) and the sex worker scene in Nullangardie has cooled considerably since HIV/AIDS and various crackdowns on street work. The tense structural relation between homosexuality and heterosexuality is not rendered asunder by the efforts of Harriet and friends. This sexual (dis)order is clearly built on ever-shifting sands. Yet it continues wantonly, and only the very skilled know how contingent any moment actually is. For chaos has structure too:

> I had just had my tits out and I got booked through an agent, right, to do a strip up at [military base] for the Sergeants Mess, when one of them was goin' to get married, right, or goin' away or something. And I said, well okay, but [the agent] sort of explained to them that a drag queen was goin' to do it, [because] they couldn't get a girl who would do it for 'em. "She's a good stripper, looks good," and all that sort of shit, and they said okay. Anyway, so I took a friend of mine with me, who did my sound and lighting for me. Anyway, [we] arrived on the base and got through the thingybob [security] and got checked out—not bad! So I finally met the guy who organized it all. Well, I was para [paralyzed with fear] see. So I said: "How do I look?" He said: "Great, lovely." I thought, oh that's nice. So I did this whole thing for 'em. I did VD Polka from the Andrew Sisters—ever heard it? (No.) It's really good, about VD. Um, and then I did that and I think I did "You've Gotta have Boobs," which is a bit of comedy. And I think I did "Let Me Entertain You," which was a strip routine. Anyway, I ended up draggin' a guy on the—and they were sus [suspicious], right, but they didn't know

[Harriet was a drag queen]—so I ended up gettin' the guy who was there and sort of unzippin' his fly. And they told me that one of the bigger bosses was there so I avoided playin' with his dick. So I unzipped it and sort of walked away during the number, and then I dragged him out on the floor and sort of sat on his face. And he got up and said: "She ain't got balls!" And it went over really well, and I was para because, thirty or forty guys, all in the army. And after the show had finished and they all clapped and screamed and all that sort of shit. And I particularly remember slinking back to the dressing room with nothing on but a feather boa wrapped round me neck [laughing]. I know how to do it. (What did you do about tits?) I didn't have my tits. (So you just used the feather boa?) Yeah, but you sort of lean forward and you see a little bit of sag sort of thing but you cover it with your fanny. You've got a fanny [merkin]. That's what they'll look at.

It is perhaps this final quote that reveals fully the extent of sexual (dis)order that Harriet inhabits and constructs. This notion of a (dis)order is not a claim for universal bisexuality or some other such essentialism; nor is it to be confused with the gay liberationist trope that every man can be had given the right circumstances. The male sexual (dis)order revealed in Harriet's story is not a majoritarian practice. And it need not be, for quantity is not the issue. It is not a question of how many homosexual men there really are, or of how many men have dabbled in male-to-male sex, or experienced desire in response to homoeroticism, or even of how many have partaken of the poorly disguised delights offered by Harriet. In the working-class city of Nullangardie—and who knows where else—it is the category male and the idea of a singular masculine sexuality that Harriet and his partners destabilize.

Sexual expression between men in this city is a major preoccupation for many, and the opportunities afforded by the historically produced sexual (dis)order provide the means whereby (homo)sexual encounters are readily available. It is not surprising then that Nullangardie does not experience high levels of gay bashing. After all, other men in the study reported that their school friends told each other of the places to get sex with other boys and older men.

In assessing Harriet's sexuality, it becomes clear that such a sexual (dis)order provides one important ingredient for the construction of a desiring self developed from multiple sources. Harriet's body has certainly experienced the sexual possibilities of this (dis)order more extensively than most, and his sexual sense of self is a product in part of that experience.

But another major aspect of Harriet's subjectivity is the culture of the gay community of Nullangardie, its particular style and rituals. It is this wicked and willful sexual culture that formed Harriet, that offered him sexual definitions and opportunities, gave sexual validation and satisfaction, in and with which he developed his sexual subjectivity. And he in turn has helped develop the community not just through his drag performances and his voluntary HIV/AIDS work, but also with his sexual activity.

If Harriet teaches us anything at all, it is that sexuality as a field of social inquiry needs to be more "warm, moist and human,"[2] if it is going to uncover the kind of depth and complexity revealed by the lives of the men of Nullangardie. Sexuality research clearly needs to be more empirical and to adopt these kinds of close-focus research techniques if sexual cultures like Nullangardie's are to be understood. Nullangardie tells us something important about the countless possibilities of an endlessly destabilizing sexuality. Harriet knows the extent of such possibilities only too well: "You shake your arse—they'll faint. Most guys do."

## Gender

There is no escaping the complexities usually collected together under the rubric *gender*. There are profound consequences for persons and societies in the arrangements within which sexual difference is understood and encoded in practice. There is also a long history of the validation of gender as a conceptual category in feminist analysis, progressive social science, and psychoanalysis. There is also an increasing concern about the concept and its theoretical culs-de-sac. In feminism itself, writers like Judith Butler (1990) have been demanding that we rethink its use, and others are questioning its privileging as a conceptual or structural category over sexual object-choice preference (Watney 1986).

What gender as a concept undoubtedly offers is a grasp on the profound consequences for each person in his or her assignment in any society to one side of the binary—men/women—on the basis of a biological characteristic of being declared male or female. This is the territory often sketched out as the sex/gender distinction, which is increasingly subject to dispute (Gatens 1983; Pringle 1992; Rubin 1993). Despite science's claims to have irrefutable proof of this biological sexual difference, Foucault (1980) questioned the process whereby this "proof" is applied with arbitrary imprecision in the

---

[2] I am indebted to Bruce Parnell, a long-time Australian HIV/AIDS educator, for this phrase.

case of the hermaphrodite *Herculine Barbin*. The certainty of these proofs was being questioned also with reference to sex testing in sport, amid concerns about transsexuals infiltrating women's sport, and so on.

Gender has also been used to cluster various, seemingly disparate social facts and processes together to enable analyses of the gross social, political, and economic inequalities that exist in almost all societies between men and women. Connell (1987) offers a complex attempt to define gender as a structural category worthy of consideration on a par with that other powerful conceptualization, class. He traces with great precision and care the evolution in social theory and politics of the concept, gender, in the first part of *Gender and Power*. Nevertheless, I am not convinced it is appropriate to incorporate things sexual within gender, as Connell does, via what he calls the "structure of cathexis" (1987, see part 2).

Watney (1986) argues that gender, particularly in its less sophisticated usage as part of sex role theory, is a profoundly *heterosexist* concept; it privileges analyses of the social order on one axis, involving the male/female, men/women, masculine/feminine binaries. Gender is by definition preoccupied—nay, consumed—by the dilemmas of heterosexuality, and in its analyses of the relations between women and men focuses on those men and women who have sex with each other and very nearly ignores those who do not. When those not heterosexually engaged are examined, it is usually in comparison with heterosexual configurations of the issues. Although most men and women in Australian society have sex with a member or members of the opposite sex, most daily interactions between men and women do not involve sex directly.

This is not to deny the sexual construction of social relations investigated by Pringle (1988); nor does it attempt to categorize as "sex" only those activities that involved clearly genital activity. What I want to distinguish is an investigation of sex and sexuality that recognizes templates for analyses other than those derived from patriarchal heterosexuality—the phrase most often used in the dominant paradigm of the gender debate. It is possible to investigate the sexual behavior that occasionally occurs between women and gay men, for example, in terms other than those of sexism and male penetrative dominance. Similarly, it is clear to those familiar with the research done on pedophilia that the preoccupation with power-suffusing analyses of heterosexual sex can do a serious disservice to studying intergenerational sex relations and offering informed assistance to those engaged in them.

Gender analyses, particularly those dominated by the concerns of heterosexuality, have a remarkable blind spot when it comes to men's sexuality. A classic example is the alignment of men-who-have-sex-with-men, men-who-have-sex-with-women, and those who do so with both on some absurd continuum (namely, men who have sex), ignoring the tense structural relations between these categories, the subordination of homosexuality to heteronormativity, and leeching sexuality of all substance and meaning beyond the biological sex of the sex object.

A second example of the consequences of gender dominance is criticism of imagery used in gay community safe sex health promotion interventions in the United Kingdom by Tamsin Wilton (1991). Relying as she does on analyses that bracket male sexuality as a continuous sexual domain, Wilton mistakes the penis for the phallus: gay male representations of gay men's bodies and their imaging of gay men's desire are read with women's eyes. The erect penis is seen as the dominating threat to the passive anus (read as an analogue to the passive vagina). That gay men may not read the anus as passive or regard the erect penis as dominating in anal intercourse is put to one side (see David McDiarmid's painting *Friends of Friends* reproduced in *Art and Text* (1991: 110), and ask Harriet about penises and passivity). That the interchangeability of position in homosexual intercourse renders the application of the readings as extremely suspect is ignored. Gay men's reading of these images is deemed secondary to this kind of feminist reading. The definition of issues, bodies, and meanings related to the problems of heterosexuality are privileged over those relating to gay men. The penis is seen essentially as a phallus and its deployment can never be interpreted otherwise.

Such preoccupations with heterosexuality are replayed in those configurations of gay men as either more polymorphously perverse (that is, as having escaped the deployment of sexuality), or as having regained a liberated position in the face of unbelievable odds in a homophobic world—a kind of structure/resistance binary. I do not deny that these analyses have something to offer, but neither accommodates the historically constructed experience of living a gay life. Harriet shows that whatever these determinative analyses may offer, the agentive production of a sexual being may be a more powerful contribution to the process than the discursive frameworks themselves.

Gender's incapacity to step outside the heterosexual domain as *constitutive of all else* must force us to look elsewhere for conceptual tools to unpack these complex relations of sex and sexuality. At this point I want to take as given a set of processes, *social* processes, wherein each of us is declared male or female and must make sense out of that declaration thereafter.

Certainly some of these are related to heterosexual patriarchal structures. Rosemary Pringle (1988) has discussed her subjects' employment of family images to describe working relationships as shaped around mother/son, dutiful wife, mistress, father/daughter "scripts" (in the sense of Gagnon and Simon [1974]). Pringle argues that these family-derived scripts encode practices that are demonstrably not of family relations—how many corporations run their businesses the way a family runs its household? Harriet employs similar scripts to describe his relationships. Yet his relationships give us reason to question these scripts. For example, the man who finally led to Harriet's despair of relationships had previously been a preoperative transsexual drag artist. The relationship with Jim, the brickies laborer, was anything but "a husband and wife team sort of thing" as Harriet describes it. I doubt that many husbands and wives deal with their sex lives as these two did. Harriet, who was "butch as well," related a more complex sexual arrangement than most husbands and wives could deal with.

In other words, care needs to be taken with the idea that the language itself reveals the discursive structuring of experience. Practice and context also transform the meaning of words. In much the same way many gay men call lovers "husbands," thereby transforming and subverting the heterosexual meaning of the word rather than reinscribing heterosexuality within homosexuality. Scripts, rather than structuring these relations, may provide the raw materials for their own subversion.

The contrariness of practice vis-à-vis discourse calls into question Diana Fuss's (1991) idea that the transgression of homosexuality may by default bolster the heterosexual side of the heterosexual/homosexual binary. She argues that homosexuality reinforces heterosexuality's need to distinguish itself from, and achieve the subordination of, homosexuality. This subordination of homosexuality is achieved even if homosexuality's transgressive acts intend, or by default seem, to subvert their antithesis (Fuss 1991: 6ff.). Such transgressions are more subversive than Fuss gives them credit for; a lot of camp and gay language has elements of resistance, and transformations of language are occurring all the time that subvert the meanings of social relations ordinarily taken for granted, particularly when issues of power and control are at stake. The gender-inverted nature of "dragon" talk may be more than simply a parody of that certain part of women's estate which many women find self-oppressive, but it could also be read as a deliberate subversion of masculine agendas, while also being offered as a powerful challenge to femininity.

Gender may well be an act, a masquerade (Tyler 1991), no longer useful when desire plays with discursive categories in the ways Harriet reported.

But Harriet also teaches us that these gender categories are subject to deconstruction in sex itself: some like being penetrated by a fully frocked transsexual; some clients eventually do not need the drag at all; pleasure and sensation, fantasy and fixation, are the currency in a sexual economy where the sexed and gendered bodies rather than determining the sexual engagement *desire* to lend themselves to even further disintegration.

For Harriet, bending gender provided many other materials to utilize and issues to explore in the local sexual economy, engaging the (ir)resolution of others to produce an operative sexuality. Does this sexual fugue offer a temporary variation in the deployment of sexuality? Is it a place where the effects of gender can be resisted temporarily? Harriet demonstrates that what we call gender can actually be used in a *sexual* construction of the self. The displacements, the inversions, the reinscriptions, the transferences that constitute sexuality, might suggest that sexuality rather than gender is the key to the construction of society. Rather than seeking a social construction of sexuality, we need to investigate the sexual construction of society.

It is certain that concepts like sexual identity, sexual preference, gender, and gender identity no longer offer adequate analytical tools for the exploration of sex lives. The two concepts introduced by Harriet, *sexual subjectivity* and *sexual (dis)order*, may be of more use and will continue to inform this analysis in this study. Sexual subjectivity enables us to accumulate from sexual identity, gender identity, the sensations of sex, the experiences of the body, and the meanings of sex itself a deeper sense of how we know and recognize ourselves sexually. This we do with others around and in us as they too enact their desire, in evolving collectivities of transgression and transformation.

# 5

# The Pursuit of Homosexuality

Becoming homosexual is complicated. It is more often sketched psychologically or psychoanalytically, usually with a determined search for a cause, than explored through experience, least of all experiences of the body. Two men, older than most in this study, offered interesting accounts of issues involved in the process—childhood sex play, adolescent sexual experience, and, very much later, the recognition of homosexuality. A third described even more delayed experiences in his forties. The three men's accounts are filled with pain and suffering. Yet each reveals a determination to deal with his sexuality, and society's response to it, with remarkable courage and endurance.

They reveal the complexity of sexual experience, reaching beyond bodily sensation to its relational character. These men offer an opportunity to explore the relation between sexual skill and interaction, sensation and pleasure, sexual identity and social denotation, and emotion and meaning. They challenge us to rethink the relation between masculine sexual perversity and homosexuality, and point to the centrality of sex itself in the social construction of a (homo)sexual subjectivity.

## Harry Wight

Harry is a large, affable, cheeky man in his early forties who lives with his lover in Nullangardie. They are key persons in the local HIV/AIDS scene, with some responsibility for a number of gay community concerns. Harry was born in Sydney and lived there for thirty years before moving to Nullangardie. He was married for eleven years, had four children, and could have followed a very conventional life as father and husband had not he, first, become interested in sex with men and, second, met John, his long-standing lover.

Harry's mother experienced all the worst a working-class girl could. Unwanted in a large family because home-based girls were a financial burden, she was forced in her mid-teens to marry a local man who had raped her. She fled the night of the wedding to another city and joined the armed services when World War II broke out. Harry's father was brought up in outer Sydney, ostensibly an orphan. He was fostered for most of his childhood, moving from family to family, and eventually ended up doing farm work before joining up. Harry's parents met during the war and later returned to his father's home locality. In full knowledge of her marital situation, they set up house as a married couple. No one was any the wiser. Children came, the last being Harry. The father trained as a technician for the local municipal authority, and the mother worked, first in a pub and then as a cook.

It was a difficult marriage. Harry's father had been violently treated as a child and was in turn violent to his family. Harry reckoned his father was disappointed that they never became the "perfect family." Respectability was precious, and the de facto marriage and its illegitimate children were never quite up to the mark. It is a painful example of the ideology of family battling the reality of a family's life. Finally, the parents separated, and each soon met a new partner. Yet the father waited until the mother had officially divorced the original rapist/husband (so she could marry the new partner) before he legally married his "second" wife, thus preserving the outward appearance of legitimacy in the relationship and carrying the pretense through to its closure. It is called *chivalry*.

Harry found out he was illegitimate when he was twenty-five, by which time he was long married. He and a childhood sweetheart met when he was fourteen. They married when he was twenty-one and he left her at thirty-two. Marrying was what Harry expected to do:

> You see, we'd grown up together for so long, it was just expected that we would get married. At one stage before we were married I hated her. And I think it was just after we got engaged. I was all right up until then, but I really hated her and I didn't want to be in this, but I didn't know how to get out of it. So I just had to carry it through.

It was a classic case of "compulsory heterosexuality" (Rich 1980).

Harry left the local high school after tenth grade because his parents could not afford to keep him there. He worked first in a bank and started a technical college course at night to get his diploma, picking up typing along the way. This enabled him to secure entry-level white-collar work. He worked as a clerk in similar institutions and offices until at age thirty-one he joined the armed forces.

He had always wanted to enlist, but his parents would not let him when a teenager. However, this new career was cut short by a series of back injuries, which left Harry discharged from the service and on a government pension by the time he started to live with John. Nowadays he occasionally does some cash-in-hand work, some craft work and odd jobs that do not strain the back. At the time of the interview, he and John were comfortably in their own home, with two cars and a very contented life.

The armed forces period deserves a discussion of its own. Harry's career there was a disaster, and his experience reveals the income and work-related vulnerability of semiskilled working-class men to any bodily damage or ill-health (cf. Barney's situation now that he has AIDS). During initial training a fellow rookie landed on Harry's back during an exercise, breaking some vertebrae. This was misdiagnosed, and he completed a reduced training program on pain killers, exacerbating the damage. When he was returning from basic training, military personnel directed to help him failed to turn up. While carrying his heavy bags further vertebrae gave way and Harry was immobilized for a considerable period. A third accident (described below) led to a discharge and a full disability pension.

A second issue of interest is that of male physicality and sexuality. The first accident with Harry's back occurred during a complex leapfrog exercise, during which the men were crawling over and under each other. Harry was at least five to ten years older than the rest and was called "Dad," carrying all the sexual potency of a married man and a father. In a moment during rookie training while the other men in the dormitory were on leave, Harry experienced the perversity of male sexuality in all its glory and handled it with considerable restraint. A teenage rookie, a "hunk," crawled into bed with Harry and asked about the facts of life. Harry (naked with an instant erection) told this youngster (who was wearing only underpants) the full story. The youngster, pressing an insistent erection into Harry's side, wanted all the details. Harry, on completing his story, sent the young man back to his bed with instructions to masturbate. Harry, contrary to the stereotype of the predatory homosexual—he was quite homosexually experienced by this time—recognized the opportunity and forbore. He told the tale with some irony, but it says something about those times, the dangers for a homosexually active person in the armed forces, and Harry's recognition of the potential jeopardy in sex between men with an existing relationship.

A third issue from Harry's experience in the armed forces concerns homophobia. Another rookie, hating the military, tried to get out by claiming (falsely) to be gay. The military police confiscated his address book and interviewed all those listed in it. Harry had been in rookie training with the guy and was interviewed in a session which went from 8:30 A.M. until 6:00 P.M. He denied being gay but, in fact, was living with John by this time. Subsequent interviews led to a psychological assessment, but the supportive assessor did not report Harry, even though he fully disclosed his homosexuality. Harry had an epileptic fit after the stress of the assessment, and John, not knowing what to do, dropped him bodily, putting the finishing touches on the already damaged back. Harry was followed by the military police, continuing their pursuit of homosexuals, as much as a year later while the discharge and pension were being negotiated.

These experiences and the issues that emerge from them—job-market vulnerability, a certain perversity in male sexuality, and homophobia—are recurring themes shaping the lives of the men in this study. The endless and evolving interconnectedness of these issues for these men is important to note, if only to remind us that a homosexual life is not simply an issue of whom one sleeps with.

Harry started his sex life a little later than others in this study. At high school Harry had a regular thing with another boy; they would meet for a "wankette" after school and on Saturday mornings before and/or after swimming lessons. They would always strip naked at the local changing-room shed. There were other kids and similar events, mutual masturbation mainly. Then an initiation in anal sex occurred after school with an older brother of a schoolmate. It was Harry, however, who did the inserting.

About this time he met his future wife, and homosexual sex stopped for a few years. Six years and one day later they married and soon had four kids. As his girlfriend, she used to come to dinner each Sunday, and they would have sex afterward. But that was Sunday. On Thursdays Harry went to college. At age eighteen, the now-engaged Harry was going to class one evening and stepped into a toilet at a nearby railway station:

Anyway, I was standing there having a leak and this guy came in. And all of sudden it just kind of clicked. And he stood there and I stood there and I remembered what I used to do before. And he said to me: "Do you want to?"—and I'd cracked a fat [got an erection], and he said— "Do you want me to do something about it?" And I said: "No, I don't." I just sucked him . . .

About a month later in same toilet, but this time with a married man he knew, Harry accepted an invitation to the man's empty home, missing class again. This time Harry fucked the guy. This marked the first significant anal penetration on Harry's part, the previous attempts not having been terribly successful. Needless to say Harry failed his courses that year as this newfound thrill became a regular pastime. He would meet this man each Thursday and learn the sexual ropes: kissing, oral sex, anal sex. Eventually Harry let the guy try screwing him. It hurt, and Harry has remained an insertive partner ever since.

Harry also had sex with other men at the toilet, using the cubicles. He was working in inner Sydney at that time and found other beats at railway stations and public toilets, which he visited en route to and from work or during his lunch hour. He was eventually arrested, appeared in court (instead of forfeiting his fine which was apparently standard practice, but there was no one to tell him that), was subjected to a psychologist's report which pointed the finger at his relationship with his father, and put on a bond. It all happened in the inner city and no one else found out.

Harry and his wife soon lost their youthful ardor. There was the odd moment of heterosexual bliss, but he turned his sexual attentions increasingly toward men. Beat sex continued uninterrupted during the ten years he was married. He occasionally ventured into the odd social event with other homosexual men. He met a male couple and through them another married man with whom he started an affair (which he quickly ended when it started getting "serious"). He went to his first gay dance at an inner-suburban town hall—"a smorgasbord"—but experienced no sense of connectedness to what he saw there. One or two of these sex partners became friends, people to talk with about difficulties. The beats became a starting point for relations with men beyond instant sex. Harry offered a picture of the western Sydney beats not dissimilar to present-day reports of the HIV/AIDS educators who patrol them (van Reyk 1990; Davis, Klemmer, and Dowsett 1991). These venues still provide for a slow development of relations among homosexually active men, moving beyond anonymous sex toward nascent relationships, stop-start affairs, new friendships, places to meet others and just talk.

Then came Harry's first truly wonderful sexual experience. He met a near-naked man at a beat:

And I really think that was the first time I ever made love to a man.

(Really, was it just straight sex until that moment?)

It was all sex, straight raw sex up until then.

He said: "Would you like to come with me?" and I said: "Would I ever!"
He took me up into the bushes type thing in the car, and he made love.

(What's the difference? What was the difference?) John and I do it. We do
it—sometimes we just screw, just fuck, and then other times we just
make love.

(Can you give some words to describe it? I don't mean describe it like in a
sentence, but just—actually—words, like sensual, touch?)

A bit of touch, a bit of, I mean [pause] it probably might just happen in the
time of your life when you most need it. Um.

(With two people at the same moment?)

Yes. Can you relate to what I'm talking about?

(Oh yes, absolutely. I just wanted you to spell it out.)

[laughter] I mean, this guy was—although I stripped off with K. earlier on
when I was a kid, and I probably stripped off with all of them—this
bloke *undressed* me [his emphasis]. There was no quick grab hold of
your cock and wank it and get your mouth around it. There was feeling to it. There was touching to it. And did I get in the shit when I got
home, 'cause I was probably there for about three hours. And he taught
me how to kiss. He taught me how to put your tongue out, and not
leave it there, which annoys me. . . . Just took his time with me.

(The magic moment, eh?)

It doesn't happen often.

This moment initiated a transformation in Harry. It illuminated the possibilities of male-to-male sex beyond orgasm and gestured toward something
more, something indefinable—at that time. Soon, it took firmer shape in
the relationship Harry developed with John.

Harry met John on a beat after Harry and his family were posted to a
military base near Nullangardie. Harry had a rule about casual sex partners at that time: he never saw the same person more than twice. This decision was designed to protect himself from the emotional connection he
knew, by then, was possible, and it was designed to protect his marriage.
But after having sex with John, they "talked"! Talking can be so dangerous: it jeopardizes anonymity, it beckons intimacy. They met again after
work for a drink. They discovered that their situations were similar: both
married with kids, both sexually interested in men, both average "blokes"
(as Harry called them), and both were regular beat users. In penetrative
sex, one preferred to receive, the other to insert. The major difference between them was the state of their sexual identities. John's wife knew he

was homosexual, and they had managed to work out an arrangement to deal with his sexual interests. Harry's wife did not, although he had introduced her to gay men he had met, in an attempt at solving his dilemma.

Eventually this growing sense of connectedness between the two men became a relationship. They met every day to talk and have sex. John's wife seems to have known about it; she even encouraged the two families to become friendly. Finally, she made it public that John was planning to leave her. This pushed Harry into making the decision he had been putting off. His wife by then had realized that he too was homosexual. After a painful breakup Harry and John moved in together, eventually buying their house. They had been together for ten years at the time of the interview.

## Ralph Coles

Ralph Coles, when interviewed, was deputy principal in a technical college and a successful man in his late forties. He was born in the country but grew up in Sydney. His father was an accountant, his mother a housewife looking after their two children until, later in life, she returned to the workforce as part-time shop assistant. Ralph called the family "middle-class" and not the closest, although he and his sister remained close. He was educated in state schools, did well, and gained entry to a teachers college. After graduating, he taught basic trade courses, achieving steady promotion while he finished a degree. This led ultimately to his current position. Ralph was active in the inner-Sydney gay community as a volunteer in a local gay self-help group, local AIDS service organizations, and various gay social groups. Ralph died of an AIDS-related condition a couple of years after the interview.

Ralph's earliest sexual experiences were with other boys at high school, fooling around long before he first ejaculated. At seventeen, having discovered masturbation while fantasizing about boys (but still not regarding himself as homosexual), he had his first definitely homoerotic experience. He was heading home from college and entered a urinal, was picked up by a man, and had sex with him in a car a few streets away. He recalls a "tremendous feeling of relief. So I must have realized that I was different and that there was someone else like me." The very next week he returned "looking for it" and immediately after the encounter the realization dawned—he was a homosexual, a poofter!

He was devastated. He was overwhelmed by guilt and spent the next twelve months trying not to be homosexual. It was a difficult period. He continued to have sex with men, had two short homosexual relationships, was arrested by the police at a beat, tried visiting bars, and so on. Finally, in deep confusion, he requested a teaching post in the bush, hoping to be removed from temptation and to meet and marry a nice woman. No such luck. Ralph spelled out his dilemma succinctly: "I suppose it was because I enjoyed the sex, but I did not like the idea that I was having sex with a man." Rural life was not homosex-free; he had one drunken encounter at a country dance. Ralph's friends subsequently bashed up the man for leading Ralph "astray." Moreover, the incident signaled that his personal struggle was being observed.

Toward the end of this period in the country he went to a psychiatrist who put him on female hormones for about two years. He grew breasts (which had to be surgically removed ten years later) and lost his interest in sex. He thought he might be better off in the city and transferred back to Sydney. Close to a nervous breakdown, he went to group therapy sessions. While attending these and, in spite of starting to accept himself for what he was, he made one last-ditch effort to be "normal": he proposed marriage to a female colleague. The engagement ended with Ralph's confession to his fiance and his family that he was homosexual. A short time afterward he met Stewart and began to live a homosexual life in earnest.

Ralph bought his comfortable, partly renovated, inner-city home some years ago with Stewart. After twelve years together they separated. Ralph had other relationships and was involved with Dennis Partridge at the time of the interview, whom he had met six to eight months previously. They started living together in Ralph's house not long afterward. Both reported this as a very serious relationship, and Ralph regarded it as the best thing that had ever happened to him.

Ralph surrounded himself with a network of loyal and caring friends, including his sister. She was a source of considerable emotional support. She nursed Ralph through some of the bashings he endured at the hands of an earlier lover but, inexplicably, refused to support the relationship with Dennis. This hurt Ralph, and illustrates just how contingent a family's acceptance of a gay man can be. What Ralph actually received, it would appear, was conditional tolerance, not unqualified support and acceptance.

## Neil Davidson

Neil Davidson grew up in Nullangardie. His parents were born there, and he still has family there. He was educated at the local high school. His father was a blue-collar trade union official, later a long-serving member of Parliament. This was the working class made good, and Neil went on to college to become a teacher. He has one married sister. Neil inherited from this family a strong sense of the right and proper:

(You weren't in awe of your dad? It wasn't that kind of thing?)

No, but, um, for, I mean, he left school at fourteen. He gave me all the education he never had himself and, um, mm.

(Did that cause a difficulty?)

No, he was, he was very generous in a whole lot of ways, but a different generation and, um, [pause] different understandings. I wonder, for example, whether or not I would have had the strength to go through and do all the things I've done [becoming a gay man] if he'd still been alive. I just don't know.

Neil outlined the constraints of living in country towns in particular, referring to the expectation that all would get married, and it seems all did. Neil started teaching, married, and fifteen years later a university degree facilitated a move to high school teaching. Finally, the family moved to Sydney where he eventually became a Faculty Head Teacher. Neil has done all the right things, and he would undoubtedly be regarded all round as a reasonable bloke. He has a retirement plan, long service leave, and security. His has been a classic Education Department career. He may take early retirement, since further advancement will be difficult. Anyway his energies have now been diverted to his new gay life and its plans. The success Neil has experienced in his career is important. There is considerable validation for having done the right thing, having been upwardly mobile in a respectable *service*, and having become an influential (in a small way) and responsible member of the community.

Neil's wife was a country girl and a nurse. They had three children, who were in their mid to late teens at the time of the interview. It had been a successful family, contented and integrated. He was a good breadwinner, and her career significantly supplemented their income. Their early sex life was okay; he described it as somewhat "dutiful," and by his account, his wife was no initiator. The last few years of the marriage were unstable, and both went through a lot of uncertainty. He eventually told her that he was homosexual, and that was the beginning of the end of their relationship.

The separation was difficult, and Neil conceded that it was forced upon his wife. There was no easy solution; he could not stay with his wife and be homosexually active at the same time. He neither spoke badly of her nor blamed her for the sexual dilemma he faced and resolved as best he could. This was no misogynist who decorated his pursuit of homosexuality with anti-women statements. Soon after embarking on a new gay life he met John-Paul, who not long afterward moved into Neil's apartment.

There are two periods in Neil's pursuit of homosexuality. The first was one of "suppression," the term Neil used to describe the period during which he was only heterosexually active and only with his wife. This dated from his marriage to his decision to have sex with men again at age forty-eight (the second period). However, he had had a homosexually active childhood, and its memories were never too far away.

As a primary school child he and a classmate played with each other's penises under the desks. Soon after there followed sex play with a cousin:

I got into bed with him or he got into bed with me, but either way, I mean, you've got two bodies. . . . It was Christmas and, um, but, he, I mean, I was thirteen or fourteen. He would have been perhaps seventeen or eighteen and, um, all that led to intercourse.

(What kind? You fucked him? He fucked you?)

He fucked me.

This activity was repeated until the cousin found a girlfriend.

A similar story with a more emotional nuance occurred with a school friend:

I had a friend that I went to school with, who was—I was fairly close to him. . . . Then I can remember one day that we were at a, a school showing of a film. [pause] He was next to me I think. Then the lights went out. He then made the approach to me and from—that would have been perhaps fifteen or sixteen I suppose—and from that stage I had a fairly, [pause] fairly active sexual life with him, I suppose, right up to I was about twenty. . . .

(What was his approach? What did he do?)

What did he do where, in the theater? (In the theater.) Oh, I think he put his hand on my cock, I think and, and I did likewise, and he was hard and, I mean, all the signs were there. [laughs] And then the relationship was basically one where we, well ultimately, end up by fucking each other . . . he would come round [pause] perhaps once a week, but he would come round of a night. I remember him on his motorbike when he was, um, when he'd come and park outside and that was enough to turn me on. [laughs]

(What stopped it?)

Well, he, he got married as well.

Much later during his married life, Neil discovered beats. The writing on the walls, the obvious loitering with intent, the glory holes, the sex acts: all alerted him to homoerotic possibilities. For years he did not have sex with men but continued the cat-and-mouse game (with himself really) of being excited by the *possibility*. Then, at age thirty-one:

I called in on one occasion to, um, the toilet block at [a beachside sub-urb]. Have you been there? (No.) Well, there was a hole and, and I met someone there anonymously, through the wall and, um, that really, that really stirred me up, I mean, really did. I—it was amazing.

This experience remained his favorite fantasy until nine years later:

I pushed that aside again and went on for a few more years and then . . . after my father died . . . I had . . . to return to Nullangardie and . . . I went to a toilet block there, which I knew, um, [pause] had all the signs around it, [laughs] drawings on the wall and that—and, um, I met a young guy there. And for a middle aged man to meet an attractive young guy. . . . I never saw him again. That was the end. That was it. That was personal contact, not the anonymous contact of previously.

There was one more experience that reveals something about the thrill of this kind of sex for Neil in a very frank way:

I must have gone in on the way home from work. It would have been a diversion for me because I was in [the same beachside suburb]. So I went there deliberately, I went there deliberately because, I mean, it's like going—soaking up the atmosphere I suppose. . . . There was a guy in the cubicle next to me and he put a cock through the hole. . . . It was big, it was just, oooh, just—I mean, honestly, I was, I was really so turned on, so, I mean, I, um, I had never—[pause] years since I'd touched anyone. I'd have never had oral sex and, um, although I, and I did that, but I didn't do it to orgasm for him. And the reason was be-cause, um, I, I, I only had—I just touched myself and I came. I mean, it was just such a turn-on. It was just unbelievable for me and, um, then I got frightened, I suppose [very quiet].

This level of fear and arousal continued in fits and starts, each time raising the pleasure stakes:

I suppose it was a couple of years after that that I went probably back to the same place. It was a couple of years, err, and it was the first time that I've ever had, or allowed anyone to have oral sex with me. And again that was another experience, another turn-on. I mean, I was really rather very frightened [laughs].

Neil was not proud of this sexual activity. He felt increasing emotional pressure about his wife and about his sexual interests and identity. He was panicky about STDs. A bout of hives sent him to a doctor, confessing all. The doctor did all the right things: a complete STD checkup and off to a psychiatrist. The psychiatrist stabilized his condition, for he was virtually on the edge of a nervous breakdown, and this gave him time to work things out. Neil reported this period as being like mental illness—not that being homosexual was illness, but within that trauma of dealing with the consequences of sexual suppression and resolution, he was definitely mentally ill.[1]

Eventually, he realized that he had to tell the family and resolve the issue. One major dilemma is his mother. She remains unaware of his sexuality and complains of not having seen as much of him as she would like. She calls John-Paul the "boarder," and she is not happy that the marriage has broken up. Neil toyed with this elaborate ruse to tell his mother about the lover:

> But, um—in fact I was on the verge of saying to her that, er, if she'd like to come over any time, John-Paul would be quite happy to share with me so that the bedroom is vacated for her, because the second bed—well, actually there are three bedrooms here, but one is more a storeroom— and, um, test her reaction on that. . . . Now sharing can mean sharing the same bed and that often happens in places where there are no single beds. I mean, you have to do that and she mightn't think twice about it.

This was an elaborate, somewhat pathetic ploy to nut out the problem of his sexuality and to rework his relationship with his mother.

He has been somewhat more successful with his kids. The younger two were attentive and open to it, the oldest has remained distant, but relations with the children have been getting slowly easier. Another consequence was the loss of connection with his own extended family. Since the separation he has seen less of them (maybe his wife did all the work maintaining the relationships).

---

[1] This psychiatrist, it would seem, no longer considered homosexuality itself a pathological condition. Things have changed since Ralph Coles's time. However, the trauma associated with social consequences of homosexuality, of *failing* to "come out" adequately, has now become a "mental illness" (Cain 1991).

Coming out to his wife was by far the most painful and he was already in psychiatric care before he attempted it:

I mean, I couldn't say it to her face to face. I had to stand round a corner. She was very supportive at first and then, as time went on, it swung round to, um, instead of being centered on me, centered on her. And I understand that of course, because her needs are just as important as mine, and from her point of view more so. And, um, but I've reached the stage where I couldn't live, live a lie any more, and, um, from the very first stage that I'd had—at this stage in my life anyhow—a relationship with men, I'd had no physical relationships with her at all. And the reason for that was as much to protect her as it was for the fact that I wasn't getting the satisfaction out of physical relationships with her. So she was, in the first instance, [pause] upset by the fact that these changes that occurred in our own interpersonal relations. And, um, the discussions, I suppose, that we had and the talking over the options, she's found it quite difficult, and even now she still finds it difficult, but it doesn't help me either.

This quote reveals a considerable amount about the dilemma Neil faced and his sensitivities in handling it. He recognized there was no solution that could work for them both. His decision to leave and come out increased his pain and disrupted the most important relationships in his life; that was the cost to him. He also recognized the cost to her but could do nothing about it.

Neil's pursuit of his homosexuality has occurred not just at great expense to precious relations with his immediate and extended family; there were also repercussions in his professional life. Colleagues recognized he was having difficulties. Some knew why. Some he told. Others guessed. His closest colleagues were very supportive, but he has not come out to the school or the Education Department. A whole new circle of friends had emerged from a gay social group and the other groups he attended. Gay friendships began to fill the spaces that family and friends once filled. It remains an ever-present difficulty for Neil: to make judgments about the receptiveness of his immediate networks and the world at large and to decide just how far he can incorporate his previous relationships into his new (homo)sexual life. This is a distinct difficulty for all gay people and a major part of the construction of the homosexual "lifestyle," "milieu," or entry into a "gay community."

There were other costs along the way, physical ones. He was bashed in a beat, on the way home from a meeting. He had to lie to his wife about an attempted robbery. His was a frightening account of gay bashing:

There was a glory hole. One guy put his cock through the glory hole and let me suck it for a while. Then he withdrew. I did likewise. He sucked me for a little while then, before I had a chance to move, he opened the door of his cubicle and slammed it against my cock, which was sticking through the hole. It was black and blue, I might tell you, and of course was very, very painful. Next thing, er, I had someone—'cause there were two of them and they were only late teens, I would say—um, at the door of my cubicle trying to push it, trying to get in, um, which I didn't allow them to do. But I was in a very disadvantaged position. I had my pants down round my ankles and couldn't move and couldn't get them up. And, um, next thing I had one over the top with a stick having a go at me through the top. I finally managed to get my pants up, which gave me a bit of a chance, but against two it's very difficult anyhow and I got out through the door. And then they attacked me and had me down on the ground. And the only comment I can remember was: "Get his wallet," which I didn't have on me.

It was a painful and frightening moment. Yet Neil worked his way through all of this, eventually doing what he could with honor to find a place for himself as a homosexual man. The process of pursuing his homosexuality in Neil's case is a good example of the contingent and agentive nature of the activity. It was a particularly personal account full of great pain and traumatic experience. It remains a constant process for him, yet to be completed. It is important to note, however, the social resources available to Neil and his access to them; Harry, Harriet, Barney, and Ralph had far less help.

◡

A number of issues emerge from these life histories, which I will now explore in a more comparative manner. None of these men had a "gay liberation" or "post-Stonewall" entry into homosexual sex, or adult homosexual life, although Neil obviously benefited from the effects of twenty years of gay liberation activism in his encounter with psychiatry. Whatever solutions men seek to their sexual desire, these three men have sought similar accommodations and fashioned similar achievements.

## Relationships

Each of these men ended up in significant relationships with other men, and for each this primary relationship became the centerpiece of his homosexuality. The relationships Neil, Ralph, and Harry created for themselves as they came to grips with their sexuality indicate the importance of close emotional connections in the pursuit of homosexuality.

Ralph counted his relationship with Dennis as the fifth relationship where "I really felt something significant for the person." The first was "puppy love," lasting eight weeks; the second was "real passion" lasting three years but ending badly; the third was his eleven years with Stewart; the fourth, lasting two years, was with a young man in his twenties, met through the new gay community contacts and for whom Ralph was a first love. Ralph's only run-in with heterosexuality was the aborted engagement with a female colleague.

What held Ralph and Stewart together was their "good rapport . . . even when we were arguing, we would spark off each other. We used to find it fascinating." This so-called rapport could actually be quite irritating to outsiders and marked the relationship with a stamp of a particular era and type of homosexual lifestyle, more "camp" than gay. They shared interests in the arts with Stewart being responsible for the education of young Ralph. When house-buying tightened the financial reins and Ralph's interest in things gay started, the relationship began to suffer. Sexual tensions were present from the second year, and each eventually played around on the side with casual male partners without telling the other. With the gap between them widening, they eventually separated.

In contrast, the current relationship with Dennis was reported as:

> One of the most important things that has happened to me in a long time, because I don't think I am downgrading previous relationships by saying the quality of this one is different to any of those I have experienced so far. It is quite different, in the way that I feel really cared for in a way no one has really demonstrated [previously].

Although there were some problems, it is clear that Ralph and Dennis were enjoying a very compatible and active sex life. More than that, this was a relationship of great passion, a bonding with overlays of greater meaning. Dennis was madly in love for the first time successfully; Ralph had been lonely and dissatisfied for a long time and was "joyous." But, Ralph was HIV seropositive and resigned to dying in a few years; Dennis had seroconverted as a result of "unsafe" sex with Ralph on their first night together. This added tremendous weight to their commitment to each other. Almost as a token of their love, they had given up condoms: a symbolic act that bound them together in a kind of love-death pact.

Ralph offered the following as those things he liked most about Dennis: "his innocence, enthusiasm, his determination, his physicality." Given that Dennis had spent many years working as a prostitute, is it not strange that innocence is mentioned first? Dennis was naive and untutored in many ways, but he certainly is "street-wise," and it is unusual to call a prostitute innocent. When asked how friends responded to the relationship, Ralph replied that he made it a condition of friendship that Dennis and his disclosed past were fully accepted: "Because of his background—and I have rarely hidden that, the fact that he was a prostitute—a couple of them have reservations."

This insistence on disclosure and acceptance had contributed to some distance from the once close sister. Later in the interview, when expressing concern about Dennis's well-being while Ralph was to take a forthcoming overseas trip, his first sentence was: "I am not worried that he will go back to what he was doing." A classic inversion, perhaps? It certainly appears that Dennis's prostitution had yet to settle easily in Ralph's mind. Dennis was "retraining" as a community worker, and Ralph has embarked on the education of young Dennis in a reminiscent round of arts events, new friendships, and so on. So there may also be just a small redemptive pattern in the emotional fabric these two men have woven.

Neil's relationship with John-Paul was his first serious relationship with a man: "I suppose I was ready for it anyhow. I mean, I was looking for a relationship as full on, at least up here [meaning cerebrally], if not anywhere else [meaning genitally]." The relationship is very comfortable. Neil is obviously in charge of the domestic relations, and John-Paul cheerfully acquiesces. Sexually they are quite active: a regular roll on the floor after work, lots of cuddling in bed at the end of the day. It is this closeness and companionship that seems to mark the depth of their commitment to each other. Their common interest in the arts and the considerable work they put into a local gay social club all provide more material for their bonding.

John-Paul came from a working-class background and had maintained close ties with his family. He had given up hope of ever having a lover and visited the saunas once a week for the odd bit of sexual exercise. He met Neil there and pursued him. Neil was charmed by the attention and eventually John-Paul moved in. They are monogamous, although Neil was not so sure he can contain his urge for flings now that he is finally out of the closet. He promised emotional fidelity and "safe" sex always; John-Paul is completely devoted and seems to cope with the uncertainty of Neil's very honest explanation of why he might eventually go beyond bounds.

It is a fairly intelligent resolution to the problems of developing a gay relationship between two aging men completely inexperienced at the task. What is clear is that the attractions in homoeroticism and the emotional qualities of gay relationships are not the same thing. Even though this is Neil's first homosexual relationship, he is not so foolish as to confuse the two.

Harry and John have built a relationship around sex and a series of activities and external relations: their respective children and natal families; hobbies; a network of gay and straight friends; social activities with gay and straight groups; and their considerable volunteer work for the local gay community, HIV/AIDS organizations, and with PLWHAs. This extraordinary degree of convergence in their interests welds the relationship together through shared practices and pleasures.

Their children seem, according to Harry, well adjusted to their fathers' lives. They visit and stay over, and handle the two men sleeping together quite well, although in one concession (to what or whom was not exactly clear) Harry and John do not have sex when the children are there. There have been the inevitable difficulties with Dad-as-gay at certain times. But the sureness in Harry's account of his relations with the kids was convincing. Harry gets on well with John's ex-wife; John does not. Harry regards his ex-wife as a sister; it is not clear how she feels about that.

The two men's social life was very full, consisting of the usual events with workmates, neighbors, hobby club friends, the arts, and so on. There was a lot of good-natured speculation about the sexual preferences of the heterosexual men in their circle (a constant pastime for many gay men). There were family outings with parents and siblings (mostly easy, occasionally brittle, but not directly related to their sexuality). Their work with the gay community was important to them, and they generally kept an eye on other various aspects of local gay life—the beats, the young ones—to make sure there is no real trouble. They are an astonishing pair in all of this work, true organic community leaders, salt-of-the-earth types, and in that community contribute a lot without attracting recognition or asking for credit. Were they doing all of this as "straight" men for the Scouts or the Blind Society, they would be honored with an Order of Australia medal or some such community recognition.

∽

Primary homosexual relationships are central to all these men's lives. They are also significant as a major resting point in each man's pursuit of his homosexuality. These relationships function quite differently, yet the companionship and emotional connectedness cannot be denied. They can truly be called *amici di cuori*.

They got to this point only after a struggle. None received much help along the way from family and friends, or gained support from the wider society in the form of dedicated government policies and programs (new home buyer's schemes, marrieds' taxation arrangements, Family Law provisions, and so on). There is little legal recognition as yet of these relationships in Australia (although such relationships will now be reported in certain official reports from Australia's Bureau of Statistics), and their efforts at rebuilding and sustaining relationships with their natal families or their children and ex-wives are similarly unsupported.

In a similar vein, common parlance reviles the homosexual relationship by depicting it as inherently unstable or by judging its worth against a heterosexual norm. For example, Harry stays at home and does the housework. Outsiders interpret these arrangements in heterosexual domestic sex-role terms, and deduce from this and the men's appearance and presence their sexual mode preferences. They cannot be more wrong. In a clever and willful exacerbation of the confusion they cause straight friends, Harry's rejoinder, "Being butch is such a bitch!" *consciously* plays with gender. Neither Harry nor John is in any way effeminate (although both can camp it up when they want to). Their domestic arrangements are related more to Harry's back problems and the demands of John's career than to the assumption of sex roles or to the mimicry of heterosexual relationships.

This is a good example of heterosexism in operation, with conclusions being drawn about gay men's lives based on the widespread and questionable assumption that the heterosexual relationship is a universal template for structuring emotional relationships. As ideology this assumption is oppressive and potentially damaging: many of the younger men interviewed had very conventional, traditional expectations about relationships. Many were led to believe, in the absence of any other obvious options, that the sexual and emotional turmoil generated by their homosexual interests would be resolved by that special man about to come their way. The older men had moved a considerable distance from this naive position and had created different kinds of relationships, which could offer alternative possibilities for younger gay men to emulate. Nowhere are these differences clearer than in the sexual arrangements these couples have created.

## Sex

Neil's homosexual life is relatively new and his fascination with John-Paul has yet to stand the test of time, which Harry and John have weathered so well or which Ralph and Dennis are managing with a little deception. Yet Neil was very explicit that although he is satisfied with the relationship on a wondrous number of levels, temptation is never too far away and he cannot promise not to taste it. Having finally escaped the sexual straitjacket of the previous twenty-five years, Neil is not going to be restrained unnecessarily again, it would seem.

It was Neil who pointed out that problems of being newly (homo)sexual are not restricted to the young; nor are the dilemmas facing those trying to construct their first gay relationships a youthful issue only. Safe sex in a newly explored homosexual life *no matter the age* is a serious issue. Others with considerably longer homosexually active lives are having difficulties with safe sex that Neil has yet to face (Dowsett 1993b, 1994b). Gay communities need to respond to men like Neil and develop a different outlook on gay life if they are to address his safe sex education needs adequately.

Neither Ralph nor Stewart remained monogamous for long. Ralph soon started visiting beats, at first, merely looking as he drove by, then dropping in, and finally having sex with someone. Beat sex became a permanent part of his sex life. After Dennis's arrival in his life, Ralph reduced the visits to the odd occasion, but:

It's part of my behavior pattern, but now—it is interesting—I go, I may be driving past and I stop. But you sort of—I don't stop there for long, I just check it out. That's all.

Ralph regarded casual sex as a natural part of his sex life, and he captured the attraction nicely:

You know, there are times when I have picked someone up, or I have been picked up by someone, and we have actually—it is usually second-rate sex if it is quick, or if you have it on the beat or somewhere like that. But there have been times when, when I have picked someone up at a beat or at a bar—the former happen much more than the latter—and, you know, you can take them home, you can go home to their place, and it can be first-rate sex rather than second rate. I can remember some really outstanding encounters.

Ralph was not a sauna user, and beats were his major avenue for casual sex. But many beats have been closed by local municipal councils during the last five or so years (partly in response to HIV/AIDS, partly in a general mood of financial constraint in public spending), and his beat using had become somewhat restricted. Yet the appeal remained. One "gets used to the beats. There is that element of danger [from police or bashers] . . . there is an element of risk and that, sort of, adds some spice to it."

For Ralph, sex inside his relationships was not so simple. His time with Stewart was tense: Stewart demanded sex every second day "as some sort of reassurance." Ralph was usually the insertive partner, but, in the face of such constant pressure for sex, he eventually stopped ejaculating. He reported that he perfected the art of urinating slightly into Stewart's rectum to convince the latter that ejaculation had occurred. On the day following such an event Ralph inevitably would seek insertive anal intercourse with someone at a beat, and he then made a point of ejaculating. On those occasions when Ralph did not want to fuck Stewart, he would submit to being fucked instead, usually "in a fairly punitive way." If there was no sex, Stewart would withhold his share of the house payments (quite seriously at one point): "It was extremely rare that I had sex with Stewart. [laughter] Practically never. I was having sex with the video I had seen at [the local sex shop with a back room], or with that guy I had got off with, sort of, at the beat or something—which is a pretty sad state of affairs." It appears that women are not the only ones who fake orgasm or fantasize in order to have sex. But note: it is the *insertive* partner who is doing the faking here.

Other questions come to mind. Why did Stewart want or need to be fucked every second day? How to explain the never openly negotiated casual sex, which both pursued? How would such a relationship today deal with the possibility of HIV transmission? What was so important about ejaculation that necessitated Ralph's extraordinary efforts at deception? The easy sexual flow reported by Harry is absent in Ralph's account; sex in this relationship was more contextually riddled with uncertainty, dubious motives, and strange urgencies.

Sex with Dennis, however, was a "union" unlike any previous experience. It was variously described as "so natural," "unbelievable," "it was *him* I was fucking," and "the quality of them [the sex acts], the love that underlies what's happening now just makes this different. Like I said, quite unique for me."

Harry and John are no sweet young things; they are "straight-looking," "straight-acting," "teddy-bears" (to use the terms currently fashionable). Harry reported having sex every day, nearly always with John or with John in a threesome (their preferred format), but occasionally with someone else at the beat. Their agreement was that they would go in for threesomes but no individually pursued sex outside the relationship. Neither has kept to the agreement, but the transgressions remain unspoken even though each has caught the other out on the odd occasion. These transgressions were explained away by Harry in terms of his "higher sex drive." He likes it often; John is slowing down as he gets older and particularly during winter. Even so they had threesomes two to three times a week with men picked up at the beat or in arrangements they have made with specific men.

Harry reported that he is always insertive in their own sexual activity and they nearly always have anal intercourse. He is also always insertive in their three-way casual encounters and John is the one who is fucked by the trick whom Harry fucks, sometimes at the same time. (John occasionally gets his turn on "top" with the trick too.)

Harry noted that most people, including their gay friends, think of him as the receptive one in sex; they generally associate John's larger physical and more immediately masculine presence with insertion. How what is called personality or persona and daily practices such as domestic relations are connected with the sexual interests and practices of a sexed and gendered body is a complex issue. The collapsing of effeminacy in behavior and receptivity in sex is a real trap, even though there are other men in this study, for example, Geoff Harris, for whom the receptive mode in intercourse operated within a long-term pattern of submission: "I kinda slotted into this role and I thought that's what one must do. You're either one or the other, and it didn't occur to me till much later that you can be a whole person and—and do lots of things. I thought that's what gay men do."

For Harry and John, their preferences are not simple inversions of their personalities or personae. Their central interest in penetrative sex should not be equated with some sort of heterosexual analogue. Their sexual practices are very diverse, and Harry's account of their sexual exploits, the development and utilization of fetish and fantasy, their games of seduction, and the patterning of encounters with casual and other regular partners reveals an interest and level of pleasure in a whole sexual experience, which goes far beyond the now-popular tales of heterosexual men's fixation on penetration and orgasm.

For one thing, John can only ejaculate once, yet Harry can do so many times per event. They choreograph their sexual activity around this, delaying John's orgasm until he is ready and allowing Harry to ejaculate as often as he likes. They share a fascination with nakedness, a conscious and common sense of wicked transgression and a pattern of creativity: a recent addition of sex toys, a fetishization of Speedos, and a skilled use of the hot tub (they are known locally as the "Gator Girls" [short for Alligator] because of their aquatic seduction skills).

Harry and John's arrangement with threesomes did not grow from a dissatisfaction with their own still very active sexual engagement with each other, but as a way of policing each other while satisfying Harry's desire for more sex. They gave me no account of the negotiation that occurred, but it coincided with their greater immersion in local gay community life. That they have successfully negotiated a format for multiple casual partners is an example of the subversive challenge of gay relationships to heterosexist norms; it is neither simply an assumption of male sexual prerogatives nor a mere expansion of the parameters of male pleasure. The fact they continue to cheat on each other within that agreement exposes the limitation of their negotiations so far, and their responses to HIV/AIDS and safe sex indicate the contingent and ongoing nature of this sexual negotiation.

Harry was HIV seronegative at the time of the interview, as was John. They have continued to have unprotected anal intercourse inside their own relationship. Outside it they use condoms always, forcefully dressing down casual partners, friends, or relatives who request or report "unsafe" sex. Harry has been particularly careful, checking that the condom on the casual partner was not broken when John is being fucked. They are safe sex *exemplars*. Well, almost. There are three regular partners with whom their judgment errs. One partner comes from a nearby town. They know him well and are aware of his closeted and nonexistent sex life. At the time of the interview this fellow had a lover who had tested HIV seronegative, and Harry and John had "unsafe" sex with him too, using withdrawal. The third is a married man, whom they have seen regularly for many years.

It is an uncharacteristic slip in their otherwise careful thinking in each of these cases, and this is a good example for HIV/AIDS educators to contemplate: why two such sensible, uninfected HIV/AIDS activists and volunteers cannot see the dangers. They "trust" these men. In this, they might be lucky in their part of the world, but would not be in a place where HIV seroprevalence is much higher than in Nullangardie.

Harry, Ralph, and Neil were at the time of the interview very sexually active men, all were over forty-five and all were engaged in negotiating a delicate balancing act between satisfactory sex lives within primary relationships and an openly stated desire to explore sexual activity with men elsewhere. At the same time they created homosexually active lives in relationships of resilience and strength in ways related more to their earlier individual histories than to a more recent history of coming out and being gay.

## Becoming Gay

All three men registered the importance of the gay community in some way in their lives. As he grew older the number of non-gay people in Ralph's life diminished and the number of gay men increased. Since the late 1970's he increased his participation in gay community life, but not always of the Oxford Street kind. He drew a distinction between those in his self-help group and Oxford Street men, talking of the former as those who "give something as well." He regarded Oxford Street men as not able to go the distance in volunteer HIV/AIDS work, for example. Ralph (with Dennis) did participate in the big events and the social clubs, but he was critical of those who are "fairly self-centered . . . they are out in the bars because they are looking for pickups . . . but I don't want to make judgments."

These are interesting distinctions. In one way they contain the common contrast between the committed and the hedonist. Ralph's having sex in beats is left to one side in his claim to a gay identity formed through participation in a certain set of practices, a certain way of *being* gay (a style of presentation, presence at events), while distinguishing himself from *types* of gay men (those he is not like: a "clone" or an "opera queen"). A gay identity is constructed here in part through a sense of membership of a group of practitioners with much (but not necessarily all) in common. It is an aesthetic process: learning how to be gay is about learning to participate in those practices and belong to that group.

It is also the *quality* of the relations between men that is being distinguished here. It was the development of his relations with an active group of gay men in the self-help group that widened the rift between Stewart and Ralph. Their dinner party set of camp men was not involved in either the Oxford Street scene or the wider gay community. Ralph was forty and changing his interests, becoming a "gay" homosexual man; Stewart was still in the closet in many ways. Stewart did not like these new people in Ralph's changing circle.

Ralph made this deliberate change in his life in the early 1980's. He was settled, with "husband" and hearth, a career, and some casual sex partners on the side—a reasonably safe and quiet existence. He nearly lost it all by starting to be gay. He lost the relationship, almost lost the house, later became HIV seropositive, and took extraordinary risks as an "out" gay man at work and in the public view. It is hard to say exactly why it happened. Certainly, life with Stewart was not what it had once been. Maybe it was turning forty? Whatever this transformation from a homosexual man to a gay one, it marks the culmination of a much longer struggle Ralph had waged with his sexuality.

In contrast, Harry made the transition from homosexual to gay without any difficulty. During the years of sexual exploration in the beats the question of his sexuality or his sexual identity was largely irrelevant until Harry recognized other possibilities in relations with men. With John he made a homosexual identity and lifestyle his own, and both began the slow transition toward gay as a result of new influences and new exigencies. Harry and John have changed with the times, adopting what they like (pornography, Speedos), rejecting what they don't (fistfucking). It is a conscious process of appropriation following the beacon of the Sydney gay community and its relation to an emergent international gay culture. Changing from camp to gay was not really a difficult thing for them to do at all. This was happening in the context of the emerging gay community in Nullangardie with which Harriet was contending less well.

Neil saw a difference in meaning between gay and homosexual right from the start in his visits to the psychiatrist:

I didn't even go in and say to him: "I'm gay." I only said: "Look, I'm homosexual." [laughs] I mean, I wasn't even prepared to use the jargon that's more acceptable to gay people. I mean, there's a little bit of difference between being gay and being homosexual isn't there, in the sense, I mean, they mean exactly the same thing, but it's [the word, gay] more of our own acceptance in ourselves . . . because, in a sense, I suppose I still had the hangups of being a child, expecting to get into trouble for being naughty.

These three elements of Ralph's, Neil's, and Harry's lives—their relationships, their sexual activity, and becoming gay—are the keys to the pursuit (maybe even the *achievement*) of their homosexuality, signaled in these cases by a state of relative calm after a number of years of turmoil and difficulty. Their relationships form the basis of this sense of calm. At first glance these men might look quite conventional with their lovers, houses, companionable social lives, and relative economic comfort. But the arrangements they have evolved reveal a more complex relation between emotional connection, sexual desire, and a sense of being gay in a straight world.

These stories capture nicely the very conscious and fragile process of appropriating gayness. They reveal the limitations of the concept of gay *identity*. There is a significant difference between the act of self-acceptance and the process of living that acceptance wholly and dealing with homoerotic desire itself. Being gay emerges in these case studies as a different kind of struggle, at one level more cultural than personal, more social than sexual, related to an ongoing reordering and resurfacing within larger discursive frameworks and in practices; it is of an order different from that of the pursuit of homosexual sex itself. It is a balancing act with costs and benefits.

The psychic disturbance involved in this pursuit is not simply internally anchored. It is clear that wider social relations are centrally involved, and the negotiations occur within families, among relatives, loved ones, friends, in workplaces. Precious things are lost in the process. Trade-offs are made, and the pacing is determined not just by the man himself. Progress is staggered: Harry and John do not have sex when the kids are there; Neil has yet to deal with his mother. It is also slow and can regress, as in the case of Ralph's sister. A gay life then becomes more an act of *doing*, rather than a state of *being*. And in the doing, one is judged and judges oneself; one's progress is assessed and critiques are offered. In this, the performativity of "gay" is established.

∽

The preceding outlines the struggles of three men as they came to terms with their homosexual interests and pursued them toward a resolution of their sexual identities and practices inside significant relationships. This section examines some of the features common to that struggle and pursues more theoretical consequences in terms of the body, the relations and contexts of sex, the perversity of male sexuality, and (homo)sexual subjectivities. It reinforces the need for research on sexuality to go beyond a sexological approach with its emphasis on counting the frequency of an individual's sex practices.

## Sexual Beings, Sexual Bodies

Harry's not-so-furtive youthful fumblings (they took all their clothes off) and his initiation into anal sex are examples of one theme common in the lives of men in this study; the *perverse sexual experiences* of boys. Harriet, Barney, Harry, and Neil all told tales of boys and youths experimenting sexually, exploring bodies and seeking sensations, seemingly oblivious to the incursion of specific anti-homosexual discourse. There was undoubtedly a loud and generalized anti-sex discourse permeating their childhoods; hence the secretive nature of these events. But the world of children is full of excursions into the forbidden and, despite injunctions against sexual activity generally, there is a profound silence on homosexuality spe-

cifically. That silence is broken later during the time of these adolescent experiments, but even then not explicitly. In these earlier moments the body's
sensations rule, and the privileges of a modern Western childhood—mainly
boyhood (even a working-class boyhood)—enable such sensation-seeking
to continue.

The childhood sexual activity of Neil and Harry was very similar to
Barney's experience a generation earlier. This sexual activity was not hidden from peers; on the contrary, it was an open secret that the local
boys were sexually active with each other and sometimes with older men.
Harriet's experiences were certainly part of a common homosexual frolic.
Is this early sex play in changing rooms, local toilets, sporting ovals, "training" for beat use in later life? What easy transition is provided by this kind
of experience? It is but a small step for a sexually inquisitive boy to proceed from sex with peers in the changing shed to exploring sex with older
men in public toilets. The pervasive characterization of such encounters
as "older-insertive/younger-receptive" by those opposed to either intergenerational sexual activity or childhood sex play is not always accurate.
Harry, for example, was the insertive one from his earliest encounters.

For Harry and Ralph, a second phase of sexual opportunity came later.
In Harry's beat-using days as a young adult, men taught him the techniques
of sex, in particular anal sex, and his skill and preference for the insertive
mode developed. He learnt to kiss and learnt that emotions could be involved; it was not all simply "raw" sex.

The transition from boyhood sex play was brought to an abrupt and
very serious halt with a "sex-is-serious" discourse on Harry's arrest. Ralph
and Barney experienced their first run-ins with the police as adults fully
aware of what was at issue; the young Harriet, of course, merely thought
it a game, commenting on the lights of Nullangardie as he and his father
were driven to the police station. It is doubtful whether Harry fully recognized the sexual boundaries and legal specificities within which his "toilet
tango"—to use Oscar Moore's (1991) evocative term—was pursued. Even
so, Harry was not daunted by this setback and sought even more directly
challenging activity, more sex not just in toilets but in men's homes. He
explored tentative affairs and socialized on beats, developing his first gay
friendships.

The sexual *skilling* that occurs in such encounters starts with the sex
acts themselves. It is about the physical possibilities of the body; what
hands, mouths, penises, and anuses can achieve. A second level of skilling
occurs in learning the *choreography* of sexual encounters. By choreography
is meant the subtle and nuanced movement of bodies in sexual encounters:

the stalking of partners, the shifting of attention from the general possibility of sex to the specific opportunity for sex, the inviting glance, the suggestive movements of bodies, the first contact, the sequencing of exploring bodies, and so on. Beyond those sensate discoveries it involves a familiarity with the context, the local sexual economy; a recognition of sites for sex as being not limited to their defined purposes and subject to certain rules of conduct.

Ren Pinch described such a choreographed event with his usual perspicuity as follows:

I was at [a beachside park] late one night. It was warm, and the moon was really bright over the headland, and it made the beat look just stunning. I walked round for a bit checking the place out—I always make sure it's safe. There were a few guys around and I saw one really cute one wearing nothing but board shorts and a singlet, bare feet. And I kinda let him know I was interested . . .

(What exactly did you do to let him know?)

Well, I walked past once and just briefly looked at him, you know, out of the corner of my eye. Then I walked back past him again and looked for longer and waited to see if he looked back. He did for just that little bit too long, you know. (What do you mean?) If they look away quick, you know they're not interested. But if they look a bit longer and meet your eyes and stay looking for a few extra seconds, you know you've got 'em.

(What happened next?)

I headed off down the rocks—there's sort of rock steps leading off the path to under where the rocks overhang. You can't be seen by anyone unless they know where to look. I've had sex there before. I checked back to see if he was following and waited to see him move to come after me. Then I went to this part of the overhang where there's a flat rock you can sit on. I sat on it with my hand sort of just holding my crotch and waited. He came down and stood a bit away near the overhang and looked at me for a long time and I looked back and sort of rubbed my lunch a bit, as a signal, you know.

(You hadn't said anything to him at all?)

No, not a word. It's better when you don't talk. (Is it?) Yeah. (Why?) I dunno—it just seems the way to do it.

(What happened then? Can you tell the rest of the story?)

Well, we did this a bit and then the guy slowly opened his fly—it was velcro and you can always tell when they open their flys when they're velcro [laughter], it's a dead giveaway. Anyway, he slid his hand inside his pants and started playing with himself. He had a hardon, you could see that as plain as day. I did the same and changed position on the rock so he could see me, you know, opened my legs a bit, sort of face on. You're enjoying this, aren't you? (All in the name of science. Do go on.) Well, I played with myself and then slowly pulled my cock out of my pants and started rubbing myself a bit. He could see my dick easily. But he still didn't come over, you know—he sort of waited there, playing hard to get, sort of, and I thought: "Right, you bastard, let's see how good you really are."

(What do you mean?)

Well, he was playing poker. You know what I mean? Upping the stakes, making it more, sort of, not just exciting, ah, more tense and more titillating by holding off and going slowly. Fine by me! (What did you do?) Well I thought I'd see just how far he was prepared to go, so I slowly took my shirt off. I was only wearing a T-shirt and jeans and thongs. No jocks. I never wear jocks to the beat; too hard to get them on again if you need to in a hurry. Anyway so I took off the shirt and he then did the same a few minutes later, all the time playing with himself inside his pants. Me—I'm waving my cock around like it was semaphore you know! [laughter] Then he undid his shorts and let them drop, stepped out of them and stood there stark naked in the moonlight. I was on the rock, it was under cover a bit, you see, but he was still out in the open a bit. And he just stood there and stroked his thing slowly in full view and looked at me. Fuck! By this time I was really hot and ready for anything, so I stood up on the rock and stripped off and we faced each other naked like, I dunno, like um, like not boxers, but like, shit, who knows? Anyway at that point he walked toward me and I slid off the rock and we did it there and then in the middle of the rocks.

(What did you do? I warned you I was going to ask explicit questions?)

Yeah, you did, didn't you. We fucked. (Straight away?) No. We kissed first, and rubbed and wanked, and then we sucked each other for a while, and then I fucked him until he came and then he fucked me until I did. It was great, a long smooth slow fuck, me bending over the rock. And then we kissed, again real slow and deep, you know, and he got dressed and took off up the rocks and disappeared. I got dressed and left. Never seen him there again.

(Did you ask him his name or anything?)

No, we never spoke. (Not a word?) No, didn't need to.

This is what Ralph meant when he said casual sex could be "first rate." This so-called anonymous or impersonal sex is anything but emotionally cold and un-involving. The sexual satisfaction is not simply a direct product of orgasm, although that counts a fair bit. Such encounters are sexually fulfilling for both partners. Each is sexually validated by their success in performing well physically and emotionally. The moment is a highly charged one, and the elaboration of the ritual carefully draws on previous experiences and recognized processes and elements. But the *frisson* derives from the overall event not just the sex. The possibility of such complex satisfactions becomes a central feature of such sexual adventuring.

Almost all the men in this study reported having to learn these skills. Geoff Harris learned at the hands of other, older guests in the gay boarding house in which he first lived when he came to Sydney as a teenager. His was a classic apprenticeship. The significance of such sexual training and skill-building lies partly in producing sexually proficient men—and encounters such as those described by Ren Pinch do demand proficiency in mutual pleasuring—but also in producing men skilled in negotiation beyond sexual technique. There is a significant lore to be learned about male erotics, the sensuality of the specifically masculine, the similarities and differences in sexual pleasure between men, the seeking of the self in another and noting the other within.

Sexual beings, capable of judging what pleasures oneself and others, who know how to make both happen in an encounter, must be created. It is an uneven process: Stewart apparently never learned its possibilities; at least they were never transposed into his sexual activity with Ralph. Harry and John specialize in this kind of activity. The Gator Girls have developed sex-in-threes to a highly skilled performance.

There is a resonance with John Rechy's *Sexual Outlaw* (1977) in the accounts of these men, the same praise for the sexuality of gay men and the capacity for and love of casual sex. There is transgression, a little recklessness, real danger, the heightened sensation that accompanies risk and fear, the pleasures involved and potentially available in each encounter. It is the sensation of an affinity between sexually aroused men and the capacity of each to read arousal in the other and match it. Within this choreography of sex it is important to think of casual sex in part as a particular sex practice and not just as a description of partner choice.

Undoubtedly part of the frisson in casual sex is derived from its transgressive qualities. The messages men receive about such sexual possibilities (as a child in talk of sex, public toilets, and "dirty old men") are subverted by the potential pleasures to be had. The messages received as a small child about penises; the chastisement received on being caught fiddling with the boy next door; Harriet's police encounter; the wrongness verified by the need for secrecy which surrounds circle jerks, fucking peers, reading pornography, and so on: all these constitute the general framework within which sex and sexual pleasure are defined and classified as transgressive. Yet its specific attractions outweigh these general costs; the payoff is regarded as greater than the risks.

One should not ignore the recreational aspects of this kind of sex. The habitué knows that sex is available at any given moment or place unbeknown to the world at large. This is also sex as *art*: the art of the perpetual seduction and pleasuring of men by men. De Sade comes to mind fleetingly; the elevation of the profane to art is not dissimilar. This is sex as *sport*, as hobby, as pastime. There is no less dedication, preparation, or even obsession, than in weight-lifting or marathon running. Indeed, the combination of jogging and stopping off for a quickie in the local dunnies is not uncommon among married men, according to gay men who do beats. So casual sex is not only a sex practice, but also a learned set of sexual relations. It takes practice, intuition, experience, and skill to operate on a beat effectively.

These sexual interests of homosexual men cannot be explained away as a product of the male capacity for ready erection and quick orgasm. What seems important is the reciprocal nature of the encounter, the easy exchange of pleasure rather than its "taking." In this way homosexual sex establishes yet another discontinuity with the discourses and practice of a unified male sexuality.

The fascination beats hold for these and many other men is interesting; there is a sense of *preoccupation* in these instances, something similar to the fascination in a cobra's swaying to bewitch its prey. The beats are not only sites of endless promise, but also signifiers of and venues for exploring the elsewhere unattainable or unavailable, of pursuing the fantastic. There is a strong bodily pull in beat sex; the fantasizing body displays or enjoins a "disembodied" (yet, at the same time, palpably corporeal) penis in the glory hole, under the partition; eager anonymous anuses are read like braille in the darkness.

Other forms of casual sex (sex-on-premises venues, saunas) are less frequented by many of the older men in the study. Perhaps, the stakes are different. Some men (e.g., Ren Pinch) note that the nudity of a sauna betrays the sagging tummy of the over-forty. For Ralph, the classical beauty of a young male body was well and truly a thing of the past and this increases rejection in such places. To be passed over when taking the risk of offering an overtly sexual proposition to another man is hurtful. He called it "disrespect," and issued a call for sexual acceptance in what he saw as a community becoming increasingly preoccupied with the youthful and fashionably desirable. To have one's sexual desire acknowledged by other men was important to all the older men in the study, and this issue must rate as one on which modern gay communities are failing in their challenge to more general sexual conventions.

Do heterosexual men ever put their sexuality on the line in such ways? Sexual rejection happens to many. But straight "singles" bars lack the same explicitness and directness as gay bars, where the emphasis is on sexual relations among homosexual men, particularly in casual sex. If one prefers specific sex practices, these too are often on display (one man in this study, Robert Cusack, proudly wore his leathers around Sydney for many years), but as a consequence can be rejected directly. Attraction is more consciously acknowledged. Desire is more explicitly engaged. Therefore, rejection hits harder.

Ralph claimed it is even more hurtful to be rejected anonymously; the more anonymous the sex, the less justifiable its rejection. A glory hole in a toilet wall reveals only penises. Yet, as he noted, sometimes the person on the other side will cover up the hole for no explicable reason. While such occurrences made Ralph feel lousy, he exhibited an interesting lack of self-awareness. He, too, rejected in similar circumstances, but justified his behavior by arguing that he is better mannered—he simply walked away!

This is part of the psychological risk attached to casual sex. For a man who visits the beat every day (such as Harriet), risks, both physical and psychological, are being taken that require a different perspective on sex. Ralph was not often successful in closer encounters. He reported that he had never met sexual partners through social organizations (with one exception) or classified ads, clubs, and so on. He was better at succeeding on beats and that was where he always returned. Ironically, he met Dennis in a sex-on-premises venue.

## The Public Nature of Sex Between Men

Such male-to-male sex occurs in a context of permanent *surveillance*. The existence of constant surveillance, and the awareness homosexually active men have of it, colors the sex right from the start. Consequently, sexual skill becomes only one component of the skill needed to pursue pleasure. Perversion is never secret; it is widely recognized but mostly unacknowledged. Far from marginal, it is present in all men's consciousness.

With downcast eyes they screen out or attempt to ignore the graffiti in the urinals, meaningful glances in bars, unnecessary touches in gymnasiums, highly charged nudity at swimming pools and saunas, and tumescent exhibitions in changing rooms.

Harry's account is that of a youthful adventurer, somewhat unaware of this sexual economy, its illegality, and the impact of systematic suppression of such sexual activity on the pursuit of sex between men. This surveillance is manifested in many ways: indirectly, by cut-off toilet doors, signs about loitering, threatening anti-gay graffiti, and closed toilet blocks; directly, through police entrapment, raids, gay bashers, and murderers. The so-called anonymous sexual encounter is in fact taking place before an audience of many individuals and institutions, not least the nonparticipating men, for they too are subject to the same surveillance and regulation.

Neil's bashing incident is one dangerous example of this surveillance that raises an insistent and nagging query about masculine sexuality. How did these young men, the bashers, account for the sex that occurred between one of them and Neil? How does the one whose presumably erect penis was sucked by Neil and who sucked Neil in turn account for this to the mate outside the door waiting for the right moment to start the assault? The particular brutality of the act of slamming the door on Neil's erect, protruding penis is frightening. Yet the basher himself put his own penis through the same hole, risking the same brutality. Did the thought not occur to him that Neil might be up to the same purpose? He could not be unaware of the correspondence in the action, in the same way that someone who rapes a man must recognize the possibility of being raped himself. In this way, surveillance of homosexual activity is a permanent reminder to all men of an erotic possibility.

All relations between men (including sex) are situated within a daily regime of immediate regulation and suppression, one that, in fact, grants little access to the explanatory discourses of gay liberation. If Foucault (1978) was right in talking of sexuality as an encoding of elements of dispersed social forces and discourses into consolidated and cogent arenas for the extension of social control, this daily public surveillance of homosexual activity is a good example of how it works.

However, one should remember Foucault's aside vis-à-vis the French working class when he conceded that they long escaped the effects of the deployment of sexuality:

If it is true that sexuality is a set of effects produced in bodies, behaviours, and social relations by a certain deployment deriving from a complex political technology, one has to admit that this deployment does not operate in symmetrical fashion with respect to the social classes, and consequently it does not produce the same effects in them. We must return, therefore, to formulations that have long been disparaged; we must say that there is a bourgeois sexuality, and that there are class sexualities. Or rather, that sexuality is originally, historically bourgeois, and that, in its successive shifts and transpositions, it induces specific class effects. (1978: 127)

Foucault was speaking of the French working class in the nineteenth century. It is clear that today's working-class heroes such as Harry are keenly aware of the "deployment of sexuality," but only as it is experienced in practices such as the interference of the state (that is, the police), peers (acting as police in a way), and bashers, rather than as an issue of subjectivity within discourse. Self-policing is undoubtedly one consequence— Neil's cat-and-mouse game during his married years illustrates this—but there remains a tenacious and persistent pursuit of these pleasures even when the dangers are known, experienced, and obvious. Ralph even argued that this tension added to the occasion.

It may be that the operation of discourse in history is transparent to the subject. Harry is not aware of any historical construction affecting his sexual exploits, contextualizing his explorations within a vast technology of regulation, or hegemonizing his comprehension and experience of pleasure. Those "in the know," of course, do comprehend this vast framing of the sexual domain. What Harry experienced was a growing accumulation of instances of activity, opinion, and attitudes in his milieu, which, as he grew to adulthood, formed into a patchy prohibition against male-to-male sex, one he systematically ignored. The "deployment of sexuality" is still uneven. On the one hand, Harry and Neil did get married after all, noting that everyone did or was expected to. On the other, their homosexual interests were subject to less specific shaping; discourses of prohibition were inconclusive and partial.

Harry offers an example of what is amiss with this kind of discourse theory, particularly in its deterministic and more structuralist versions. Harry is left with nothing more to defend himself than something like a new, even wordier account of "false consciousness," or "limited penetrations" (to borrow Paul Willis's [1977] disturbing term). It is assumed Harry is unable to recognize as counterfeit that which he experiences as an enacted policing of sexual boundaries. Yet Harry has pursued his sex life through an authentic experience of homosex. He sought its sensations and therein divined its truths, and still does so because of the *fit* of those sensations within an evolving sexual subjectivity; and he did this despite the discursive "deployment of sexuality."

The actual sensations of sex between men are what contribute to the counterhegemonic capacity in homosexuality. This calls into question the notion that it is gay *identity* that is actually subversive—a notion privileged in much sexuality writing. Only sensation—the bodily sensations of sex— have the power to contradict prohibition. Earlier sensations and experiences—"all of a sudden it just kind of clicked . . . I remembered what I used to do before . . . and I'd cracked a fat"—confront and often overwhelm prohibitive discourse: "He said: 'Do you want me to do something about it.' And I said: 'No, I don't.'" But he did.

There is further mileage to be gained in exploring the diverse transgressions available in the male (homo)sexual economy. The working-class men in this study are perpetual larrikins. Barney told of wartime trysts at the beach pavilion with men in uniform. Harriet told of the remarkably enduring homoerotics in Nullangardie. A number, like Dennis Partridge, prostituted themselves. Geoff Harris by his early teens was involved in ongoing sexual relationships with a number of schoolmates. Martin Ridgeway started doing the local beat regularly at age twelve. Harry's lover, John, was masturbated in the cinema by his older brother's mate while his brother got off with a girlfriend in the row behind.

There are discourses on boyhood that on the one hand, are continuous with "hegemonic masculinity" (Connell 1983, see chapter 2) in certain ways (adventuring, rule-breaking, testing new sensations, particularly proscribed ones—smoking, wanking, drinking, fucking, stealing) and, on the other, disruptive of it (becoming known as a cocksucker, getting involved in pedophile relationships, falling in love with another boy). Harry brought to his exploration of homosexuality all the energy and brashness of boyhood. Harry was not simply an unknowing subject of hegemonic discourse, but was practicing elements of competing and disrupted discourses of masculinity, in particular with reference to its physicality. In his case there is sufficient contradiction between the prohibition on homosex and the license granted males for him to continue his exploration with far more certainty than some others in the study.

Hegemony and counterhegemony should not be seen as competing blocks of forces, ideologies, and intentions. Setting aside for the moment the possibility that counterhegemony may be a tautology anyway, it is important to seek some fragments of homosexuality's subversion both of hegemonic masculinity and compulsory heterosexuality in the accumulated bodily experience of homosex. It is here that any counterhegemonic potential is found in male homosexuality. Its challenge is to other men, masculinity, a unified male sexuality, and heterosexuality (for it offers to women a critique of the shaping of their sexuality, too; feminists should therefore not assume that male homosexuality offers no challenge to gender). Gender, to be of any use as an analytical tool, ought to be defined as the structure of relations between *and* within the sexes, not just between men and women. Harry offers glimpses of a multifaceted spectacle of the homosexual challenge.

These sexual games of boyhood become problematic as time goes on: more incisive and explicit discourses on sexuality enter, defining various previously unnamed pleasures, practices, and events as homosexual and framing these activities within the unnatural, the deviant, the immoral, and (in the case of Ralph's hormone treatment) the physically defective. In his second beat encounter, Ralph was suddenly constituted as homosexual, as a poofter, a pervert, a person of illicit desires. In part he constituted himself as such. It is an astonishing moment to witness so clearly. Heavy social disapprobation landed on Ralph in a single instant. The stereotype of the child molester then took root in his head, making him fear for himself even though he had no history of such sexual activity to warrant this alarm.

This is an important and difficult moment in the formation of a sexual identity; yet it is actually a moment of *disintegration*. The public imaginary of the homosexual is imposed internally (whether or not an external event has occurred, such as an arrest). It is a process of suddenly recognizing oneself as a different being and then having to incorporate that being into a new self. Dr. Jekyll discovers he is Mr. Hyde—the person everyone, including himself, fears—but in this case the mirror reveals no external changes at all. The process involves standing outside oneself, examining the whole being by focusing on sexual matters. From then on, even for men in the closet, being homosexual is actually a public state, a discursively formed condition. The pink triangle is worn not on clothing but on the psyche. Private homosexual acts are always "observed" thereafter. Any attempt to confess the crime, to expiate, manifestly compounds the problem; for gay men never control the terms of acceptance (repentance?).

Few heterosexual men need to do this, unless they sexually abuse others or find themselves caught in a web of other paraphilia[2] and thereby face social condemnation and marginalization. Otherwise, heterosexuality—if it is thought about at all by heterosexual men—is experienced as comparatively continuous with the self. It is a recognition of sexual interests and

---

[2] Yes, there is a sanitized but still pathologized term, of which Stoller says: "*Perversion* is a sturdy term, throbbing with assumption, while *paraphilia* is a wet noodle" (1985: 6).

their expression in a way that expands and rounds out adulthood in this society.

Ralph, going through this in the 1960's, had an extremely painful and damaging experience. He confessed to his mother when he was caught by the police in the beat, but not to his father. Hers was a case of where did we go wrong? His response: "I am what I am" (another example of anachronistic motif in such memories, and of the pervasiveness of that wretched song). He is not sure when or how his father found out, but when Ralph and Stewart broke up, the father's response was that gay relationships did not last long. Ralph reminded him of the sister's two marriages and put paid to that fallacy. But the terms on which Ralph's sexuality was to be dealt with were no longer of his making; he was now publicly homosexual and would forever engage the oppressive if uneven discursive framing of his sexuality fortified only by the authenticity of his erratic sexual experience. And trumpeting one's last tryst in a toilet is hardly a winning weapon!

In spite of this, the pursuit of the homoerotic is remarkably resilient. Men contrive to return to beats, backroom fuck bars, saunas, and sex cinemas to seek pleasure. Part of the reason for this is that there is more to this exercise than the sex acts themselves.

## Sexual Relations and Sex Practices

Sex does not exist only as an individual experience; it is also social, and as such is constituted in relational and contextual domains. There is an element in sex with casual partners that illustrates the human side of such encounters. First, feelings are involved; it is not a case of men treating other men as men are often accused of treating women. The ritual interplay differs from that of heterosexual relations, just as the ritual interplay of sexual relations differs from culture to culture.

Second, for some men using beats, this kind of interaction is but one of an array of sexual relations constituting a sex life. It is important not to deduce a simplistic, singular conceptualization of enacting desire in casual encounters on the beats. Not only do the relations and practices of casual beat sex differ, but the positioning and importance of beat sex differ from one man to another.

Ralph was asked if certain sex practices were reserved for casual sex and others for sex within relationships. There is some connection here between experience and maturation. Ralph's sexual repertoire developed as he aged, became more sexually confident, and expanded his experience beyond primary relationships. For example, his first experience of esoteric sex—he had fisted only a couple of men—was not a real turn-on for him, and he did not want that kind of practice for himself. In fact, he reported that these activities took place only because casual partners wanted them, and that the real thrill for him invoked a quite different dimension of arousal: "Yes, I fistfucked him. I fucked him and that was quite a turn-on—the fact that my cock was in there where my hand had been—but it [the fisting] didn't do anything really for me."

Another example of a sex practice and its relational constituent is Ralph's inability to ejaculate in sex with Stewart, in particular, the story about faking orgasm with a small amount of urine. This example would indicate a possible distinction between penetration and achieving orgasm for at least some homosexual men, namely, that ejaculation may not always be the sole goal. A man may fuck another until the receptive partner comes, and the insertive partner may then choose to reach orgasm another way, maybe by being fucked himself. Alex Lawes, a married, openly bisexual man, adopted a similar technique in sex with his wife: he would penetrate her only until her orgasm; he would then withdraw, preferring to reach his orgasm by hand. Perhaps not all men are as fixated on penetrative sex as one might expect.

Ralph and Dennis shared another version of this. In anal sex Dennis is the one who likes being fucked; Ralph was the insertive partner more often than not. He did not always cum when he was fucking Dennis; he preferred cumming in Dennis's mouth, inserting his penis just at the point of orgasm. This did, however, mark a change in practice for Ralph. In his younger days: "I probably would be more passive than I am, because through the sixties I can remember some memorable times of being fucked . . . [He liked the feeling of] a couple of guys who were fairly large and I managed to accommodate them, just again feeling the cock inside you and feeling someone was there and being really intimate with you." The importance of the sheer physical nature of sexual engagement is important to note here; as is the measure of competence. Ralph did not judge his sexual prowess on the strength of his penis.

This mention of intimacy in anal sex occurred in many other interviews. This is another element of the communicative function of homosexual sex noted by R. W. Connell and Susan Kippax (1990). It contrasts strongly with the (not-unchallenged) feminist critique of vaginal intercourse as an exercise in domination and, possibly, misogyny. Is it simply that men can be both insertive and receptive? If they are in the habit of using both penis and anus for sex, does the issue of power in penetration, as defined in heterosexuality, become simply irrelevant in homosex?

On this uniquely male sexual possibility, Peter Standard argued strongly for "double the pleasure," the sensation of a stimulated prostate gland adding to that of an aroused and stimulated penis. Reciprocity is an important feature of male-to-male anal intercourse. But then so is the ambiguity in that interchangeability. One of Harriet's specialties as a sex worker (remember, he usually did "anal," that is, receptive) was fucking those tricks who prefer to be penetrated by him (or "her," if in drag).

Neil Bartlett in his novel, *Ready to Catch Him Should He Fall* (1990), captures beautifully the contradictory dimensions of this reciprocity in homosexual sex, where active and passive as sexual mode and meaning collide:

> But for the men I know and for myself certainly I know that it usually comes out as *fuck me, please fuck me*, though that may not be exactly what you mean. I mean it is not necessarily about wanting to be actually fucked this feeling. It's more to do with the way women friends use the word "fucked," when they say, *I fucked him*, or *I didn't want to fuck him*—for us it still means literally I fucked him, he got fucked by me. What I mean is, sometimes you are on top of him you have the back of his neck in your teeth, and you still find yourself wanting to say to him, fuck me, go on, go on, even though you are on top. (p. 109)

Privileging an interpretation of anal sex as an exercise of domination can be a trap; if only because in gay pornography, for example, the macho top, energetically rooting his groaning partner to the slick dialogue of "Take it, take it. You like that big cock, don't ya, you faggot," is almost certain to bend over in the second reel and be "serviced" himself. Domination between men may in itself only be fantasy, after all.

The S/M ideologues argue for the performative attributes of their activities (discussed in Weeks 1985, chapter 9) and offer thereby a recreational view of power in sex: it is interactive and agentive. Even in oral sex (according to Connell and Kippax [1990: 177] the most frequently practiced orgasmic homosexual act) the meaning can vary. In contrast to the intimacy of anal intercourse, Ralph Coles and Peter Standard both regard sucking as an act of domination/submission: the sight of the penis so close/the person kneeling below. Yet mutual sucking—the famous 69er—requires reciprocity (not to say skill and timing), and it would appear the domination and the submission occurs more at the level of fantasy than as an intrinsic product of the practice itself. Gay men refer to it almost always as "cock-sucking," implying that the *active* partner is the one with the mouth; it is rarely referred to as "mouthfucking."

Sex practices are undergoing transformations. It is not that much of what we do sexually is so different from that which Chaucer or Boccaccio or Congreve playfully discussed. But anyone who has had sex with eight other men on a twelve-foot circular waterbed must recognize that sex itself is changing. This may simply be sexual *fashion*. There are plenty of examples of the external image of desire being manipulated: Rubens's chubby women versus Twiggy; the flapper's flat chest versus women's conical breasts in the 1960's; codpieces in Henry VIII's time and the return of the tight "packed lunch" jeans in the 1970's and 1980's; heterosexual swingers clubs in the 1970's, gay jack-off clubs in the face of HIV/AIDS in the 1980's.

These changes go further than in the images of desire or the arrangements for sex; sex acts themselves change in meaning and order, and sex itself is a historical production (see, for example, Lillian Rubin's discussion in *Worlds of Pain* [1976] of the incursion of popular discourses on oral sex in the 1960's in a working-class community). HIV/AIDS changed oral sex again in the 1990's. One does not swallow semen any more. As Dan Berger noted, among homosexual men this would once have been bad manners: "The way I was brought up, it was important . . . in the etiquette of the sixties . . . swallowing, I mean. If you spat it out, that was very bad. It's really rude. It's like you downgrade the whole activity."

Sex practices and sexual relations are mutually constitutive. Practices may be segregated, that is, devoted to one type of relations and not another ("I never *fuck* in beats"), or they may be practiced across relations of many types. They carry meanings constructed in those particular relations or carried to them from elsewhere ("I loved being sucked off by blondes"). The same practice, for example, anal intercourse, may be vastly different in sensation and meaning. Ralph fucked both Stewart and Dennis, and he rarely ejaculated in either; the reason, organization, and meaning of that fact was vastly different in each case.

It is this relationship between sex practices, relations, and meanings lying at the heart of sexual experience that in the face of an intolerant and oppressive society, offers a major mechanism for creating homosexual subjectivity. The homosexual self is rooted relationally in desire articulated, desire experienced, and desire embodied.

What is more difficult to piece together is just how much of the present practice of negotiated nonmonogamy among gay men (Vadasz and Lipp 1990) grew out of previously existing homosexual subcultures (Bell and Weinberg 1978), how much out of the dominant discourse of male sexual behavior in general, and how much out of sexual liberation ideology. Such sexual permissiveness is likely to have been produced through an interaction of all of these. Certainly, Barney offered a glimpse of pre–gay-lib days. So these kinds of sexual agreements did exist before, and there is verification of this in the growing stream of biographies and historical accounts of the lives of gay persons.

Beyond the Gator Girls and their threesomes, other interesting sexual possibilities occur, for example, in Ralph's sexual interests, his main fantasy—having sex in groups. In this he refers to what happens in saunas and backroom bars:

> At the old Club 80, there were two very attractive men . . . totally naked just, sort of, fucking each other in one of those cubicles, three or four people watching. It was really a turn-on.
>
> (Do you like being watched?)
>
> I do not mind. It doesn't worry me.
>
> (Has it happened often, in the sauna or at the beats?)
>
> Not all that often, you know, it is a bit of a turn-on when it does happen.

The interaction between exhibitionism and voyeurism is neatly captured in Ralph's account. All fantasies should be so harmless and achievable. But it is worth noting how transgressive these mild fantasies really are in a society that exacts severe punishment from anyone, gay or straight, who has sex in a public place. Gay men in these events are certainly challenging something, though again, from what motives other than pleasure, it is unclear. Pleasure itself may be enough. Why should sex always be deep and meaningful?

John Rechy's argument about sexual outlaws seems somewhat contrived at this point, and the framing of such sexual activity as refusal (Weeks 1985) or realignment (Bristow 1989) seems more a strident protest from those wearing the mantle of the "oppressed" than a realistic assessment of the sexual moment and its motivation. After all, neither Harry, Neil, nor Ralph had their minds on challenging the sexual or social order when they frequented the beats.

Much of men's capacity for multiple partners is attributed to some essential characteristic of male sexuality; one that has considerable sociobiologistic support. For example, two psychologists on the Australian Broadcasting Corporation's *Health Report* on Radio National sometime in 1988 argued for natural polygamy in humans. They called it "xenoeroticism"! They argued that there was a correlation between size of (male) genitals and the *need* for multiple partners. Elephants have small penises, rapt listeners were told, in relation to their body weight, and they mate for life. Working one's way through the primates, it appears that animals become more promiscuous. The human (male) genitals are extraordinarily large in relation to body weight, hence as a species we need (that word again) multiple partners.

One might logically ask if those with the largest penises are entitled to a greater number of partners? We were left to presume that the human vagina is extraordinarily large too (to accommodate these large penises) and, therefore, women are probably also naturally xenoerotic, although this was not made clear. It could also be concluded that those men with very small penises are more likely to be monogamous; therefore, women who want faithful husbands should do some measuring before they tie the knot!

Discourses on male sexuality always try to explain away men's philandering in the face of the none-too-serious social disapproval accompanying male heterosexual activity. Various discourses are invoked to support or oppose this philandering: once it was sin, the work of the devil; now it is instinct, or even liberation. Those seeking a "natural" cause often have difficulty handling cultural variability; more so when it comes to homosexual activity than heterosexuality.

These conjectures betray yet again the paucity of the sexological approach. Sex is reduced to its acts, the fit of vagina and penis. The relational character of sex is ignored, and the relation between meaning and enactment is neglected entirely.

## Cathexis

Sex can move beyond its subversive physical and relational elements to challenge emotions as well. A good example is Ralph's first visit to a backroom fuck bar:

> And I walked in and within ten minutes I was kissing this man. It did not stop. The first kiss did not stop for at least half an hour. That was wonderful.

(And you had never met him, before, not spoken to him?)

No.

This was an important moment. Ralph had a soft spot for kissing and said of an earlier lover "he kissed beautifully," in a manner that suggested he was giving a character reference. But this moment in the fuck bar went further; the man he kissed was Dennis. This was how they met. It was a moment in sex which Dan Berger called "a very sudden intimacy," when it all shifts gear to become something more. It would appear that the stakes were raised in that first sexual encounter. Their connection moved almost instantly to intimacy.

This qualitative change emerged in Harry's encounter with the nearly naked man when they "made love." Something more than physical pleasure occurred; here we have *cathexis*. Connell (1987) uses the term to refer to the *structure* that organizes the "construction of emotionally charged social relations with 'objects' (i.e., other people) in the real world" (p. 112). He is claiming a systematic ordering and determination of "sexual social relations"; these relations are not random or accidental, even if they are experienced as such by the actors.

In Harry's example, part of this construction is available for scrutiny. First, Harry's beat encounters occur within a broadly defined frame. One does not flash erections at other men in urinals, and one does not have sex in public toilet cubicles. There are laws about it, and at Harry's age at the time, his recognition of the transgressive quality in these acts would have been reasonably clear. Second, Harry was having sex with his fiance at the time, heading toward validated heterosexual married life with only a little chafing at the bit. But within this broad frame there were other elements and sensations informing his response to these homosexual possibilities. His memories of early sex play combined with the physical sensations of the accumulating sex acts with these men in beats, homes, and elsewhere to delineate a different possible sexual trajectory. Third, Harry noted certain connections: the nakedness was no longer just boys taking their clothes off, itself a transgressive act, but "he *undressed* me." This was a transformation. This event revealed the possibility of something beyond "straight raw sex," thereby challenging and finally subverting Harry's experiment with compulsory heterosexuality.

The new sexual skilling involved in the event not only invoked memories of past discoveries, but also transformed these once familiar sensations of the body into something hitherto not even hoped for. Harry had, and had been, kissed before, but not like this, "He taught me how to kiss," and not at the hands of another man. This event prefigured Harry's later life with John, opening the way toward an ongoing sexual *and* emotional connection with another man. This was a moment with its suspension of time that could possibly only occur in special moments in a life. These events were lifted out of the purely physical and deposited into a psychic domain.

These elements are at one and the same time conformist and subversive, revealing a process of structuring fraught with tension and contingency. The frisson, the allure and thrill produced by nakedness for Harry, John, and Ren Pinch, was never clearer. Getting naked seems a significant element in a number of men's stories. Our culture specializes in frantic eroticizing of the body, especially by regulating its exposure to the eye; but for men to grasp the body-erotic potential of their own sex is strictly frowned on. (For women the injunction is less absolute.) Under that prohibition, the body itself becomes for men a secret item of wonder; the genitals may absorb most of the intensity for some eventually, but it is clear that the erotic attractions are broader than just the genitals for these boys in their early sex play and as young men.

It is the body in *context* that adds spice. Nakedness in a bathroom is quite different from nakedness in an inappropriate place where by stripping eroticism is conjured. Children are often keen on such exhibitionism and soon learn to explore clandestine venues where such activity can happen. Going beyond those venues becomes erotic in its own right—the key is transgression. Exactly what nakedness represents is an issue worth pursuing: the risk/delight in public nudity is a feature of our society despite the general prohibition against it. In changing rooms, public saunas (not gay bathhouses), male bodies are exposed to other male bodies in a context of an active prohibition against erotic responses.

Yet Alan Cunningham reported initiation rites in his factory and acts of anal intercourse in the shower rooms enacted as a playful challenge to masculinity. Other writers report similar homoerotic activity among men in such environments (for example, in factories, Willis 1977; in mines, Couch 1991). Pornography, particularly straight pornography, enables heterosexual men to see other men's bodies in a genuine state of arousal and climax. (They see women's bodies in [often] a faked state of arousal and one harder to identify anyway.) A visit to any sex shop with video cinemas or booths will find men having sex with each other while watching heterosexual pornography. What or who exactly is the subject of the male sexual gaze in such moments? This capacity in many men for erotic responses to varied stimuli raises again the issue of a perversity of male sexuality. Dollimore quotes Freud as follows: "One does not become a pervert, one remains one" (Freud 1953[1905], in Dollimore 1991: 172), but goes further to argue that perversion is "insubordinate" (p. 181). One thing is certain about the men in this study: the subversion of sexual rules and proprieties becomes an intrinsic part of the sexual excitement itself. "The social pattern of desire is a joint system of prohibition and incitement" (Connell 1987: 112). In this sense Foucault (1978) was correct in talking of the "incitement" to sexuality, but perhaps Harry, Ralph, and Neil's "toilet tango" was not exactly what he had in mind!

This capacity among men is not just sexual libertarianism or undifferentiated polymorphous perversity; there are some caveats. To position oneself sexually as *passive* (and I do not mean receptive in terms of penetration here), that is, to receive from another man the skilled lovemaking that

Harry recounted, is also both conformist and subversive. It is *men* in conventional masculinist sexual discourse who are the sexually skilled, taking pleasure or, in these more modern times, giving it as well. Modern heterosexual discourse rarely positions the man as receiving pleasure — taking it, yes, but not receiving it (except as consumers of women as spectacle, as Sex personified, as prostitutes, and so on). Men are active in sex, not passive. Harry experienced passivity (in this sense) quite powerfully in this encounter; he received pleasure in a way he had not experienced before. He experienced male sexual pleasure both actively and passively, narcissistically, with his image and pleasure mirrored in the other, the same.

In the context of the mutuality of pleasuring between men, passivity becomes subversive of masculine desire. That configuration is clear in the accounts of Ralph's, Neil's, and Harry's beat sex. But Harry's special moment of lovemaking was not simply desire in operation but desire in *transformation*. It was happening to a married man in his mid-twenties with four kids; to a man experienced in homosexual sex as a technique leading to physical pleasure and orgasm only. This time Harry "gets fucked" (in Bartlett's sense), although he was undoubtedly the insertive partner.

This moment is neither a resolution of Oedipus in early childhood, nor a significant adolescent disruption of a heterosexual trajectory — those moments in some theory wherein homosexuality is "made." Homosexuality is made in sex itself, in this kind of moment of transformation in an adult's existing practice. This is a moment when the process of the construction of "emotionally charged relations" has moved beyond the sexual as purely physical to the sexual as redemption, as salvation, as resolution. This construction of homosexuality through practice occurs simultaneously in the emotions, physically and psychically. And therein, subversion of masculinity is possible; the counterhegemonic capacity of homosexuality lies both in *homosex as sex* (its inversions and its reconfiguration of bodies and their appropriate fit) and *homosex as the transformation of relations between men*.

## The Process of Becoming Homosexual

Becoming homosexual is problematic in our culture, with reference both to discourses on sexuality and in daily life. Homosexual men often report seeking out information in books, dictionaries, indexes of psychology books, and checking it out with doctors, psychiatrists, and so on. Depending on the era of their self-discovery, sexual experience precedes, follows, or accompanies this reflection, this searching, this turbulence. For Ralph Coles, this was a painful and physically damaging period. The contrast with Neil Davidson's experience is marked; the latter's is an example of the specific contribution of significant changes in the recent past to that same process, particularly in psychiatry.

Entry into a homosexual subculture and nowadays a gay community involves learning a lot of social skills as well, for instance, loving Bette Davis and Barbra Streisand, buying Art Deco or postmodern furniture, cooking well, and learning to tell tall tales and true from one's legendary past. The process is one of *enculturation*; a process in many aspects at odds with the masculine culture of most men's upbringing. Heterosexual masculinity becomes a distant context, articulated to the daily life of homosexual men, and yet increasingly tangential to gay community–attached men (Dowsett 1993a). Although maturation always involves interaction with the broad cultural dynamics of a given society, for homosexual men the process involves an arresting awareness of *difference* as well, a recognition of oppression (usually experiential, sometimes discursively grasped), experiencing a new kind of sex and a conscious coming to grips with the self. It is not just problematic; homosexual men have to *problematize* it deliberately and consciously in order to get a handle on it at all.

It is a mistake to line up male homosexuality and male heterosexuality as too rigidly parallel: two equal options, two possibilities. This is where ideas such as "everyone is basically bisexual" lead. Sexuality becomes a simple option or choice, differently valued by each society. This is where a gender-privileged analysis deposits homosexual women and men: aligned with their biological sex category rather than prioritizing their sexual interests. One consequence of such an analysis is that it obscures the increasingly divergent paths emerging in male sexuality/ies.

A practice-based theory of sexuality perceives desire as complex, inconsistent, contradictory, and changeable. There is no single explanation for any sexual expression. Beats, for example, are not frequented only by those unable to negotiate sexual interaction in social settings; beat sex is not a substitute for real or meaningful sex. There are as many socially proficient men using beats as there are any other type of man. (One obvious problem is the danger in the use of "types" of person in this field.) In pursuing sex at a practical level, homosexual men have a different and varied set of sexual opportunities to negotiate and choose from: backroom fuck bars, sex clubs, saunas, beats, as well as the more socially proper opportunities. It is not just the issue of the sex of the object choice that distinguishes gay from straight!

What is of chief concern is how the process of discovering, expressing, understanding, developing, and elaborating homosexual relations and practices dominates the lives of the men it involves. The structuring of a life with homosexual desires is the *homosexualization* of that life. Sex becomes not just the binding activity, the common focus, the registering of similarity in the face of others; it is the lingua franca of gay life. No wonder it becomes an obsession for the men involved at the level of sexual expression and liberation politics. This may be part of the reason why other major social structures, such as class, seem hard to dig out when researching homosexuality in Australia:

For many gay men, fucking satisfies a constellation of needs that are dealt with in straight society outside the arena of sex. For gay men, sex, that most powerful implement of attachment and arousal, is also an agent of communion, replacing an often hostile family and even shaping politics. It represents an ecstatic break with years of glances and guises, the furtive past we left behind. Straight people have no comparable experience, though it may seem so in memory. They are never called upon to deny desire, only to defer its consummation. (Goldstein, quoted in Hurley 1992: 144)

The lives of these three men illustrate the remarkably diverse and complex enactment of homosexuality and its position within the development of a multifaceted sexual subjectivity. Their pursuit of their homosexuality has many similarities and significant differences; each has found a resolution of sorts that, inter alia, includes the building and development of primary emotional-sexual relationships with other men. But primary relationships are not the only way to develop a homosexual life. Each of these men has participated to a different extent in a gay community, and Ralph, Harry, and Harriet have made significant contributions to those communities in their own ways. They in turn have been affected by changes in those communities over the last two decades, some not without cost. Barney's growing and inexplicable isolation is the most painful example of this. Harriet is feeling growing rejections of his form of gayness. Neil watches the Mardi Gras parade, but that is all. He and John-Paul regard Oxford Street as a young man's scene. Even Ralph had his distancing, his various disapprovals. There are other men who embrace a gay community as a way to engage with their homosexuality and they pursue that option to the full. It is to this embrace that this study now turns its attention.

# 6

# Gay Community

One of the concerns of much HIV/AIDS social science research is to monitor behavior change among gay and homosexually active men in response to the HIV epidemic. The different approaches used in seemingly comparable studies often produce different "readings" of the process and character of the extensive behavior change found in these types of studies. Although some of these differences are related to method and sampling, the major differences are derived from the studies' theoretical and conceptual underpinnings. The first major Australian survey of gay and homosexually active men, the SAPA study (see Kippax et al., *Sustaining Safe Sex*, 1993, discussed in Chapter 3), differed from much psychosocial work on HIV/AIDS elsewhere, and perhaps the most important difference lies in its conceptualization of *gay community*.

I was part of the research team that undertook that survey—a team, whose membership of gay men and non-gay men and women, academics and gay community activists, university-based researchers and representatives from the AIDS Council of New South Wales, in part led to the study's distinctive research design and conceptual framework.

At the time the study started in 1986 there was no doubt in my mind that the efforts of the gay community to convince men to adopt "safe" sexual behavior were paying off. As the findings came in, we were able to offer a sophisticated account of behavior change that pointed conclusively to the contributions of the gay community to that success. Using single-item variables, such as "membership in gay organisations," and scales measuring exposure to educational materials and programs produced by the gay community, the analysis confirmed there was an important and complex relationship between prevention and gay community (Connell et al. 1989; Kippax et al., "Question of Accuracy," 1990).

This analysis was based on a large range of questions about social, sexual, cultural, and political practices, such as: How often do you go out with gay/bisexual/straight friends? Where do you go out with gay friends? Where do you go to seek sexual partners? Are you a member of, or do you go to, gay sporting/social/cultural/political organizations? And so on. These questions mapped the wide variety of *practices* (over and above the sex practices occurring in these men's lives during sex acts) that might constitute their participation in a gay community of some kind or other. As the early findings of this relationship between some of these gay community variables and sexual behavior emerged, it became clear that a more theorized starting point was required.

From the beginning of my work in HIV/AIDS research in 1986 I argued that the term, gay communi*ties*, be adopted as a starting point for unsettling the notion that there was one single, whole, and all-encompassing gay community to which gay men belonged. I knew from my own participation in the inner-Sydney gay community that there were other groups of gay men who unequivocally regarded themselves as part of the gay community but of one quite unrelated to the Oxford Street "scene." After all, columns of classified ads in gay newspapers seeking partners were and still are full of men asking for, or describing themselves as, "non-scene."

My suggestion to the research team was to cluster participation in gay community within three broad classifications: political activity; participation in the (Oxford Street) sexual scene; and social or "good times" (i.e., nonsexual) activity. The intention was to pick up on what I had observed in my own life: gay men have different patterns of participation in, and use of, the inner-Sydney gay venues, lifestyle, sexual opportunities, and activities available. Not every gay man goes to every event and not all feel comfortable with everything that happens in gay community life.

While the statistical analysis of the SAPA study was under way, I started pursuing my ideas about participation in gay community in the earliest in-depth interviews for this study, and in this chapter I pursue the issue of gay community through that interview material. Meanwhile, my somewhat sketchy idea about gay community participation turned out not to be far wide of the mark in the statistical analysis. That analysis turned up three quite distinct patterns of activity or sets of related practices: a set of items that measures *sexual engagement*; a second set that measures *social engagement*; and a third that evaluates *gay community involvement*. Together these constitute *gay community attachment* (Kippax et al., "Gay Community," 1992). A partial use of these measures in the Project Male-Call national survey confirmed their reliability, validity, and utility (Kippax et al. 1994).

The two *engagement* measures examine just that: the quantity and variety of sexual or social activities engaged in. The gay community *involvement* measure evaluated a more complex pattern of immersion in political and cultural life in a gay community and included choices to be in gay sporting or religious organizations, actions that represent a choice to relate to gay versions of activities rather than those available to the general population. Participation or membership in gay organizations dealing with political and HIV/AIDS issues, and patronizing gay businesses was also included. The term *involvement* describes more than a passing interest and gestures to a more collective enterprise.

Choosing to describe the overall term as gay community *attachment* rather than, say, *participation* was deliberate. It had been clear to me for a long time that as a gay man I had to decide to what extent and in what activities I participated within the gay community. For example, I could participate in demonstrations for gay civil rights and feel deeply attached and committed to the cause. But I could also participate in a gay dance, for example, and not necessarily feel that I belonged there. I (like many others) could be an outsider in many gay places such as bars, sex-on-premises venues, private parties in unfamiliar social-sexual networks, or among the more sophisticated, already active socially/sexually engaged and politically/culturally involved men of the developing gay community.

Attachment registers a closer, more intense, and conscious pursuit of, and identification with, the patterns of practice. In framing these interlocking sets of practices within the concept of gay community attachment, the SAPA study was not merely reflecting the intercorrelations between the three scales of practice, but offering a really viable way of analyzing the collective activity that in its overall "hum" could describe the constitution of gay community—at least with reference to HIV/AIDS and changes in sexual behavior.

But these statistical measures capture only some aspects of gay community life. For example, they omit participation in large-scale events such as the annual Sydney Gay and Lesbian Mardi Gras and the different aspects of its month-long festival. Items in the measures, such as "reads books with gay themes," barely captures an abiding interest in the explosion of gay prose and poetry, the enormous intellectual and theoretical work making up gay and lesbian studies, and the seizure of gay print by gay men the world over which defiantly relocates many writers and their work within a broad and definitively gay framework.

Similarly, "goes out with gay friends to . . ." again fails to capture the character of the dramatically refashioned lives of men in this study like

Peter Standard, Robert Cusack, or Ren Pinch, who spend most of their waking (and sleeping) hours in the company of gay men in one way or another, to the virtual exclusion of non-gay persons. And finally, the sexual engagement notion only begins to sketch what John Rechy fictionalized in *The Sexual Outlaw* (1977) or Larry Kramer in *Faggots* (1986) in the United States, and the Australian writers in *Travelling on Love in a Time of Uncertainty* (Dunne 1991) and *Fruit* (Dunne 1994). It hardly even begins to explore what Edmund White describes in *States of Desire* (1986).

It is an obvious shortcoming of forced-choice questionnaires that such measures cannot capture the process of coming to gay community, or show changes in attachment over time, or in the milieus within which it is pursued. The greatest shortcoming relates to the meaning of the activities themselves. What does it mean to be a "gay man," a "member of a gay community," or "attached to a gay community"? How is that membership understood? What is the sense in which it is declared, and why? What solutions does an intense and encompassing immersion in gay life, perhaps to the exclusion of non-gay persons, actually provide? And what happens to those with "less" attachment? How do they experience their less- or unattached lives? What prevents them from being attached or partly attached?

The SAPA study concept of gay community attachment reveals the limits of conventional data collection, but raises other complex issues. It opens up a way of documenting the lives of gay men that goes beyond the simplistic idea of "being" gay to gesture toward a way to investigate the practices of "living" gay. It moves beyond a preoccupation with identity to an interrogation of praxis—and then starts to link both. While these conceptually strong statistical measures offer a confident recognition of gay community as a multifaceted collective endeavor, it remains to be seen just how that collective experience is constructed and pursued. The original concept of gay community attachment remains an important base upon which this study is grounded. However, in order to go further into the detailed process and meaning of the production of gay community–attached lives, it is necessary to go beyond the questionnaire, however refined, to life-history work.

In order to investigate the phenomenon of gay community attachment, I present three case studies of men with significant levels of participation in Sydney gay community life. They were not interviewed with this in mind; in fact, the similarities in their lives only emerged late in the analysis. They are from three different "generations" of Sydney gay life: Robert Cusack was fifty and had moved to the Sydney scene long before the rise of gay liberation; Ren Pinch was in his mid-forties and had spent the last twenty years closely involved with the gay community politically and culturally; Richard Cochrane, in his early thirties at the time of interview, enjoyed Sydney gay life in its heyday of the late 1970's and early 1980's. What they do have in common is that they all shared in that extraordinary *sexual* adventure that is the Sydney gay community.

## The Man Who Had Ten Thousand Fucks!

Ren Pinch volunteered that his sex life was an open book, which I could investigate at will. He was not an ordinary gay man by any means. He reported having paid work for only three days in his whole life; instead, he lived off a private income. The most startling thing about him was his conscious pursuit of the (homo)sexual, a pursuit that had dominated his life. In the case of Ren Pinch this hobby was facilitated by a sense of personal power and, of course, income.

It is important to remember the privileged position Ren occupied, a university-educated man with a strong intellectual predisposition. Ren's pursuit of knowledge, of detail, was an ever-enriching and deepening source of pleasure for him. His scientific training and proficient pursuit of pleasure have been applied quite systematically to his culture, lexicon, and discourse on sex, not coldly, but in a way that has magnified his pleasure.

Ren claimed to have had sex with over ten thousand men, which probably marks some kind of maximum range of possibilities. He has also had sex with a small number of women. There was not a hint of misogyny in his accounts of these sexual encounters or of his relations with women; it was simply that he finds *men* erotic and that is that. There was also a remarkable absence of obsession in the account of his sex life; an absence that distinguished the tally of ten thousand as something to do more with the possibilities available rather than with a peculiar desire for sex. A preoccupying hobby would seem the better way to describe Ren Pinch's sexual interests.

Ren's account of his childhood masturbatory techniques was the most clearly explicated of all the participants in this study. These involved various articles of clothing, their textures and fabrics providing different stimulation. Other techniques came about as a result of experimentation with his body, exerting pressure on his penis in different ways until he ejaculated. He only discovered the word "masturbation" on the day he first ejaculated, when the intensity of the orgasm and the shock of the ejaculate sent him to a previously unread *Father and Son Movement* manual for boys. But the techniques were clearly well established from years of preejaculatory experimentation on himself. These experiences point to the importance of the body itself and each boy's exploration of it and understanding of its functions, often well before the imposition of clear definition or injunction. They could be characterized as *prediscursive* in a sense reflecting an autonomous discovery of bodily sensation before any discernible formal or informal discursive inscription, and lacking significant structural formation. I asked about how he learned to masturbate, if he copied techniques taught by others: "I can't remember anything like that, that I learned from other people. I think most of the things I did, apart from just the pure masturbation itself, which I think I learned from somebody else. . . . I think that all of those things were products of my own experimentation."

These early solitary explorations were followed at age seven by the usual sex games with another boy. There was a memory of indirect disapproval attached to this event and also to the time he and a female playmate were caught trying to have sex at age eight. These experiences of tension contrasted with the ease of most of his sex play with other boys. Before Ren could ejaculate there were a series of events with groups of boys, including his brother, such as circle jerks (masturbation in groups to see who could ejaculate first or farthest); all in all, sufficient collective sexual exercise to inform Ren of the fact that he was on the right track. By the time he learned the names for and specific injunctions against the sensual pleasures he was pursuing with other boys, the sensations of sex itself were well and truly known.

A second important feature of his sexual development was a sexual relationship with an older brother: "I can never remember him doing anything to stimulate me. And I think there were a few limited occasions where I stimulated—masturbated—him. But I was quite keen to do so. There were only a few occasions when he agreed; situations where I felt that I was able to, sort of, trespass I guess, to do so." Not a sexually abusive relationship, it clearly meant more to Ren than his brother, who was to remain an object of desire for Ren for quite some time. The word "trespass" seems a good one for Ren; it formed for him one template for much of his later pursuit of a sexual career.

In the following excerpt we can see more of an interplay between homoerotics and masculinizing processes at work in Ren's self-assessment:

> I was, you know, after that still, sort of, turned on by him [the brother]. And I was a very nonphysical sort of a person, in the sense of not active in sport or anything, I was intellectual, sort of thing, and he was a competitional swimmer and I used to be quite turned on by the physicality of his body. I can remember he used to have his own room downstairs

and the rest of the family lived upstairs, and I can remember peeping outside at night into his [room] trying to catch him changing clothes, trying to see him naked.

This would fit with Connell's analysis of the part played by older brothers in the masculinizing of men, especially where the elder brother as a sporting success represents "hegemonic masculinity" (Connell 1990: 458).

The specific bodily character of Ren's attachment to and admiration for his older brother was significant in shaping not just his sense of self physically as a male, but his sexual desire as well. There is evidence for this in Ren's adult sexual practice, which indicated an adoring gaze on, and an emotional charge connected with, highly masculinized object choices. But it would be foolish to propose a direct or determinative connection between this early sexual interest and adult object choice.

Asking the right questions to figure out what it was about men that Ren found sexually attractive proved difficult. The first thing he mentioned, which should come as no surprise, was men's buttocks ("buns" to use his phrase), a major attraction particularly if he was doing the fucking. But he immediately stated that there were many other turn-ons: "I've got very wide tastes [laughter]. I find it very difficult to explain why I look at somebody and think they're sexy and another person, who would perhaps be described in exactly the same terms, I don't." He nominated age as generally unimportant, but preferred men of his own age for their experience. A large penis was important in principle, if not always in practice. There was a stated interest in nice hair, hairy legs, and hairy chests, but not all-over hirsuteness. He did not like redheads, people who dyed their pubic hair, and beer guts. There was a kind of aesthetics of sex being offered, warranting investigation and differing from the idea of *fetish*, with which such sexual interests are often linked. This aesthetics goes beyond the simple taxonomies of sexuality in most sexology and sex research, which start and end with the notion that desire merely equals the chosen sex object.

What is clear about Ren's object choice, particularly when he talked about his relationships, is that it was the overall *masculinity* of men which interested him. The men in his life with whom he has built significant relationships were given to sports and other strenuous pastimes, intellectually rigorous occupations, strong political convictions—a masculine physicality in presence and preoccupation. He was not interested in hairdressing, fashion, night-clubbing, and drag parties. He did not despise the campery of gay life, but was far from effeminate himself.

There are many other stories from men in the study about older brothers, cousins, playmates, and even men in the neighborhood playing a formative sexual part in their early experiences and in their self-assessment as males and as sexual beings. This intermingling of sexual pleasure and masculinizing processes is central to the making of these men. But few announced such a singular style of sexual interest. Ren's sexual interests and his success in their pursuit have provided him with an enormous source of success *as a man* and fulfilling sexual pleasure; his sexual skill with men is *his* measure of himself as a man. The idea of object choice suddenly appears performative for the subject, rather than being merely a characteristic of the object himself.

As in the reports of Ralph Coles and Harry Wight, sex between men includes more than physical sensation. There are other aspects of Ren's further sexual encounters with boys in adolescence that have a more distressing emotional flavor. There were two serious love affairs with boys his own age, one in early high school and one during Ren's later high-school and undergraduate years. The first happened before Ren began engaging in male-to-male sex with casual partners on a steady basis. The second occurred well after the beginning of Ren's more adult-like sexual career.

Ren "was pretty emotionally keen on" the first boy and their single sexual encounter, at Ren's instigation, caused strong guilt feelings (in both, it appears), since it was "not mentioned between us." This contrasts strongly with the earlier encounters with other boys and points to a change in character in the sexual encounters of adolescence. Other meanings, beyond orgasm, beyond play, become attached to sexual activity during these years. It may be that one basis for this deepening of sexual meaning relates more to the greater emotional isolation in which boys are expected to pursue their adolescence and manhood. It is a period when our culture fairly systematically ignores boys' needs for emotional support, touch, and security.

Ren's second sexual relationship was a very important one. The two young men were constantly in each other's company for four years, virtually lived with each other's families, and were so close that: "I'm quite sure that, for four years, the relationship was so strong and involved together, that I never once repeated myself, never once said the same thing twice, because I could virtually remember everything I'd ever said [to him]. And although there were only two incidents that involved sex between us, it was basically a real love affair." One is reminded again of an *amico di cuore* dimension in this account, illustrating complex elements in male friendships in practice. Although Ren initiated the first sexual encounter, the friend actively encouraged the second. They were twenty at the time, and well beyond childhood explorations; Ren reported that his subsequent guilt was related not so much to the acts of sex themselves but to the recognition of the "terribly, terribly strong" feelings associated with sex with the man he loved.

Ren was becoming clearer in his own mind at this time that he was genuinely interested in men sexually, and had already been through the stage of considering himself "bisexual": "I think I thought it was probably a reasonably trendy thing in some circles I mixed in to admit to." He remembered being aroused by "heterosexual turn-ons," which should remind us of the wayward nature of sexual responses in youth and the arousal capacity of things generally sexual, irrespective of their object-choice focus. What is also clear here is the importance of the emotionality of these relationships. They were not just physical; they involved significant emotional connection, comradeship, closeness, and communication as well as a sexual charge. This relationship can be likened to Harry's cathectic moment when he "made love," a clear registration that men can respond to each other in a manner that transcends the merely physical.

These emotionally charged relations with peers coexisted with Ren's pursuit of sexual trespass elsewhere. He started doing the beats when he was fifteen. An older man convinced him that he would be a good clothes model and would he just come into this public toilet and have his measurements taken! Ren knew the score anyway, having read the graffiti on toilet walls, and was soon stopping in at the local beats every day on his way home from school. A little later he started sneaking out late at night, because there was more action at that time. A driver's license facilitated a wider circuit of beats: "I hate to think of how much petrol I spent getting from one beat to another!" By his late teens Ren's experience of his homosexual interests was not simply confined to peer explorations. He had a keen awareness of a wider world of sexual opportunity and a disturbing recognition that there was more to sex than the "plumbing."

Ren's first chance to fuck another boy came with another schoolmate already known as the school "poofter." Ren was fucked in turn and did not like it. A few subsequent attempts proved more successful but the practice never really grabbed his sexual interest. He quite liked fucking other men in the beats, and with that experience in mind, he discovered an interest in getting fucked only within his first adult and serious relationship with another man.

As a university student, Ren pursued these sexual explorations, gaining skill and forming tastes, but the range of experiences was somewhat limited. His was a very ordinary sexual repertoire in the main and was only transformed significantly when he moved to Sydney. Even in this later milieu Ren has not sought to pursue sadomasochism, scat, watersports, body-piercing or shaving, and has "no desire to be dominated by anybody else and I have no desire to dominate anybody else." Mutual pleasuring, that is, reciprocity, figured highly in his accounts in sex and counted for more than particular practices in themselves.

I find masturbation pretty unsatisfactory.

(What's missing?)

The social aspect. You know, as far as I am concerned, sex is something you do with somebody else, not on your own. See, I'd probably masturbate more if I hadn't found it easy to have sex with other people . . . throughout my life.

Further:

(What constitutes a good fuck?)

Um, if only we knew.

(Well, if you don't, nobody does.)

[laughter] There are so many types of good fuck, really, but one of the things about good sex as opposed to a good fuck, for me, is a, sort of, total body arousal more than just strictly genital sort of thing. And I have, at times, and [I] can reach a state of arousal or stimulation or whatever, where lots of other parts of the body are exquisitely sensitive and pleasurable. And I find orgasm after that state much more emotionally satisfying, you know, than just a quick fuck.

(Can you explain that sense of emotional satisfaction a bit more?)

Um. [pause] Well, I guess it means that it's more pleasurable in my biological definition that I learned when I was doing biology—in terms of being more likely to result in a repetition of that experience—so I guess, in a way, it means more bonding on a personal level.

This relationality challenges the accepted wisdom about the self-ish and alienated nature of male sexuality. The other person is a human *presence* for Ren, not just a vehicle for his own pleasure. This is more than the reciprocity noted earlier in sexual practice; it is another example of "communicative primacy" (Connell and Kippax 1990: 180) as a second dimension of sex for gay men, even in casual encounters.

An important aspect in the relationality between men is the collision of *bodies*. There was a revealing moment in Ren's account where the sensations of the body and its capacity for erotic pleasure make us reckon with the meaning of experience, again devoid of heavy, discursively defined meaning. Ren talked of his experience of multiple orgasm, a phenomenon usually regarded (see Masters and Johnson 1966: 131) as exclusively female:

> The orgasm tends to last longer and a heightened sensation. And some-times there is a really long, you know, immediately preorgasmic phase where, you know, you are at orgasm and there is nothing that you can stop to change that, but that pleasure state lasts longer before [ejacula-tion]. And the other thing is that there have been a number of occasions I might—in which I have had true multiple orgasms. . . . I'm not talk-ing about ejaculation, I'm talking about the orgasms. And you know it seems to be multiple orgasms just as it's been described as normal for women, in that you go off it and then come up to it again with-out any—I've forgotten Masters and Johnson terminology now—but without going back to zero, sort of thing. And I think those have been associated with, sort of, state of total body arousal.

I asked about the difference between ejaculation and orgasm, and Ren clarified his understanding of the experience:

> Well, [pause] you can have ejaculation induced by prostate stimulation that's—while it's not devoid of orgasm, it has some of those [qualities]. But I mean, it can occur at a very low level of arousal. That doesn't in my mental conception constitute an orgasm. And you can similarly just have, by pressure on seminal vesicles, the seminal fluid expressed without any of that—I mean, there is a trickle and not in spurts, for ex-ample. But can you repeat the question again?

I did.

> Oh it's rare, but certainly I've experienced that. I mean, the multiple orgasms that I was talking about were associated with multiple ejacu-lations. I didn't mean they weren't. But it's just that I think the ejacula-tions derive from the orgasms rather than the orgasms derive from the ejaculations.

The language is so deliberately explanatory, and cast in terms so scien-tific as to argue for a specific discursive formation of understanding. But this is actually an attempt to make sense of sex *after* the event, to reach for explanation and meaning after sensation. The sensations themselves were undoubtedly shaped by the context of the encounters, the choreography of the sex, and the "chemistry" of the partnership. But these physical sensa-tions when originally experienced altered his perception of sexual reality.

In Ren's case of multiple orgasm, the experience contradicts the later-received prevailing notion of a more limited male sexual capacity. Again, the term "subversive" comes to mind to describe the contribution of the body to sex.

In a number of interviews men reported their experience of orgasm in anal intercourse, which challenges the received wisdom of its beastly nature. This experience of sensation and pleasure, that is, the *practice*, would seem to contradict the prohibition in *discourse* on anal sex between men. The body subverts the mind; experience contradicts hegemony. It is for this reason—their actual experiences of sexual pleasure—that many gay men believe they know something about men and male sexuality that exclusively heterosexual men may never discover. These sensations and experiences constitute homosexuality in a way that inhibits (at least at first), then contradicts or resists, the smooth operation of prohibitive discourse. It is for this reason that the early gay movement claimed all men can be or are gay; it recognized the potential in such sexual pleasure.

But bodies collide in context: on beats, in beds, and with other forms of more "interior" decorating. Ren had considerable experience of anal intercourse both receptively and insertively, and reported mediocre satisfaction with the activity until he started using drugs in sex, particularly marijuana and amyl nitrite. It was the physical relaxation these drugs produced that enabled Ren to enjoy receptive anal sex. From that time on he became far more focused on that particular practice, but in a different sex culture, which initiated a new pattern of sexual encounters. Subsequently, Ren's participation in the sex-on-premises venues of Sydney's inner-city gay community led to a pursuit of other esoteric sex practices, particularly fisting, and to his inclusion in a quite distinctive sexual subculture within the gay community in the late 1970's and early 1980's.

While his pursuit of sex was facilitated by initiative, experience, opportunity, and a private income, it was assisted by a fairly strong-minded belief in being gay, to which gay liberation politics spoke readily in the mid-1970's. There was a strong discursive overlay and reformulation of his sexual subjectivity as a result of this participation in gay politics. He has also traveled a lot and pursued his sexual adventures when and where he could. He is a very *practiced* sexual adventurer.

In a very real sense Ren Pinch experiences the world as one of rampant, ever-present sexual possibility. To achieve a tally of ten thousand sexual partners (not events) requires a keen eye for a likely candidate, savvy in recognizing a propitious moment, deftness in leading another less courageous man beyond his fears, experience in identifying settings for sex readily, and a well-defined sense of colluding in an extraordinary domain of forbidden delight. For Ren, this homosexual domain was like the world's largest clandestine Masonic club; except it is not hands that are secretly shaken. His homosexuality is just not a personal attribute but part of a collective, verifiably human capacity and expression.

Ren started the interview with a declaration that we all needed to be far more open about sex and our lives, if things were to change. It was clear from then on that he was a gay man, strongly identifying with the gay community and its project of liberation and community building:

I tend to think there is a certain sensitivity and a certain amount of socialization in a sense that . . . I think they're [gay men] less inclined to form isolated family units, sort of nuclear family style thing. Um, [pause] I'm not sure whether there is a true difference or just a perceived difference in terms of promiscuity . . . the number of persons with whom you have relationships that are sexual.

The terms here are relational first, then sexual, but the connection between the two is firm.

Ren pursued these ten thousand partners in the context of four main gay relationships that dominated his adult life. They provided the emotional context for all his other sexual experience. They were the earliest sites of experimentation with more esoteric sex practices, confirming the SAPA study finding that regular partnerships were more likely than casual sex to be the site for the exploration of esoteric sexual activity (Connell and Kippax 1990). This again supports the argument for the strong relational base to male homosexual behavior. Two of these relationships were quite long-term, the most recent had lasted over a decade. Yet these were never monogamous relationships. Like Harry Wight, Ren Pinch has managed to negotiate quite open relationships in which the sexual explorations of other partners are not just approved but part of the mutual recognition of the other's sexual needs or prerogatives.

The literature on gay relationships, though small, uniformly reports extensive nonmonogamy (Bell and Weinberg 1978; Silverstein 1982; McWhirter and Mattison 1984; De Cecco 1988; Vadasz and Lipp 1990), indicating that such patterns are far from related only to gay liberation. However, gay men like Ren have substantially shifted the ground on the definition and terms of emotional-sexual relationships with reference to fidelity, monogamy, and openness. Even if pre-Stonewall homosexually active men were equally nonmonogamous, what is clear is these relations have received considerable shape and legitimacy in post-Stonewall modern gay communities and among their members.

There is, for men like Ren, now over twenty-five years of gay liberation and gay studies literature debating sexual relationships, monogamy,
recreational sex, sexual practices and meanings directly, and an enormous
body of fiction in English (or translation) published worldwide that indirectly informs gay men's sexuality. This literature has offered a challenging
critique of and created a powerful counterpoint to an ever more restrictive
sexual discourse carried by mainstream media and straight society, a discourse that has markedly stiffened since the onset of the HIV epidemic (see
Watney 1987b). As Peplau (1988) notes, suggestions that homosexual men
use heterosexual relationships as role models must give way in the face of
long-standing evidence and of current, collectively acknowledged and consciously pursued practice to the contrary. For highly cerebral and intellectual men like Ren, this countervailing discursive framework has contributed to his sexual development for most of his adult life. And its locus in
practice and principle is now firmly embedded in the gay community.

Ren happily accepts the mock derogation, "slut," a recognizably gay
appropriation by which Harriet and Richard Cochrane also defined themselves:

I can remember coming from [northern suburb] to Sydney and calling in
    at a series of beats on the way, and getting screwed eight times and just
    loving that. This was the pre–safe sex days. . . . I can still remember, part
    of the deliciousness of it was the feeling of cum dripping out of my arse
    and the slipperiness of my cheeks moving past each other as lubrication.

There is more than a hint of "trespass" here—walking around the streets
silently bearing witness to male-to-male sexual transgression, lots of it and
in public places too. Having another man's semen inside one's rectum is an
insistent motif in much gay poetry and fiction, and its forfeiture is a serious issue to deal with for safe sex education. It would appear that women
are not the only ones with worries about wet patches, and that there is a
greater dispersal of pleasure in male anal intercourse than is captured in
the idea of "genital primacy" (Marcuse 1955; Connell and Kippax 1990).

Ren exhibited a remarkable degree of openness about the unseemly side
of sex. It was almost a challenge to the listener. At the same time there was
a very studied quality to Ren's interest in sex, unlike Barney Sherman's
wicked earthiness:

For me there are lots of forms that sex takes, that I can take. It's sort of an
    analogy, you've music but then you've got jazz and you've got classical,
    et cetera, et cetera. And not one of them do I say I like best or worst
    or whatever, but different times different ones appeal to the mood at

the moment. Now, within that context, the being passive just absorbing the sensations and the stimulations, et cetera, getting the most out of that is a sort of mental state thing. And the drugs can become a factor in that for me. And one of the things that I do really enjoy is being fisted. A big part of that is sort of getting into a mental state, I think it's like some people feel about yoga and things like that, you know. You're concentrating on one half on the sensations but also on being totally relaxed and allowing your body to relax completely to where you can accept this, also a tremendous intensity and the sensations and stimulation you are capable of getting higher up in the intestinal tract.

Being fisted takes skill and experience and, clearly, drugs as well. Not to mention trust. To attain that skill is no simple matter of drive or instinct. Fisting is a very clear example of the progress of sexual practice and the transformation of desire and pleasure, again through a social process.

A second feature of this sexual progress is its reliance on subcultural opportunity. Ren's initial explorations on holidays to Sydney as a teenager were sexual, not social—visiting the bars, cruising the local inner-city beats, being picked up in the street. There was no clear-cut gay precinct at that time; Kings Cross and Oxford Street were part of the overall inner-Sydney "bohemia" with nightclubs, illegal casinos, sex venues of various kinds, and brothels. It was the era of "R & R" (Rest and Recreation leave for U.S. troops fighting in Vietnam). The visiting servicemen created a boom in "trade" of all kinds in the area for a number of years (see Wotherspoon 1991, chapter 4, for an account of this era). But Ren's real adoption of Sydney's sexual offerings awaited his permanent arrival in Sydney in the early 1970's.

Throughout the 1970's Ren explored the growing sexual opportunities of this increasingly gay precinct. A sexual community was being developed centered on a certain level of infrastructure and a common set of sexual interests amid a growing, newly shaped sexual identity. By the time Ren started being fisted in the late 1970's, there was a large, definitively gay community established in Sydney, increasingly connected to a gay liberation project in some ways, and by then centered on a series of backroom fuck bars, fisting venues, and a burgeoning, definable, clone-centered gay culture.

Fifteen years later, sex for Ren was less easy to come by, partly because there was less of it going on, he thought. Speaking of the saunas, he said: "It's just that people are not doing things the way they used to. . . . I'm being less choosey than I used to be. I think I've got a fairly accurate self-image thing of where I—who's more attractive than me and who isn't. I'm prepared to go a fair way on the negative side for a good time, but I get turndowns from most of them." Ren was experiencing what Barney had faced a decade earlier, and it was not a nice feeling, particularly for a man who saw himself as having given a great deal to this sexual community.

Ren still participates in the gay community extensively; his friends are largely gay men, he belongs to many political and cultural organizations, and he and his lover are always at the major social events. To that extent, Ren Pinch regards himself as a fully-fledged member of the gay community, even if a central form of engagement—sex—is now slowly diminishing. But just how far this sexual community of interest has turned into a gay community, inclusive of all its participants and its other creators, in ways other than through their sexual pursuits, is yet to be determined.

No one is born into a gay community—except as the offspring of gay men or lesbians—and a gay community is not at all like an ethnic minority in the new multicultural Australia, for its culture does not migrate here in family units from elsewhere. Gay communities have to be constructed, made, willed into being; they are products of enormous effort. Australian gay culture, whatever its influences from a world of instant information and mass communication, is a locally grown product. Where there is a similarity with the notion of minorities, it lies in the fact the members of a gay community "migrate" to it. But there the similarity ends, for gay "migrants" do not bring very much "culture" with them of direct use in the making of gay communities.

Ren is just one example of this migration to gay community and his participation illustrated the development of a modern homosexually active man from a patrician background to a gay man living in a gay community. Well-educated and perspicacious, Ren entered a nascent gay community with considerable sexual experience and presence of mind. He continued to develop as a highly sexually active and adventurous man and was an activist concerned with gay rights and, later, HIV/AIDS as that community itself developed. Ren is clearly recognizable in the pages of books such as *The Gay Militants* (Teal 1971), *After You're Out* (Jay and Young 1975), *Coming Out in the Seventies* (Altman 1979), *States of Desire* (White 1986), and so on. In this sense he may be a typical member of a gay community, even if his sexual achievements may be atypical. But other men migrating to gay communities were not so noticeable, so committed to liberation, and their experience of gay community was different in some important respects. Their experience revealed other aspects in creating a gay community life out of a homosexual desire.

## Richard Cochrane

Richard Cochrane was born and bred in Nullangardie and hated it—
"the biggest hole on this earth!" In 1988 he returned there with AIDS to die.
His family—mother (home duties), father (a retired delivery van driver),
and three siblings—took him in, rarely ever mentioning AIDS or gayness,
and looked after him until his death at age thirty-two, about a year after I
interviewed him.

Richard was educated at the local state schools until the tenth grade and
then left to be a sales assistant, a job secured for him by a relative. Richard
had been overseas for two extended periods in Europe: the first trip came
as a teenager; the second happened in his late twenties and lasted a few
years. He spent the time in between working around Australia, on farms, in
bars and pubs: "My whole life's been on the road. I've never settled down
anywhere." A considerable number of the Australian years were spent in
Sydney where he was part of the Oxford Street scene.

Richard's working life was organized more around where he wanted to
be than what he wanted to do. He mainly worked in the hotel industry,
doing everything from bar work to deputy shift manager in a big hotel.
This is the closest he came to a career. It is certainly not a trade, but it is an
industry with plenty of job opportunities, and the skills acquired are trans-
portable to anywhere on the planet. It is also an industry that attracts gay
men perhaps for that reason, and perhaps because it is safe to be gay there.
It certainly facilitated the gay life Richard led.

Richard had his first sexual experience at age twelve with a man aged
twenty. The older partner was a nurse at a hospital where Richard was a
patient. He reported that they almost seduced each other in the ward, but
then arranged to meet for sex after he was discharged. Their first encounter
was rather unusual by Richard's telling:

Ah, we fisted for four days.

(This was when you were twelve [says the incredulous sociologist]?) Yeah.
    (Good grief!)

He sort of led me slowly into it. It took four days to get there. (But he was
    fisting you?) We were fisting each other. But it took four days for him
    to get there, you know. So it was done slowly, it was done properly.
    And with him being a nurse, he knew what he was doing. So I never
    had any fears there.

Richard retained a liking for fisting, particularly the insertive mode, as he
got older.

His teenage years were filled with the usual opportunistic sex, with a cousin, with men he met here and there, with a group of older mates. It was a very sexually active time, but one in which the action, Richard insisted, came to him. As with Harriet and Alan Cunningham, there seemed to be plenty of opportunity in the sexual (dis)order of Nullangardie for boys to obtain sex, to obtain it when young, and continue to find it if they wanted. There is some evidence of networks of friends admitting to homosexual activity or informing each other of its availability, and, as we know from Harriet, these anarchic clusters of sexually active youth soon connected with networks of men in the homosexual subculture of Nullangardie.

Such exploration might be described in individualized terms: "Oh yeah, I was a slut. Yeah," said Richard. But, the opportunities these youths explored were too systematic for that simplistic explanation. How far these experiences can be generalized to the male population of the region is difficult to assess. But the steady availability and experience of homosex for the male youth of Nullangardie requires a historicized rethinking of the structure of the sex lives of men and boys in that town; one that might confirm Kinsey's findings on homosexual activity and lower socioeconomic class (Kinsey et al. 1948).

Richard left Nullangardie for Sydney and was very sexually active there, often seeking and obtaining multiple partners in a single night. It was a classic "fast-lane" mode of inner-Sydney gay life at that time: "I've gone up to guys in a bar and said: 'Take me home and fuck me.' Some of them have fled in sheer horror, that somebody had the boldness to come up and say that to them. Or they've either picked me up, thrown me over their shoulder and taken me home and fucked me. Or they've fucked me there, then and there at the bar." His tendency to exaggeration began to throw doubt on the story of his sexual initiation and on many of the other tales he told of his sex life. He referred to yet another "four-day fuck" when asked about his most eventful sexual experience, raising further doubts about his accuracy and revealing an audience-related aspect of his sexual subjectivity. He covered his tracks with a second claim to being a "slut," illustrated by being fucked by multiple partners in saunas. But it was an obvious slip. Something more vulnerable was revealed in that moment. Richard's pursuit of the sexual had a tension to it. His was not Ren Pinch's easy embrace of every opportunity.

For Richard, his men had to be:

Big, beefy guys. I cannot stand loud-mouthed obnoxious queens . . . good looking. . . . Rugged good looks, really, a natural thing . . . (Tall, short?) Doesn't matter. (Hairy, not hairy?) Doesn't matter. (Blond, dark?) Doesn't matter. (Big dick, short dick?) That matters! [laughs].

It is a distinctly nonfetishistic objectification, almost catholic in its obviousness and its lack of focus. This, with the loathing of "queens," can be read as: an identification with Oxford Street men of that particular time (literally, his sex objects); a device to distance himself from the provincial Nullangardian style; and a modern image of gayness as a claim on masculinity.

He spent some time in the leather scene, arguing that the smell of it enhanced the masculinity of the man who wears it. But he was not into it any more: "I've been there, done that. Now it's a case of just get in there and have a good time. Forget the games, you know, gets you nowhere. Waste of time when you could be fucking." The change partly stems from the fact that he had had no sex for the previous four years. He feigned a lack of interest in sex generally and ascribed it to his antibody status. He had been on AZT at one time, which can depress the libido, and at the time of the interview he had treatment-resistant ulcers and thrush and was not too steady on his feet. All of this contributed to his lack of interest in sex.

Richard's first sexual relationship also occurred at age twelve and lasted about three years. Later, three or four "loose ones," that is, short-term and not serious, led to a four-year relationship during Richard's second trip abroad. There had been no relationships after that. Richard was monogamous in two of these relationships. Were he not, he recalled, in one he would have lost the lover; in the other (with the European) they had an arrangement. When they were together in the same city they were monogamous; when Richard returned for a time to the United Kingdom each was permitted to have sex with others. As with Ren Pinch, this arrangement captures nicely the extent to which gay men have negotiated their own new sexual politics: "That's my idea of monogamy. I mean, you can screw around or you can be on with a guy here and you can be on with a guy there. . . . It doesn't mean that you're screwing around. You're in a one-on relationship with that guy. Then you come back here and you're with that guy. So, you're in a one-on relationship with that guy."

The second "guy" was, as it turned out, HIV-antibody positive. At that time Richard found out he too was infected. He did not regard this man as the source of the infection, but rather looked at his whole very sexual history in Australia (in Sydney particularly) and abroad as the source.

Richard regarded his sexuality, his gayness, as something that was there:

From the word "go."

(What made you realize it?)

That I liked men? Let's say it was a recognition of that. It didn't strike me as being not normal or normal or anything like that. It was just the way I felt.

(And did you know anyone else that felt like that until you met that man?)

No. I didn't ask anyone else how they felt about it. It was just an accepted thing.

(Did it ever occur to you that it might be a stage that you were going through, that you might grow out of it?)

Well, I'd heard about that. I didn't believe in that. I don't believe in these stages. I didn't give it time to sort itself out because I enjoyed what I was doing. So the stage never had a chance, if you know what I mean.

Richard may have been wiser than he realized. This is yet another example of sexual skilling through practice and pleasure led by the body, with discursive imperatives running a ragged second. Yet I suspect we are also hearing another example of reworked material, of sense-making again in hindsight. Richard was simply too busy having sex to hear anything.

It would be wrong to configure Richard's boyhood sexual pursuits as resistance to discourse in the sense Weeks (1985) often ascribes to adult gay men. After all, boys like Harriet became marginalized from working-class masculinity quickly if they adopted a homosexual life as a resolution to their sexual interests. Although many of the local boys knew what was going on and there was a level of open discussion between boys, the sex was still hidden. But this hiddenness does not reflect a determination to resist; it simply reflects that such sexual adventuring occurred in what might almost be termed a *discursive silence*, a place where substantive definition had yet to occur.

This sexual activity did not lead to Richard's inclusion in these local homosexual networks, as it did for Harriet. He chose instead to explore the gay community already available in Sydney and abroad. In retrospect Richard was scathing about the old Nullangardie homosexual subculture, calling them "gutless," afraid to speak out, and "snotty-nosed." This last epithet referred to the upper-class set of "social queens," the "fashion set," the "screaming queens" with their offensive "peacock" parade and characteristic laughter. Richard had a greater sense of class differentials than Harriet, and of his place within them. He did not mean drag queens by this; he liked drag shows and had a few friends into drag. Richard also rejected my thinly veiled attempt to label him macho by pointing to his earrings.

These distinctions, apart from their daily value as the stock-in-trade insults of a "bitchy queen," reflect a more significant historical transformation. The perceived differences between gay men point to an ongoing dynamic of identity reformulation being played out within homosexual subcultures. Richard left Nullangardie before gay really happened there. Now, as the gaying of Nullangardie undermines Harriet and reinforces Richard's kind of gayness, it is too late for him. These transformations are not simple descriptions of behavior, subcultural patterns of acting, or superficial group activity; they are related to more profound historical processes at work within male homosexuality.

Richard also had a great deal of resentment toward younger gays, regarding them as enjoying the good times without acknowledging the efforts of older gay men to bring those good times about, and to that extent he aligned himself with an undefined liberationist sector of the gay community. In fact, he stopped short of active involvement in gay political demonstrations, only joining in if he felt like it. Although he was sexually and socially engaged in gay community life, he had little involvement in its culture or politics, and referred to political gays as "them." This confirms the SAPA study finding that the three statistical measures of gay community attachment do operate with some independence.

Richard regarded the Sydney gay scene as a real gay community, but as having deteriorated from its heyday; it was never anything like London, and neither city met Amsterdam's attractions. There was much "street credibility" to be gained from these overseas travels to gay meccas; a claim to be among the supremely gay, with which to soar above not only Nullangardie but to leave Sydney and Australia behind as well. The Australian "cultural cringe" has undergone a gay reworking here.

For all his braggadocio about sex, Richard lacked the sexual self-confidence of a Ren Pinch. Their sexual domains overlapped considerably. They were both very active in Sydney's gay community during its pre-HIV/AIDS sexual heyday. But Ren continued to pursue and develop his sexual interests; they constitute a life and an achievement of gayness. For Richard there is a distinct sense of failure. The sexual community in which he explored himself and others has disappeared, for him. Those familiar and anonymous men who populated his fantasy and his daily life were no longer there. Richard's return to Nullangardie was evidence of his failure to develop relationships in the Sydney gay community that could sustain him during his illness. Richard never really fully belonged to the gay community in Sydney. He fucked his way through it and had a good time. But unlike Ren he was not able to constitute his social relations to achieve the status and benefits of a fully attached man. His partial engagement with one aspect of gay life—its remarkable sexual opportunities—did not a fully gay life make.

It was this bitter Richard I met, one disappointed that he was not surrounded by the Sydney gay community and its HIV/AIDS services and programs, by friends, "fuck buddies," and a sense of being in the thick of it. Instead he was with parents, poor after a working life of low-paying jobs, being supported by the gay community of Nullangardie, those very "queens" he'd longed to leave and loved to loathe. No matter what they offered, they were simply the wrong gay community.

Another man, ten years older than Ren and almost twenty years older than Richard, illustrates a more successful movement from a poor rural working-class background into a homosexual community that was transforming itself into a gay community. His story offers a glimpse of consequences of the HIV epidemic different from those of Richard. He too has experienced the limits of gay community.

## Robert Cusack

If not a broken man, Robert Cusack was certainly a severely depressed one. He lived in a small inner-Sydney flat, surrounded by memorabilia from past glories as a key person in the leather bikie scene in Sydney's gay community. Many of his friends were dead, and his social life consisted only of occasional dinner parties of reminiscing queens. Yet he was only fifty at the time of the interview, HIV seronegative (he regarded this as miraculous), and employed in a secure if mundane clerical position. He could retain a central place in a substantial social and sexual network within the gay community if he so chose. Instead, he was planning to take early retirement and return to the country to look after an aging parent. The ennui that suffused the interview was saddening. There was little sense of the vigorous man of a few years ago.

Robert was born in a country town. His large family were local people, poor, working-class, and most still lived in the area. He was educated at local schools, but left early and entered the public service. This was a classic trajectory for the postwar years for working-class Anglo-Australians— advancement for the younger generation was understood as moving from "blue-collar" to "white-collar" work. He eventually relocated to Sydney and, after some exploring, lived in the geographic heart of what was to become some years later the Sydney gay community. Family ties remain strong, though at a distance, and they do not know he is gay.

Robert had read Freud or a commentary on Freud and has a clear lay explanation for his homosexuality based on psychoanalysis. It goes something like this. Robert found out as an adult that his mother had borne him out of wedlock and that his stepfather had "adopted" him. The rest of his siblings were therefore half-brothers and -sisters, and this, he believed, had led to his different treatment at the hands of his mother and stepfather. His mother appeared to believe that he was her responsibility alone. She kept him from the stepfather and overprotected him (he was a sickly child so the story goes). During the early years the stepfather was off to war, and Robert grew up with a longing for this man, a longing never satisfied. Whatever the family dynamics were—and poverty did not help—Robert's unsatisfactory relationship with this man was, to his mind, a significant part of his being gay.

This is reminiscent of Neil Davidson's formulation of his homosexuality around the figure of his father and a powerful example of the discursive formulation of one part of a sexual subjectivity, a formulation assembled much later than the experiences he was seeking to explain.

Robert recalled that sense of difference from others so often reported by men in this study: "I think I knew I was gay from about twelve year old, I think . . . 'cause it was what I used to like. . . . I think I was seduced at that stage by a nineteen-year-old nextdoor neighbor." This experience with a youth who was "notorious" in the town grew from considerable earlier sex play with other kids. There was a good-looking "exhibitionist" mate, some sexual experience with girlfriends, and continuing sex with schoolmates, followed by a religious period trying to fight the urge to have sex with boys (helped by a homosexual priest). The "notorious" nineteen-year-old was known to be homosexual in the town (it was unclear why), and Robert was warned about him; yet they had a six-year sexual relationship. Robert was fucked by this youth at age thirteen and soon returned the favor. The sex ceased when this youth told his mates that Robert was available for sex and a group of them raped him one day after school—yet another, if more disturbing, example of a collectively and consciously pursued masculine sexual (dis)order.

Later, out of school and in the workforce, Robert's early trips to Sydney led to the discovery of a now-defunct steam baths and a recognition that there were others like him. Many others, it seemed. He was like a kid in a chocolate shop: "It wouldn't be uncommon for me to, sort of, get with about at least seven or ten people each night I used to go there." His job allowed for transfers and he soon obtained one to Sydney. There he spent the 1960's and 1970's in a zealous pursuit of sex.

Robert listed (and frequented) each and every bar, drag show, sauna, beat, sex club, and back room in Sydney during the next twenty years:

I used to pick up numbers of [men in the] toilet up in [park] and, um, pick
them up at the [monument] or something like that. It was just, you
know, it was like sex whenever I could get it. [pause] It's quite amazing
to sort of go back on my life now. . . . I've been lucky I suppose. . . . I've
been to America what, three times . . . I did the whole thing. I did—yes,
as I said, [I've] done all sorts . . . of sex . . . and things like [this] and
that sort of thing. I [was] at one stage heavily into the, um, the S and M
scene. I've given all that up [laughter]. Everything now.

Given that for Robert "it's much easier being screwed than being the aggressive partner," he is remarkably lucky to be HIV-seronegative. He went
on to speak of good sex as being with someone who knew what he was
doing and who was passionate or sexy, thereby gesturing toward the more
relational aspects of sex.

Sex for Robert may have been easy to find, but it was always difficult
emotionally. His sexual explorations were pursued singly throughout his
life. Robert had but one short-lived relationship, which started the day his
father died. He presented this as part of a deep-seated need to deal with
the death. Robert preferred pornography featuring a father/adult son relationship but not pedophile pornography. He offered this reflection on his
sexual needs and object choice, cast again in a pseudo-Freudian mode:

I'm starting to become the father—the thing that all my life I knew what I
was looking for. I was always looking for that father image. And I think
most of my sexual partners were always older than me. Maybe because—this is going back to what, what happened and how I first came
into sex . . . with a person six years older than me. And, um, it's funny,
you don't think of those as you grow up, but as you look back on life
you sort of—there is, there is a definite, definite pattern there. And I've
always looked for that form all—er, mostly father, father-image person. But now I, I sort of realize now that to a lot of people I am, I am
that, that image of that they—that I've been looking for. I've only just
found sort of realized.

This is yet another example of the post hoc framing of experience to
which Robert was prone. This Catholic-raised man clearly has spent a
considerable time searching for explanations for his sexuality. In the era
during which he was exploring the sensations of homosex, the prevailing
discourses were far less sex-positive than they were to become ten years
later for Ren Pinch. He had no liberationist perspective to counter his
more morbid and despairing discourse. His was a sexual subjectivity full

of doubts and fears: of late he even masturbated before going out on the town, to keep himself from getting the "urge" to play around.

Robert was instrumental in helping establish the 1970's gay leather scene in Sydney and, though he had left it, he still participated as an "eminent person." A trip to the United States had led to his first eye-opening experiences with leather:

> Yeah, the leather scene was just really rife then and, er, all that was just the "in thing," I think, over there . . . and that's where all the sexy men [were] and that's what they, they used to all do, sort of, and, er, I was with these people and I took a fascination, and they dressed me out in leather one time and put me. . . . I was riding a bike and everything. And I was, I was won over from there on, sort of thing. So I came back . . .

> (What did you feel when you got all dressed up in leather that first time?)

> You feel, um, [pause] a different person, I think—just to say, um, like another fantasy. But [pause] it's the old saying, I think: "The clothes make a man" . . . asking people why, why do they like me dressed in leather and they say: " 'cause I look so sinister" . . . that's the part of my life where, where I did become very aggressive sort of thing.

This is a revealing account of sexual *fashion* in operation. The sexual activity in the leather scene in the United States offered at that time a tempting encoding of sexual desire for Robert. The homosexual meccas of the world experienced by Robert and others like Dan Berger in New York during the same decade were eye-openers. Dan talked of men openly cruising the streets of Greenwich Village, inviting sex from attractive strangers at the drop of a hat, day and night. By the 1970's these places were exploding with highly sexualized masculinity among gay men (see Levine 1992). These attractions of homoerotic fantasy (dressing-up?) were particularly strong on the West Coast of the United States, reflected, for example, in the films of Kenneth Anger, such as the ironic essay on the pouting bike riders, aping James Dean, in *Scorpio Rising*, or the desirable sailors and the narcissistic eroticism of Anger's own homosexual body in *Fireworks*. The artist "Tom of Finland" was drawing his imagery from, and reflecting it back onto, North American gay culture from the 1960's onward, encoding a masculinist representation of homoeroticism for appropriation in image and in sexual practice; all in the context of a growing sexual liberation ideology and against the general background of sexual permissiveness.

Australians were not immune to that sexual and cultural influence. Many traveled to these gay meccas, appropriating the image and style, copying the sexual choreography, and learning its repertoire. There has been little reflection on these influences on gay life in Australia.[1] In spite of concurrent general debates in Australia about American "cultural imperialism" amid the aftereffects of the Vietnam War debacle, there was a curious lack of critique of American influence on sexual desire and representation. Somehow, sexuality was regarded as an arena in which the progressive elements of the broader social struggle in the United States were still being acted out. The second half of the title to the hardcover edition of Dennis Altman's (1982) book (but subsequently left off the paperback), *The Homosexualization of America—The Americanization of the Homosexual*, possibly reflects an early awareness of this influence.

For Robert, this debate was little more than a backdrop for his unfolding sexual drama. From these early trips to North America onward, he pursued every aspect of esoteric sex that came his way. Yet his reflections on it were apprehensive:

Oh, oh, I have done—I've dabbled in all of it. . . . I have dabbled in bondage and all that but . . . after I went into [leather]. I learned the scene, yeah. But I don't, I don't particularly like—I mean, it is a turn-on but it's also dangerous I think. Um (In what way?) Well, I mean, it all—unless, I mean, the fantasy's gone. I mean, the, it, it, it is a sort of fantasy. But if you pick up a person that—and try to have, to have a fantasy, right, with leather and bondage and that, it's, you know, just doesn't work. . . . It's gotta work with a complete stranger. And then again they, they've got to be able to portray that part that makes you frightened. But then again, [pause] when are they acting and when, when are they serious? 'Cause, I mean, you pick up papers and, and you read all these sort of people who trust people and then, then they've been murdered.

It is an extraordinary account from a man with over twenty years experience in the scene, a founder and leader of a well-known leather bikie club and a world-traveled, sexually very experienced gay man. The loss of nerve stands out. There is palpable fear in the last sentence; the hesitancy, the broken syntax, the justification exposing his turmoil keenly.

---

[1] From the distance of the 1990's, the early Australian debates such as in *Gay Information* (Johnston 1981, 1981/82), though sophisticated theoretically, seem remarkably inward-looking. They are centered around the rise of the new gay communities from the gay movement, the social construction of gay men, and issues for debate between lesbians and gay men about the new "macho" imagery of gay men. They are remarkably devoid of references to the impact of this emergent international gay culture and its American hegemony. Altman (1987) is a rare exception.

He certainly *learned* the scene, and skill reigns supreme in understanding and acting out a sexual partner's fantasy. This is "sex-by-numbers," in the sense that perfect strangers must understand the choreography; they must recognize the same code, the meaning of image, style, sequence, and language. To do it well, without preliminary explanation or a crib, is the mark of a true "top." Robert could be either "top" or "bottom" depending on the partner. But it did not always go smoothly:

> I've had it at the stage where I, I sort of, you know, I was being choked and I couldn't get out of it. But I sort of—and, um, I just sort of went calm and said [to himself]: "Just, just control yourself." 'Cause, I mean, this person is going to let you go sooner or later, you hope to God, you know. And, er, and that's when—I think it was after that experience that I, that I will do any[thing]—but I will not have my hands tied.

As he says: "Everyone meets their match after a while." Fisting followed leather, again a taste newly acquired in the United States. He preferred to insert but, again, his courage has now failed him, and he talked immediately of its dangers.

Life for Robert was not all dressing up in leather; he also dressed up regularly for a local amateur musical society, a hobby shared with gay friends throughout his life. He has done his bit of traditional drag, borrowing Mum's "best black" for the odd ball, fundraiser, and party. But the leather scene, its bikes, its sexual practices, formed the deep core of his sexuality. Or did it?

> (Can I ask a bit about [the bike club]? Is it because you ride a bike that you joined?)

> No, I've never ridden a bike. Although I've been, I've been virtually all over Australia on the back of a bike with other people. (But you don't actually ride one yourself?) I have ridden a bike; I've ridden my brother's bike. But I'd never actually buy one for myself, 'cause living in this area, that's just—would be suicide!

There would appear to be not a little masquerade here.

There is no doubt that the leather bike club offered Robert many things and helped make his life an adventurous one. In the public service he remained a lowly clerk. But after work a transformed Robert and his club would take bike rides into the country, go camping, hold barbeques, organize sex events among members, and seek and find casual partners among the group. It was a far cry, though, from the raunchy stories of gay bikie clubs often told in pornographic magazines in Australia like *Ribald* and *Gay*:

> Ah, I think a lot of it, lot of that was a lot of fantasy. But, I mean, I'm not saying that there was no sex on runs; there was quite a lot of sex, but it was all to do with the individual persons. And I think any of those [sexual] initiations were like another hit theater show. It was, er, was for entertainment for those, those poor unsuspected, um, visitors who didn't, who heard all about these notorious people and. . . . That's my, that's my opinion, and maybe that's not right. . . . There are people still in the club scene [who] take it all so very seriously and, er—I, I did take it very seriously.

(What does that mean: "taking it seriously"?)

> Oh, I mean, that was the ultimate thing. I mean you, you wore the colors and you wore the leather and all that, and it all meant that was the only thing. . . . But that's not the way, you know, there are other things in life. I mean I, maybe, maybe that's why I ended up resigning.

Robert's interest in the bikie group did not preclude other interests. It was he who drew the winning tickets in fundraising raffles, made the thank-you speeches at social events, gave out prizes in local gay competitions. Like the mayor of a small town or the president of a local cricket club, Robert was a minor official of the community in his own right. In addition to these more mundane daily aspects of gay community life there were nights of great glamour, and others of downright sleaze:

> I don't even remember going to the sauna—went with a friend. I was told I promptly went into one of the cubicles and went to sleep and was woken up at a quarter to six next morning. I woke up one time and there was a couple having sex on, on the floor in the cubicle and I thought "Oh, ugh" and promptly went back to sleep again [laughter]. . . . I had a frightful hangover next day.

To capture a complete sense of these twenty years in so short a time is difficult. There was a great deal of good humor in the telling of these tales, yet so often he ended on a note of regret, of loss, of nervousness, of fear.

For Robert, unlike Richard, there was a complete move into the gay community. He became a significant part of it, sexually, socially, and culturally, although, unlike Ren, there was no hint of a political perspective on gay rights. This appropriation of gay community was won on its sexual fringes, in a sexual subculture within it, and raises the question: which gay community are we talking about? What really constitutes the gay community? Robert experienced his attachment as total; yet he would not come within a bull's roar of Ren Pinch in the absorption of gay culture, its literature, theory, sensibility, and its keen political edge. Rather than hone his skill and pursue his immersion in gay life further during the HIV epidemic as Ren has, Robert has almost completely lost sight of his gay life.

> I've got to go to another funeral on Wednesday of someone who died on Friday and, um, there was a couple last week. And, er, this is just getting regular, 'cause of that circle of friends I used to have. Not that I've always had, had sex with um all of them. I didn't—well mainly I didn't have sex with any of them I don't think, but I mean they were close, you know, and in the same circle. . . . It also makes it hard at work too, because you've got to get to the stage where you have to explain to bosses why you're having all this time off.

The epidemic has taken a tremendous toll on Robert and he is foundering in its wake:

> So, er, I mean I, I sit here and proselytize [*sic*] and think: I just can't understand, er, why was I sort of [pause] saved. 'Cause I mean, I, I did all the wrong things in my life. [very quiet] Maybe I did all the right things but I don't know. [laughter] But I've had people . . . like this in hospital who're dying and, and they looked at me in the eye, straight in the face and said: "Why, why am I here dying and you're as healthy as anything?" I just said: "Well, I can't answer that question." I said but, um: "I don't know." I said: "I can't answer that question." I said: "If, if the Lord wanted to take me," I said, "in your place," I said, "I'd be happy to go but—" because, you know, [it] wasn't my time.

For all the leadership he has shown in his part of the gay community, Robert still thought there was something wrong with being gay, that he had some hidden emotional-psychic disturbance. There is a definite limit to Robert's liberation. Now with the epidemic decimating his sexual and social circle, the weight of this puzzlement and doubt about his sexuality has overwhelmed him:

> I go to [sauna], um [pause] but, I mean, the opportunity's there but I mean I seem, I seem to freeze this time of—when it sort of comes to sex I mean, I will, I'll play around sort of thing and, um, as far as anal sex and that, I have had [anal sex] with condoms but, it just, I just sort of go cold. I don't know—can't explain why. I suppose I can explain why 'cause

of maybe, you see, a mental block in your mind because of AIDS, and 'cause I mean over the last few years I've lost so many friends of AIDS.

(How many? Do you know the number?)

Oh, [sigh] um, I'd say at least about twenty, I'd say.

This level of despair means that Robert cannot even be bothered getting dressed up in leather any more. The masquerade itself now takes too much effort. This raises a question about the common configuration of leather as fetish. One would usually regard someone like Robert as fixated on a characteristically fetishized sex practice. Yet he gave it up rather easily, passing it off almost as Richard did as no longer worth the trouble. These sexual interests were not heavy sexual fixations. Their presence in his sexual repertoire can be explained more in their moment in history; they were the excitements of that time. They provided a steady supply of sex partners, as well as a social milieu. The leather held no strongly obsessive sexual interest; it was something he chanced on, was good at, enjoyed in an amicable milieu. He belonged, and was proud of having contributed to building something.

Robert was about to retire "on his laurels," and he stated that it would be nice to have a relationship; in the same breath he lamented the state of affairs for younger gays coming out in the middle of the epidemic. His current sex life consisted of the odd tense trip to the sauna. Socially, his life revolved around a few long-standing friendships, dinners, trips to the theater (musicals), and the occasional gay community event. He kept up with gay affairs by reading the gay newspapers, but did not approve of all he saw there, for example, the gay "nuns" such as the Sydney Order of the Sisters of Perpetual Indulgence (an effect of his Catholic upbringing, perhaps). He mourned the loss of the local beats and the predominance of the rent boys on the scene nowadays, where it had once all been available for free. His distance from the gay community that had dominated nearly thirty years of his life was steadily increasing.

∽

It was not my intention to portray the gay community in depressing terms, but to investigate living within a gay community in ways that do not look as if they simply come straight from the pages of *Christopher Street*, *Outrage*, or the *Sydney Star Observer*. It is important to remember that the inner-Sydney gay community of all the Australian gay communities has been the most devastated by the HIV epidemic. This gay community has experienced the worst of the early illness and death before the onset of antiviral interventions and other helpful treatments. Somewhere between 1000 and 1500 gay men have died so far in Sydney. This community also contains the largest number of HIV-infected persons in a given geographic area, with a possible eight to ten thousand HIV-infected gay men attached to this community in some way. In that environment, it is not really anomalous that two of the three men in this chapter have been infected with the virus and one has died. Nor is it surprising that someone like Robert has been to twenty funerals in recent years.

## The Sexual Construction of Gay Community

> His bare torso tight
> hands rubbed
> nipples erect
> (no Dali time-piece here).
> Time even said that
> I was hot.
> Light hands
> placed headily
> pleasured
> on my cock and
> hell I can't think who
> chimed louder
> lusting
> thrusting moans.
>
> —Kurt Joseph Schranzer, 1991

These three men, like Harriet, Ralph, and Harry before them, identify with gay community, and have been active in it either socially, politically, sexually, or in all of these ways. Were we to apply the SAPA study's statistical measures of gay community attachment discussed earlier, these men would obtain slightly different but equally high scores. They have lived their lives deeply involved in the development of their community and have grown sexually with it. Each has been part of the daily activity that makes for the overall presence of a sense of community in the daily lives of gay men. They kept organizations going; they worked behind the bars and waited on the tables, opened fetes, raised money for HIV/AIDS, and fucked like bunnies all along the way.

This is a far cry from the glossy photographs of nearly naked "young-men" (as Rechy [1977] calls them) dancing till dawn, which fill the pages of gay newspapers and fashion magazines, along with their tempting travel offers, endless classified ads for sex worker services, and, more recently, cars specifically marketed for gay men (see *Outrage* March 1992: 53ff.), and new apartment blocks specifically targeting a gay market—"You don't have to be a rich bitch"—(*Capital Q* 1995: 13). Their lives also contrast with the endless supply of glossy photographic essays on the gay male nude besieging the coffee tables of inner-city flats or the extraordinary amount of imagery dominating the gay community as a result of HIV/AIDS.

These men reveal the less glamorous daily chore of living a gay life, a life suffused with HIV/AIDS in an everyday grind of pain, loss, and hope. In their own ways, they represent what is happening to those whose efforts built this now large well-known community; whose successful work to stem the epidemic must rate as one of the great community-based public health actions of Australian history; but who, to a marked extent, are quite worn out by it.

There is no doubt that the idea of gay community attachment helps us understand what is now called gay community. But there is a lot more to living within or as a part of a gay community than the statistical measures assess. The process of living a gay life, of creating one's gayness, is a complex and highly contingent process. It is this more complex picture of gay community which these case studies reveal.

Gilbert Herdt and Andrew Boxer (1992) in an attempt at a more structural account of gay community foreground the cultural aspects of gay life, stating that "gay culture is a perspective on human nature and the world, not just on sexuality and consumption" (p. 4). Furthermore, gay "signifies identity and role, of course, but also a distinctive system of rules, norms, attitudes, and, yes, beliefs from which the culture of gay men is made, a culture that sustains the social relations of same sex desire" (p. 5). I am not so sure I agree. There is a danger in this kind of convergent search for order, in conceptualizing the gay community as a unity, a "distinctive system." After all, Robert, Ren, and Richard illustrate that "the fact of being gay is not the same thing as living one's life openly as a gay person and a member of the gay community; the ultimate arrival point, however, depends on social status and culture" (p. 7). If participation is stratified at least on "arrival" by "social status and culture," then the different patterns of attachment noted so far must be taken seriously as a possibility of a more fractured gay community; not just as gay communities—Nullangardie, Sydney, New York, Amsterdam, Berlin—but as dissonant yet overlapping sets of social networks intersecting with competitive commercial infrastructure, and suffused with differently appropriated cultural and political interpretations. Neither gay identity nor gay community life is a *singularity*; each must be conceptualized as a *multiplicity*. Gay community attachment cannot be a quantity of more or less engagement and involvement; it is a tense conjunction of seemingly contradictory practices and often competing subjectivities. Robert, Richard, and Barney are deeply ambivalent about gay community. Similarly, Harriet and Ren, in spite of their remarkable efforts at community building, experience considerable frustration and at times isolation within their highly committed gay lives.

What would happen if the three men being discussed here were to meet now (Richard's death notwithstanding)? How would they recognize their similarities, their differences? Robert's shining days were the 1960's and 1970's; Ren accumulated his astonishing record of sex partners in the 1970's and 1980's; Richard arrived on the scene in the late 1970's, early 1980's and was dead by the end of the decade. During that nearly thirty-year period, but particularly in the last twenty, they individually (maybe even together for all we know) contributed to the building of a remarkable sexual culture.

Inner Sydney had long been the site of a sexually liberal culture and a place for the sexually "deviant" to come and live relatively unpestered (see Wotherspoon 1986, 1991). But what these men participated in was something different again. The opportunities for sexual exploration and the accumulation of skill and experiences in sexual acts only dreamed or even unheard of had not been seen in this country before—at least not since World War II.

Much of the influence came from overseas. Robert and Richard were but two of many gay men who visited the United States and Europe, enjoying there the developing gay communities and the sexual opportunities travel offers. But much was local product as well. The gay liberation movement in Australia was a strong national movement for much of its short time in the limelight. The gay movement was built on the back of a progressive student movement in the heady atmosphere of post-1960's permissiveness, the emergence of second-wave feminism, and a post-Vietnam era of social change ushered in by the defeat in 1972 of the conservative political parties that had governed Australia for over two decades. From 1975 on, the gay movement, in its national conferences, debated sexual politics and practice, and the activism and leadership that emerged led to the legalization of male homosexual sex in most of the country by 1991.

By the late 1970's, the movement began to give way to the development of gay communities amid much debate (Sargent 1983; Johnston 1981; Cozijn 1982), again learning from the North American experience along the way (Johnston 1981/82). These debates were already wrestling with an existing and evolving phenomenon: the "community" was already there,

claiming loyalty from its participants/members and providing a burgeoning range of social and cultural services and activities. Oxford Street had
already made itself "the Pearl in the Oyster," as Wotherspoon (1991) calls
it. The sexual arena that Richard entered in the late 1970's was already far
more sophisticated than it had been even five years earlier. Robert, Ren, and
their intimates had already made their mark. The highly elaborate sexual
culture that emerged in inner Sydney was unparalleled in Australia (and
to a certain extent still is). It was not necessarily a "sexual community" in
John D'Emilio's terms (1983), for it was not yet a political community—
the gay *movement* and the gay *community* were not the same entity. But a
sexual culture it certainly was.

It would be incorrect to privilege the political activities of gay lib-
erationists in their attempts to elevate to respectability the deviancies of
homosexuality and to claim rightful places as full citizens, the plotting of
which preoccupies the recounting of gay history. While the meetings and
demonstrations were happening, many other men were sucking each other
off under lush trees and fucking in dark moist places. After the meetings
and demonstrations, large numbers of activists were also heading off to
sex venues, dropping their pants in pick-up places, or jumping into each
other's beds to do the same. It was the desire of these men, their ardent
pursuit of sex when and wherever they pleased which produced this sexual
culture. This *sexual construction of gay communities* must become a central
component of our understanding of gay community and much-neglected in
the story we often tell. It seems the gritty bits are often left to the poets,
fiction writers, and pornographers.

One of the most provocative pieces in the preconference papers for the
first Amsterdam conference mentioned in Chapter 1 was "A Retrospective Ethnography of the Mineshaft" by Joel Brodsky (1987). It did not
make it into the published collection of papers (Altman et al. 1989) possibly because it was light on theory. But it was one of the few papers that
even began to talk about the sex. Speaking of the front bar at the Mineshaft, Brodsky (1987: 49) reported: "Occasionally it became the scene for
a variety of simple activities that used the pool table or the bar as props:
people would bend over the pool table, sit astride it, or stand at the bar,
while their partners would penetrate or fellate them. It was especially appropriate for those who enjoyed a sense of public spectacle, exhibition, or
humiliation." Sydney did not have a Mineshaft, but it did have Club 80
and others like it, and Ren and Robert were among their frequent patrons.
Ralph Coles talked of men "totally naked just, sort of, fucking each other
in one of those cubicles, three or four people watching," reminiscent of the

scenes in New York gay bathhouses described in Michael Rumaker (1982). In the absence of bodies—their sweat, smells, and semen—from many gay history accounts of the era, it seems important to say out loud that *there was a lot of sex going on.*

As gay men collectively exercised their desire and enacted their fantasies on and in each other's bodies, they drew on resources and stimuli from their sex lives to date, from their experiences in country towns, within families and among neighbors, among schoolmates, with the local men of their area, and in toilets at railway stations, parks, beaches, and pubs.

This sexual engagement with the growing gay community in Sydney is something Ren, Richard, and Robert had in common even if they were exercising it differently. There was a determination to pursue sex anywhere; but beyond that they contributed by their exertions to the creation of sexual opportunities of the Sydney community itself—and thereby reworked their own desire and remade themselves. It is important to acknowledge this process of sexual construction, the collective toil in a willingness to help break the rules, to shatter the boundaries of privacy in sexual expression. As dedicated, if often unwitting, transgressions of the law (narrowly) and discursive frameworks on sexuality (more broadly), such sexual activity seems central to any discussion of gay community, of gay culture. Yet on this point even gay theorists are silent. There is more to the construction of gay community and gayness than sex, but gay sex itself deserves more than just a moment in the spotlight. It significantly modifies Herdt and Boxer's configuration to a sexual "culture that sustains the social relations of same sex desire."

The development of the leather scene, which Robert led, offers an example of this dynamic in the developing gay community: a very distinctive sexual subculture focused on a delineated range of practices and symbols could lead also to a *sexual construction of sociality.* These men (and occasionally women) created out of their growing common sexual interests a club with a clubhouse and a program of social activities where sex was neither peripheral nor central but suffusive. The sexual purposes and commonalities were quite explicit; in this these gay bikies are remarkably similar to Connell's (1991) heterosexual bikies. But Robert rarely ever rode a bike. And there is a strong sense that the determined obsession with bikes for which bikie clubs are usually noted was not the raison d'être for many of Robert's intimates. Their interest was symbolically represented by leather and the imagery of bikes.

In this Robert and his friends masquerade as bikies: they wear leather as drag, as easily removable as taking off one frock and putting on another.

Indeed, the potential of taking it off, partially or fully in sex, is part of the attraction. But is their leather no more than costume? The direct connection with a specified range of sex practices and sexual meanings ought to alert us to more significance. Within gay and lesbian studies, its theory and popular writing, there have been remarkable claims made for S/M and leather sex around issues of empowerment, power-sharing, living life with greater sexual intensity than "vanilla" sex offers, and so on (Preston 1981; Rubin 1981; Califia 1982; Andros 1983; Scoville 1985; Weeks 1985; Macnair 1989; Scholder and Silverberg 1991). This masquerade should not be dismissed as acting or pretense; the meanings associated with the masquerade are real—at the time. Yet Robert and Richard simply stopped doing it when they lost interest in it.

There is a tangible overdetermination in much discussion of these sexual proclivities, discussion captured by an almost obsessive psychoanalytic gaze. The appeal of the heavily cathected, the unconsciously driven, the discursively determined in sex in general, homosex specifically, and the paraphilias in detail, in much modern and postmodern writing about sex never ceases to amaze. This is not to deny the powerful point made in psychoanalytically inspired writing of the part played by the deep and meaningful; rather, it is an attempt to register that not all sexual motivations are always so complex.

There is a significant degree of sociality and sexual fashion involved in Robert's and Richard's interests. Opportunity and history combined to offer a range of explorations previously unavailable or unthinkable. Dan Berger reported that "it was like some sort of enormous power is out there that comes out of you." But the idea that "coming to leather" always involves a taking-on of a deep-seated, psychically structured obsession and the finding of a truer sexual self is as essentialist as the idea that one is born gay. We should be suspicious of the discursively burdened explanations of those pleading leather's cause as some expression of intrinsic sexual self, for Dan went on to say: "I'm also not very creative, I mean, I can't do all of that, and the dialogue is so terrible. I mean, [a partner] is into that 'fuck that arse, man'. . . . I mean, it's all so trite—not that I expect Hemingway." Dan recognized the masquerade and the fashionable side of such encounters, its very real pleasures and its performative aspects. Beyond the fun and games of sex itself, Robert's inexpert use of the pseudo-Freudian absent-father complex as an etiological gesture should be sufficient warning.

Undoubtedly, leather does represent sexual interests and does conjure and encode possibilities for different kinds of pleasure. The widely seen program *Sex*, shown on commercial television in Australia in mid-1992, featured an investigation of leather sex. The program narrative outlined in fairly light-weight terms the potential offered by leather for enhancing sexual practices in specific ways. Although the commentary did not mention gay men at all, the screen showed only gay men in leather. The key difference between this image and the non-sexuality-specific commentary was the collective character of the gay men's interest; they were in groups, laughing, kissing, arms around each other, in public places (it was the 1992 International Leather Pride Week). There was clear evidence of a collective sexual subjectivity, beyond an identity as gay men, and larger than an interest in a particular set of sexual practices, though related to it. This was an image of a public sexual proclivity, not a private shameful craving.

Compare this with an article on "Fetishism" (Tabori 1978) in a special edition of *Forum*,[2] which discussed leather among a range of items: "hair, physical deformities, blemishes, dolls, bald heads, feet, shoes, high heels, breasts, anti-breasts, urge to destroy, arson, tattoos, transvestism, corduroy, fur, silk, female underclothing, perfumed handkerchiefs, velvet, boots, corsets, tight clothing, long gloves, whips, leather, and rubber" (p. 115). Paul Tabori encodes these items as interchangeable props in a sexual pathology. The article, despite a libertarian posture, is riddled with psychiatrists' advice, gruesome tales from Havelock Ellis, and a cacophony of "paraphilia-gone-wrong" stories to the effect that the "main problem for the fetishist, which technology can seldom solve, is the feeling of isolation, the conviction that he [*sic*] is unique" (p. 119). Robert's twenty years in the gay leather bikie scene contradict this, as do the images in the leather segment in *Sex* mentioned above.

On the same night *Sex* was being screened, the Australian Broadcasting Corporation televised an episode on gay men of the British-made *From Wimps to Warriors: That's Masculinity!* series. It centered on two leather queens (definitely queens). The similarities were obvious. Viewers saw these older gay men in leather, bald or with as much facial hair as they could still muster, cruising a torrid back room—camera angles temptingly oblique and fragmented—intercut with direct face-to-the-camera explanations of their sexual interests. A parallel set of contrasting images was offered: a light-hearted chat (replete with giggling, tale swapping, and recognizably gay, even camp, dialogue) at the bar of the venue between those

---

2 *Forum*, although a popular magazine rather than a journal, was widely read in the 1970's, and numbered among its editorial board prominent academics, doctors, counselors, and psychologists. It took seriously its task of sex education in a changing Australia, then emerging from a conservative period.

just seen strutting their stuff so seriously in its back room; next, a scene of comfortable domesticity with the leather queens fluffing pillows in an immaculately decorated bedroom and laboring in their carefully tended English garden.

To the outsider masquerade looks like pretense, incongruity, even farce. Are these leather men "hustlers" or "homemakers," "macho" or "mary," "fetishists" or "fantasists"? The correct answer is "all of the above." The sexual subcultures that constitute a significant aspect of this sexual community called the gay community are not simply sites of singular manifestation, lone searches for insatiable consummation; rather they are significant collective constructions, which cluster desire, interpret it, mold it, and manufacture it anew.

However, the presumption that the be-all and end-all of gay men's desire is comprehended by positing a democratic diversity of masquerade, experiences, and sensations and a collective history of pursuing sexual possibilities can lead to its own essentialism: we end up merely with a plurality of gayness, of homosexual*ities*. This liberal urge obscures the unseen, the divergent, the contradictory, the not easily assimilable. It relegates homosexualities to an anodyne postmodern relativism, yet another minority to be added to the growing list.

Will the notion of a multifocus sexual subjectivity help us better comprehend and define these desires? It will do so if the tendency to depth is decentered. The sexual subjectivity of the men in these sexual communities involves paradox. One can be a leather queen and sing in amateur productions of *Oklahoma!*, Robert Cusack did; one can be a beat queen and collect porcelain, Ralph Coles did; one can belong to a gay church and cruise hitchhiking surfies for sex, Jack Sayers did; one can spend the afternoon being fisted like a handpuppet and attend demonstrations on gay rights, Ren Pinch did; one can perform fully frocked to raise money for HIV/AIDS and suck off a few straight men in the local toilet on the way home, Harriet did.

A more disaggregated conceptualization of gay sexuality is needed, if this apparent paradox, this counterpoint in concupiscence, this evolving erotic fugue that fashions the sexual, social, cultural, and political lives of men attached to gay communities is to be understood. And fashion is a key word here. In this sense a sexual subjectivity is a light construction, superficial, fluid, impressionable, mutable, and plastic; the indicators of sexual desire may be only masquerade.

It ought to be clear by now to any sexuality theorist and researcher that we need to go well beyond the analysis of sexual identity as being primarily constituted by the biological sex of one's sex object. The challenge offered by Michel Foucault (1978), Jeffrey Weeks (1985), and Diana Fuss (1991) to the homosexual as a discursive sexual category must be accepted here. The homosexual/heterosexual binary is truly misleading; its day is over.

That does not mean gay departs with it. Sexual identities perform valuably for men in this study, whether they are interchangeably gay, homosexual, or camp (as for Harriet) or strongly declaratory (as for Ren Pinch). These are not simply individual sexual identities. They are profoundly collective constructions, whether that collectivity is recognized in the sexual possibilities of beats, which held Neil Davidson's attention for so many years, within the old homosexual networks of Nullangardie, or in the modern gay community of Sydney. Regardless of the terminology used by these men, or whether they regard their sexual identity as genetic, organic, psychologically derived, or socially constructed, the increasing performativity of a collective gay sexual identity cannot be ignored.

Beyond the contribution of sexual identity we have also seen considerable input to a sexual subjectivity from the physical, from bodies exploring each other in acts later inscribed as transgressive or deviant, which in turn spurs further pursuits of pleasure. The sexual (dis)order encountered by the men in this study has at its roots a deep physicality, an embodied ambivalence to sexual prescription, and a daunting capacity for dispersal of pleasure, for inversion, displacement, and "transgressive reinscription" (Dollimore 1991), but this occurs in the practices themselves.

This sexual construction of the gay communities must take a prominent place in the theoretical arguments of the future. Documentation of the social construction of homosexuality has concentrated its efforts on discourse and identity, on rediscovering gay history, on the search for Boswell's "gay persons," on the politics of struggle with sexually oppressive practices in law, medicine, education, and the interrogation of literary discourse. Fine. Indeed, they are fine, but at the curious neglect of sex itself. After all:

> Writing about sex is one thing.
> Writing erotically is another.
> Licking is something else.
> (Hurley and Hutchinson 1991: 19)

Sex has been treated as serious business, as the site of only complex, far-reaching, heavily laden, and therefore often structuralist determination. There needs to be more consideration of sex as frolic, fashion, flimsy foment—a bit of fucking about for the fun of it with a few friends. The gay communities, by removing perverse sexual interests and practices from the individual closet to a collective, public sexual culture, have achieved some "liberation" after all.

The sexual construction of gay community and the sociocultural way of life that emerged from the efforts of men like Ren, Richard, and Robert are neither fixed nor forever. Robert, ultimately, saw a certain senselessness in it all and talked of "settling down." Inexplicably, life seems to have passed him by. Ren Pinch, dogged by deteriorating health, is experiencing a shrinking of his arena of action with some frustration. For him too there have been significant losses to AIDS, and HIV/AIDS politics in the gay community is a draining and difficult arena in which to sustain an energetic contribution.

Overall, the social engagement of each of the three men was crumbling at the time I interviewed them. Richard's was the most distressing example. It was clear that the relationships he had formed in the Sydney gay community in his heyday could not withstand the pressures of his illness. His attachment to the gay community was only ever partial, largely sexual in fact; when more was required of his friends and associates, it was not forthcoming. Ironically, the gay community in Nullangardie did rally round; yet he had nothing but disdain for his local "queens." There was a brittleness to Richard's overall attachment to gay community; a sense that for all the fabulous four-day fucks, he had never truly belonged there.

There is no denying the tragic effects of HIV/AIDS on Robert. Uninfected though he is, his miraculous salvation was severely compromised by the continuing attrition of the sexual and social intimates with whom he has made his life. The fear of sex, his rejection of leather, the confusion and despondency, reek of despair. No combatant here, Robert now finds that nearly thirty years of investment in gay life has led him to a country retirement cottage looking after an ailing parent.

Ren was by far the best placed of these three men, having developed in his years in Sydney a network of friends, a brotherhood of queens, which served purposes similar to—but constituted a different formation from—family. Like Ralph Coles and Dan Berger, his networks were often based around organizations and causes. However, these men are all middle-class, and this figured significantly in their facility in developing these new relationships.

Ren noted that he had first met many of his friends in sexual encounters, something which was playing less of a part in his social world of late.

Dan Berger was having difficulty reconstructing new friendships in the aftermath of the end of a long-term relationship. This was complicated by the difficulty he was having obtaining sexual encounters that went beyond a single, or often merely promised, event.

The gay community attachment measures are beginning to look a little shaky; they seem to capture better the making of lives, not their unraveling. The sexual engagement measure captures a dimension markedly different from the social engagement or community involvement measures. Interconnected they may be, but sketchy they remain. Not only do they neglect to assess the effort involved on the part of the men themselves, but they fail to register the differential character of such attachment.

The sexual construction of gay life to which these three men contributed with their sweat and semen is a brittle thing. As if to add to this depressing picture, it is important to note what has happened to these men's sex lives. Richard had not had sex for years, a plight many seropositive men report and rail against. Robert was fearful in all sex now. Ren, in uncertain health, refused to have sex with other seropositive men if they were in any way symptomatic, seeing in them a reflection of his future. Both men were sexually less sought after by the endlessly younger others. Ren's sauna stories reflected a frustration that this once sexually voracious man must now summon his proclivity for rationality to aid in understanding and accepting rejection. Robert invited those in need of a fatherly touch, but these were passing fancies (exactly whose is unclear); the need for a relationship was starting to press more as the prospect of a lonely old age dogs him.

∽

There are issues about being part of this sexual community that go beyond a simple participation in fun, good times, and transgressive behavior. The lives of men in this study reveal the formative nature of early sexual experiences and meanings. There is no doubt that sexual motivations permeate the life decisions they made. This is significant at a number of levels: the oppressive impact of the master discourses of law, medicine, science, and religion; the deployment of power by institutions such as the state and the labor market; the negotiation of the self within the framework and practices of hegemonic heterosexuality determining the assumption of masculinity.

A second feature of these men's lives is the impact of sexual experience itself. A third feature is the collective nature of their sexual enterprise. In light of the experiences illustrated here it seems foolish to analyze sexuality as an *individual* unfolding of desire or as the construction of a singular subjectivity, since it is when that singularity ceases to exist that desire is transformed into a collective enterprise. There is then a structuring of sexuality in the gay community undertaking, which though ever-shifting and evolving, performs for those who engage it, offering a far-reaching solution to homoerotic desire. That undertaking has yet to offer complete or permanent sanctuary, but the edifice constructed by gay men in their pursuit of sex and homosexuality has dramatically transformed the relations between homosexually active men.

## The Active Anus

> I moved my thumbs into his mouth.
> He moved his mouth to mine.
> He pushed fingers into me.
> I was held fixed.
> He moved his fingers and I came.
> His spit dribbled down my thumbs.
>
> —Hurley and Hutchinson, *Two Timing*

Ren, Robert, and Richard expressed a decided preference for receptive anal intercourse; they enjoyed being fucked. It is apparent from their accounts and those of Ralph, Harry, Barney, and Harriet that the sensations of anal sex are learnt, and not always easily. It takes practice, experience, and often skilled guidance. Sodomy, though once a crime against nature irrespective of the sex of the anus involved, is now regarded largely as a synonym for male homosexual sex, and we must acknowledge the very special place it occupies for gay men.

A number of men nominated intimacy as an important aspect of anal intercourse, but the act is not a singularity. Its meanings vary not only in the differences between men in relationships and those engaging in casual intercourse with perfect strangers but, as Ralph Coles indicated, from relationship to relationship and from moment to moment. The practice itself combines a capacity for physical sensations with relational meanings, against a backdrop of considerable discursive derogation. But the partners are capable of swapping position and replicating the other's pleasure and sensations, a factor that registers it as a deep, mutually shared experience; the sexual partner is not Other at all. Anal intercourse between men is redolent with such significances.

There is no denying the acute physicality involved—"double the pleasure"—and Ralph Coles and Ren Pinch both recalled the exquisite pleasures gained from multiple insertive partners in beats. Ren Pinch also talked of considerable fulfillment from pleasuring others. Harry Wight gained pleasure from the sight of his lover being fucked by "trade" and then fucking the "trade" as well. Dan Berger noted a more abstract pleasure in "riding" a sex partner in a soft-ish S/M scene, and Barney Sherman gained wicked pleasure in ensuring he got to do the fucking in the parks of inner Sydney in his youth. These men reported that casual sex, far from being impersonal, can actually be a remarkably emotional moment of sharing pleasure with great skill and consideration. The choreography, though an enormous part of the pleasure, is not attached to a singular meaning or pattern of practice in the sex acts themselves.

Even pornography offers multiple interpretations of meaning and choreographies of practice with reference to anal intercourse between men. This should warn us about too much meaning too soon, or too little meaning too often. Samuel M. Steward, as his pen name and alter ego "Phil Andros," concentrates the action on his macho hero always being a "top"; except of course when he turns soft and bites the pillow to help some guy out or when some "stud" gets the better of him. These are always good-spirited, only vaguely reluctant moments of submission, often with wry humor at the hero finding himself in such a position (see Andros 1983). On the other hand, the once-reigning star of West Coast United States gay pornography, the remarkably endowed Jeff Stryker, specializes in taking advantage of every available bent-over man in sight; but he never takes it himself. That moment is awaited worldwide, and its actualization will constitute one of the great legend-making moments of modern gay life. Let us not forget also that there is a game being played here: a market for what will probably be the world's fastest-selling gay porn video is being created, and we should not be fooled into thinking that gay men are unaware of that.

Stryker would appear to confirm Robert J. Stoller's "desire to harm" (1985), an antagonism structuring sexual activity that seems to verify certain feminist critiques of pornography as an enactment and representation of men's desire to subjugate others in sex.[3] Certainly, Stryker's sex scenes are based on his sexual domination of other men, brutish language, and strenuous insertion. But there is a counterpoint in the partners' capacity to "take it." Many a porn star accommodates Stryker's appendage, and his manhood is enhanced thereby; he becomes a bit of a hero, a star in his own right (reminding us of Ralph Coles's pride in being able to "accommodate . . . fairly large" men).

The industry specializes in fantasy; the men swap sexual positions, constantly unraveling who is "top" and who is "bottom," dispersing pleasure

---

[3] For a critique of this position, see Segal and McIntosh 1992 and Rodgerson and Wilson 1991.

from anus to penis, from genitals to nipples, from hands to tongues and lips. This is sex as sheer performance, devoid of any deeper motivations and complexity. These men are constituted as always sexually active, whether they are receptive in penetrative acts or not; that is, they are *phallic* representations, they embody desire in action. What the anti-porn crusaders seem to forget is that the penis cannot subjugate by definition where there are two penises present and where pleasure is allocated evenly between the men—they both come, something that cannot be faked by male porn stars—and dispersed among penises, anuses, and other body parts. In gay porn then, the narrative is as discursively informed by, as it is formative of, the designation of anal intercourse between men as democratic and immensely mutually pleasurable.

There are other meanings attached to anal sex beyond pleasure and intimacy. The novels of Gordon Merrick, for example, *The Quirk* (1978), offer highly romanticized and explicit accounts of anal sex between men; pleasure and emotion intermingle in an eroticism that heterosexual romance novelists barely echo. Romance is woven out of emotional intimacy, sexual pleasure, and the exposed vulnerability of men in sex. Neil Bartlett updates Merrick's romanticism in *Ready to Catch Him Should He Fall* (1990), picking up more ambiguity in sex, recognizing its apparently contradictory moments: "Boy began to think there were two kinds of sex: the kind of sex where you say *do this, do that*, or you manoeuvre yourself into position for a particular kind of pleasure; and then there is the other kind of sex, where you want to say, *do anything. Do anything you want to me, you can do anything you want, I give you entire permission over me*" (pp. 108–9).

Some psychoanalytic writing seems to lock sex into singular, almost functionalist meanings. Freud's "Wolf Man" and the passing of the stool at the primal moment springs to mind (1955[1918]). Although Freud usually distinguished between receptive and passive, his followers did not always do so. There is no doubt that these interpretations of anal sexual interest and pleasure are useful and challenging. Their singular focus is less than adequate in the face of the multiple meanings the men in this study associate with the practices and relations of sex, and in the face of a growing sophistication among gay writers and artists in representing gay sex.

A much-praised safe sex campaign in Sydney in the early 1990's featured the work of local well-known gay artist David McDiarmid. The five posters were based on previous paintings—thematic investigations by McDiarmid of gay erotics and HIV/AIDS (see *Art and Text* 1991: 110; also Gott 1994: 154). Prominent in these posters were two images of male homoeroticism that repositioned male-to-male anal sex, in particular, as confronting. The first featured two stylized bodies fucking, the receptive partner bending (beckoning?) toward the viewer, the insertive partner standing behind. The receptive partner has the words "safe-lust" written on his chest, the insertive partner has "safe-love"; intimacy and pleasure were thus partly disaggregated and allocated inversely. The only penis in view is that of the receptive partner, un-erect and partly out of frame. The other poster featured a view of a naked man's back arched to emphasize his buttocks, his un-erect penis dangling between his legs in the background. His hands pull the cheeks of his buttocks apart to expose his anus beckoning the viewer, with the words "deep" and "heat" tattooed on the knuckles. They are provocative reminders not to misread the penis as phallus; more important, McDiarmid is claiming a central place for the desiring anus in gay men's transgressive and collective sexual subjectivity.

Ren Pinch's story of the semen dribbling from his anus and the sensation of a forearm in his rectum during fisting can be situated within this frame. The desiring anus, far from merely and passively responding to the insistent penis, must be reckoned with in any reconsideration of gay men's sexual subjectivity.

In a sustained attempt to do just this, Leo Bersani in "Is the Rectum a Grave?" accused much of the canon on gay male sexuality of conventionality (1988). He offers a critique of affirming interpretations of homoeroticism, the kind of pervasive analysis that, he says, grows out of the work of Weeks, Watney, and others concerned with positioning homosexuality *within* the overall scheme of things, even if as a response and challenge to history. Bersani rightly accuses these writers of doing a cleansing act on sex, refusing to recognize the "big secret about sex," which is that "most people don't like it" (p. 197).

Bersani accuses such writers of failing to recognize sexual subjectivity as formed within powerful frameworks that may take many forms. He argues that underlying some feminist distrust of the wholesomeness of heterosexual intercourse itself, there is desire for a definable and delicious, yet strangely essentialist (in this case women's) sexuality; a search Bersani calls the "redemptive reinvention of sex" (p. 215). Bersani sees in the post-Foucauldian redefinition of pleasure and of the body's multiple possibilities for erotic response a kind of liberal *pluralism*, a plea for diversity, for an anodyne expansion of sites of pleasure, a continuance of the theme of human sexual liberation.

More radically, he proposes that it is the sexual which produces the social, arguing that during sex the anatomical possibilities of the body, in particular the disintegration of the psyche that accompanies orgasm—Bataille's "little death" (1989)—offer the denial and destruction of the self, a loss of its power, and by definition something masochistic. In taking it up the arse, not only do gay men symbolically divest themselves of their power as men, but in their very avid pursuit of these mutual pleasures, in their multiple encounters, they refuse to enact power in sex by "re-presenting the internalized phallic male as an infinitely loved object of sacrifice" (p. 222).

Bersani next argues that the logic of homosexual desire includes a loving identification with the gay man's enemies:

An authentic gay male political identity therefore implies a struggle not only against definitions of maleness and of homosexuality as they are reiterated and imposed in a heterosexist social discourse, but also against those very same definitions so seductively and so faithfully reflected by those (in large part culturally invented and elaborated) male bodies that we carry within us as permanently renewable sources of excitement. . . . If as Weeks puts it, gay men "gnaw at the roots of male hetero-sexual identity," it is not because of the parodistic distance that they take from that identity, but rather because, from within their nearly mad identification with it, *they never cease to feel the appeal of its being violated.* (p. 209)

That violation has two aspects. Gay men realize/embody men's capacity for anal eroticism, and, as women do, "gay men spread their legs with an unquenchable appetite for destruction," "to be penetrated is to abdicate power" (pp. 211–12). Bersani also claims homosexuality as subversion, but it comes from elsewhere—the loss of manhood, the loss of self; it comes from being fucked.

While attempting to distance himself from lauding (homo)sexuality as redemptive of human sexual potential, Bersani ultimately redeems gay sex as a primary site of self-discipline, the place of denial where the powerful self loses "sight of the self, and in doing so . . . proposes and dangerously represents *jouissance* as a mode of ascesis" (p. 222). This individualized vision condemns the relational character of sex to a "struggle for power" (p. 218). Yet the men in this study would indicate a mutuality constitutive of a recognition of collective sexual possibilities.

Bersani accuses Foucault, Weeks, Watney, and the "gay activist discourse on gay male machismo" of belonging, ultimately, to a "pastoral" impulse. He seeks to undo the pervasive account of homosexuality as resistance, as rebellion against oppression, as a radical politics offered by Weeks (1985) and Watney (1987a) and others.[4] Bersani argues that macho

---

[4] Bersani disagrees with Weeks's argument that the difference between gay and homosexual is that homosexuality is about sexual preference and gay is about a subversive political life. The men in this study reveal that radical politics and rebellion are to the fore only in a few men's minds, and rarely when they have sex.

gay is not subversive and to claim that it is is ludicrous. He suggests that macho gay, rather, is and is understood as "oxymoron" (p. 207); it may unintentionally validate heterosexual men by proving after all that they are the objects of gay men's desire:

The very real potential for subversive confusion in . . . the signifiers of machismo is dissipated once the heterosexual recognizes in the gay-macho style a *yearning* toward machismo, a yearning that, very conveniently for the heterosexual, makes of the leather queen's forbidding armour and warlike manners a *per*version rather than a *sub*version of real maleness. (pp. 207–8)

What of the collectivity of the gay masculinity, its claim to sexual space, to public sexual identities? Is there no subversive potential in gay community in its structuring of collective sexual relations among men? As a disturbance of image, collective clonedom, or any other form of gay masquerade for that matter, may indeed subvert, as might making public what is expected to be private—sex.

In the British TV program already mentioned, an ex-army gay man retells with pride the effect of new macho gay bodies on straight men: as a group of scantily clad muscle queens left a cab on their way to Heaven (a London gay disco), one of a group of straight men nearby was heard to say: "Look at the size of those fucking faggots!" There is certainly a recognition of implicit desire ("fucking") as the exposed bodies ("size") challenge but are written off ("faggots"). Or are they? The undercurrent of ambiguity in the men's remark reveals not only a permanent and great fear but also a perceived proximity. Perhaps, Bersani's singular *per*version is on the way to becoming a collective *sub*version after all. Although it was as oxymoron that the British TV program presented leather gays (the cushion fluffing in contrast to the backroom sex venue), for the men themselves there is no problem of inauthenticity or instability. Robert, the clerk, and Robert, the leatherman, appear incomprehensible to those outside the milieu. But the gay communities comprehend these authenticities readily. The oxymoron exists only in the eye of the beholder; when writ large it begins to look far more stable and integrated.

Stephen Schecter, in an essay in *The AIDS Notebooks* (1990), criticizes the "undialectic" adoption by Bersani of the demolition of the self as the only outcome of sex. He regards the redemptive project as more subversive than Bersani gives it credit, and particularly in reference to anal sex, which is

Thus also an indictment at the very level of the body upon which is condensed and displaced the neurotic energy that drives our social setup. As pleasure, anal sex thus questions the value of the sacrifice we make to keep the dynamic going, suggests that the sacrifice in the end is worthless, misplaced, a "pile of shit," that in the end we might be better off playing around in other people's assholes. (p. 105)

The men in this study deny any particularist definitions of intent and meaning and offer a more diverse engagement with anal sex in a constitutive transformation of collective homoeroticism over time. They reveal a lighter, more agentive relation to their desire, enacted in a collective enterprise where meaning and pleasure are continuously redefined. There is sufficient evidence of a concerted interest in macho, leather, and esoteric sex to warrant an invocation of weighty psychoanalytic formulations of sexuality. But these fail to explain fully the assorted choreography available in the sex practices, so often discussed in theory as if they were singular actions; nor do they take into account the changes in these practices, their enactments and meanings, their fashion, over time. It is important to wed the weighty determinist or structuralist frameworks that dominate the academic discourses on sexuality (and which underlie Bersani's approach) to a theoretical grasp of more immediately tangible collective practice, where contingency and opportunity engage experience and consciousness in a quite playful invention.

There is a clear demonstration in these life histories of sex as a consciously pursued activity, a hobby almost, involving a process of skilling through accumulating experience, later embracing meaning-making discourses in homoeroticism, becoming available through the emerging and increasingly open pro-sex gay movement and the opportunities provided in its growing communities. This form of *recreational* sex is a crucial contribution to the configuration of sexual activity that gay men more than any other group pursued during the 1970's and early 1980's. White started to investigate this in his *States of Desire* (1986), particularly in the chapter on New York City.

Recreational sex describes the high profile that sexual encounters assumed during the 1970's and early 1980's, and endeavors to praise the pursuit of sexual pleasure for its own sake; to identify that part of a gay man's sexual interests which existed alongside, but not instead of, that involving primary sexual relationships entailing long-term commitments to another. It occurred as discourse and practice simultaneously. Recreational sex is sex as a hobby, a highly ritualized pursuit of sex with all the concentration of a performance and the dedication of a champion; it is sex as an art form.

Even if recreational sex might be acclaimed as revolutionary (Weeks, Rechy), one has to agree that for many it was just recreational—the pursuit of pleasure. For many gay men the world over, sex became the next most important thing in life to eating and sleeping. Many, like Robert and Richard, spent hours each week engaging in sex acts with men in clubs and bars, back rooms, public beaches and parks, orgy centers, fantasy venues, blue movie houses, private parties, saunas and steam rooms, on trains, in cars, in any and every conceivable way. The 1970's and 1980's were a moment in history when gay men had the chance to explore the outer limits of sex as pleasure, and some did so. And almost all of it was free; it cost nothing.

These three men were helping construct a sexual community of seemingly endless homoerotic possibilities. Whatever the psychodynamic and experiential underpinnings of their sexual interests, their ongoing exploration of desire contributing to a collective reformulation of sexual practice and meaning must be reckoned with by history. As a remarkable solution to the homophobic structuring of modern Western life (Sedgwick 1990), it provided these men, at least some of them, at least for a few years, with possibilities hitherto impossible to envisage.

The dilemma has become to render an account of homosexuality in the era of HIV/AIDS, where these dimensions of homoeroticism can find room to maneuver. Robert Cusack suffered in person that which the discursive framing of sexuality is suffering in general: a fear and loathing of sex as diseased, centered on the penis-in-anus, and carrying with it all the weight of a historically formed disavowal of sex and the body. Paula Treichler's "epidemic of signification" (1988) haunts all the men in this study at a very personal and basic level. Recapturing for them some sense of their sex lives as whole is vital in the face of Bersani's chosen epigraph:

These people have sex twenty to thirty times a night. . . . A man comes along and goes from anus to anus and in a single night will act as a mosquito transferring infected cells on his penis. When this is practised for a year, with a man having three thousand sexual intercourses, one can readily understand this massive epidemic that is currently upon us. (Professor Opendra Narayan, The Johns Hopkins Medical School) (1988: 197)

What these men teach us, in contrast to Bersani's disintegrative revolution, is the enactment of sex as centrally constitutive of men's sexual subjectivity. The collective pursuit of sensation and pleasure, in/with youth, with oneself and two/three/more others, the public disavowal of private sex, its frolicsome and fantastic masquerade, its sheer selfish recreational pleasures, speak to some other *con*struction. There is no need to redeem sex as pluralist polymorphous pleasure, opening the way for the transformation of antisexual societies—nice as that might be. Its recognized collective enactment, and even the inciting possibility of it, offer possibilities far more wicked and willful. Its capacity to transform relations between men occurs not simply through "the infinitely more seductive and intolerable image of a grown man, legs high in the air, unable to refuse the suicidal ecstasy of being a woman" (Bersani 1988: 212), but because men's desiring anuses know something remarkable about pleasure. Any man who has taken another man's cock up his arse knows only too well that sex will never be the same again. Any man who has done so "twenty to thirty times in a night" knows something about men's sexual capacities that cannot be snuffed out, by HIV/AIDS or anything else. The transformation in desire produced by gay communities, this collective reinscription of transgressive desire, best signified by the rapacious desiring anus, will endure beyond the epidemic.

# 7

# The Resolution of Desire

Whatever communities Ren Pinch, Robert Cusack, and Richard Cochrane constructed; whatever sexual choreography they created; whatever their contribution to the sophisticated sexual culture that is the Sydney gay community; whatever subversion their desiring anuses collectively achieved in decentering and refocusing masculine sexual potential: for them their moment has passed. The issue at stake now is how such sexual possibilities are represented to younger men about to begin their exploration of homoerotic desire. For they begin their adventure in dangerously different times. As the late Eric Michaels (1990: 192) said: "We need to take some responsibility for our own history, for conveying it to our young. It is not nostalgia. If one is going to go to all the trouble to be gay, one ought to do a more interesting and useful job of it. Models exist in our recent past. They should be recalled."

There are six men in this study who were under thirty when I interviewed them: Dennis Partridge, Martin Ridgeway, Pip Bowles, Phillip Gibbs, Simon Little, and Geoff Harris. Their experiences of male-to-male sex have occurred since the gay liberation movement started, and their sexual explorations beyond childhood also occurred within a general framework of the existence of gay men and gay communities in public discourse. For the youngest, Martin Ridgeway and Simon Little, all their sexual experience has occurred since the onset of the HIV epidemic.

These men make it possible to reexamine the themes of this study in a different light, that of the pursuit of homosexuality within the contemporary gay community. First, early sexual experiences of these younger men occurred more recently, which permits us to consolidate the analysis offered so far concerning the formative and collective structure of such events. Second, these men have easier access to a gay sexual identity, which permits us to put the notion of a sexual subjectivity to the test. Third, we can assess the contribution made by the gay community to the resolution of their difficulties in coming to grips with homosexual desire, thereby answering Eric Michaels's challenge. Last, we can examine the relation between discourse and praxis with reference to the social construction of homosexuality in the light of these young men's struggle to define, interpret, absorb, and resist their experience of homosexual desire.

## Phillip Gibbs

Illuminating a life history with theory requires a sufficiently coherent history of the life being examined. Phillip Gibbs's account of his life was choppy, repetitious, and often unclear. Phillip was a young man with a good memory, a poor education, and a limited vocabulary. He recalled his life as a stream of consciousness; he remembered its events vividly, but he had not reflected on them. It was difficult at times to differentiate the lovers from the people with AIDS, from the drug dealers, the girlfriends, and the rest of those he mentioned. The interview with him flowed well enough, but it took place at his home under the (casual) scrutiny of his family. He was wary at times of being overheard, so we ended up in the garage. But the discontinuities in his account also derive from how he lived his life— moving from one moment to the next with little forethought or planning beyond his immediate concerns.

The first problem was to get the basic facts of Phillip's story straight. The preadolescent part of his life emerged as a discrete period, bounded literally by a geographic area (one part of western Sydney) and by the constraints of childhood. In contrast to this boundedness, his early sexual activities during the same period were almost libertine.

At twenty-five Phillip could pass for twenty. He was short, thin, boyish-looking, with clean, well-cut hair. He was proud of his hair and nominated it as a feature men found attractive about him. He dressed like a "Westie"[1] (blue jeans, cotton check shirt, and sneakers), but they were all squeaky clean; the jeans and shirt were ironed and the sneakers scrubbed. The whole image contrasted with his younger straight brother, who looked just that bit more disheveled and sloppy.

Phillip lived with his family: his divorced mother (an office worker),

---

[1] "Westie" is a derogatory term used to describe people from the western suburbs of Sydney. It has a specific class meaning, as western Sydney has many, largely working-class, dormitory suburbs serving its industries.

an older brother, an older sister (divorced), and the younger brother. The father, a violent alcoholic, left the family when Phillip was six or seven. He has rarely seen his father since the divorce, and it was the mother who has worked to keep the family. The siblings are not close. Phillip and the younger brother had a closer relationship as youngsters, but that did not prove sustainable beyond early adolescence.

Phillip ran away from home first in his teens. Since then he has returned for brief periods, occasionally with friends, often basing himself there but spending days and nights elsewhere with friends or lovers, without family inquiry. His family seems permanently tense and detached; rather than close, they seem to have been shackled together by adversity.

The family house was a classic freestanding, postwar, brick-veneer, three-bedroom house on a sizable block, neat and comfortable, in a street and suburb full of the same. The suburb adjoined a state Housing Commission area, providing a distinctive identity for its inhabitants. There is little infrastructure in that area apart from schools and parks. The local business district is over thirty kilometers from inner Sydney. There is little to do; kids play in streets, ride bikes, and eventually when old enough head off to inner Sydney to find entertainment.

Phillip's life was populated with disturbed families, disrupted relationships, stories of abuse and disrespect at the hands of peers, and arbitrary mistreatment. He has lived variously in group households in the west, a squat in the inner west, a deserted government-owned house, and a Housing Commission home. He was in a reformatory for four months and has been through various government-run programs to get him back into the workforce. He has experienced the system in many of its most arbitrary forms.

A recent bashing had left him with headaches and occasional blackouts and afraid for his safety in public. Phillip was on Sickness Benefit as a result and was awaiting the outcome of a criminal compensation case. This might give him enough money to buy a block of land and a car. Then he hoped to start his own nursery, although he was untrained in horticulture. He spent a good deal of this waiting time working on the garden at the family house, which was impeccably neat and lush. Four to five months after this first bashing he was "poofter bashed" at a beat.

His whole life he has been overwhelmed by forces he cannot explain, although he tries to constantly:

I think if I'd have had a father, I would've been different than what I am now. (Do you think that's the reason you're like you are?) Yeah. (What, meaning gay, or what?) No, not actually gay, just, you know, when you've got a mother who works all the time, she can't spend time giving you love and all that. I know—I find it really hard to love people and all that sort of thing. 'Cause I haven't had much love, sort of thing. And I think if my father was with us and my mother didn't have to work, you know, she'd spend more time with us. . . . It's because of my father pissing off, my mum getting a divorce. We used to—my brothers—me and my brother never got on, sort of thing. . . . He used to, at one stage, bash me up quite a lot . . . which caused me problems at school, with headaches and all that sort of thing. . . . I think because of what happened to my mother and father, my brother took it out on me, sort of thing. It was like he wanted to, sort of, get back at my father and he took it out on me, sort of thing.

Phillip went to the local primary and high school. He did not do very well at school and in his neighborhood he was bashed up frequently. At the same time the older brother was bashing him at home. This constant theme of bashings and headaches may indicate a case of child abuse with real physical consequences, or a permanent psychological response to what was happening around him. Whatever the case, the selective processes of schooling got the better of his inattention and distress, and he dropped out in his third year of high school, undoubtedly thinking of himself as a failure, as most who leave school early do. In any case he was poorly positioned for a seriously degraded youth labor market.

As a consequence of neglect and mistreatment, Phillip has experienced life as a consistent failure to get on top of most situations. He does not fully understand the forces with which he must contend; he can ponder the problems in his family, but understanding the structural impact the Australian school system and the youth labor market have had on his life is beyond him. Yet there remained a striving to work it out, to explain, to get it clear, to find a way out. "Oppression is *never* totally internalized. It always implies an expenditure of energy, a struggle" (Connell 1983: 15).

It's an open question whether Phillip is chronically unemployed or unemployable. In his own words: "I haven't worked in a long time, you know, since—it would be about ten years or something since I sort of had a normal job, if you know what I mean." It is important to note the difference between Phillip's experience of work and of the labor market. There is no labor market for Phillip. The youth labor market in Australia had been drying up since the late 1970's, long before he left school. He was on the fringe of the labor market from the moment he left school early in an area where

there was little employment anyway, and his school history made him virtually unemployable. He has had some jobs, in order: putting badges on hats
in a factory; doing the odd bit of amateur prostitution; working in a fast
food outlet and a local grocery store; and working in the black economy
sporadically, in a cinema, doing lighting for amateur pub shows, and in a
sex shop. He was always on the dole at the same time. The Commonwealth
Employment Service (the national job placement agency) finally sent him
to a pre-employment course at the local technical college, where he chose
to study retailing and "was going to be a manager," but he has not worked
since the course.

His experiences are of mindless work and victimization. Accused
wrongly of theft in one job, he was sacked. The sex shop job depended on
his being the sex partner of a coworker. Prostitution was a youthful excitement related more to his interest in sex and was no longer attractive. The
supermarket job, arranged by the reformatory, was the one real possibility.
But his self-discipline was undermined by his discovery of a local beat, and
by an introduction to Oxford Street, which seemed far more attractive. He
left the supermarket for a job in the black economy, but the sporadic cinema
work he obtained was contingent on having sex with the cinema owner.

Work in the black economy is insecure, often mindless, and its illegality brings with it exploitation and instability that renders youngsters
like Phillip even more cynical and resentful. It also produces working relationships and a workplace culture that are marked by a lack of individual
responsibility and loyalty; one can simply leave if something better comes
up. Phillip was quite young at this time and encountered other experiences
that subverted whatever discipline might be required to sustain his participation in regular paid work. These were sex, drugs, and partying surrounding the black economy, all of which formed the collective practices
of one of Phillip's emerging social networks. With the recession of the early
1990's Phillip had little hope of making enough money to set up a nursery. Unskilled, with few resources, Phillip is destined for the social welfare
scrap heap unless his own resilience can carry him through.

Phillip began smoking the odd joint in his early teens, and this increased
as he moved into the friendship circles he was developing outside school.
At fifteen or sixteen, Phillip was introduced to Oxford Street and there he
tried amyl nitrite. About the same time he met a drug dealer at a western
Sydney gay venue, and this marked the beginning of more systematic use of
drugs: "I, sort of, not fell in love with him, but fell in love with the drugs."
Next came tripping (it is not clear on what) and eventually "speed" at age
seventeen or eighteen (though not injected). While he smoked cigarettes

during this time, and still does, he did not drink and there was no indication of any trouble with alcohol.

His pattern of drug use paralleled his developing friendships and relationships. Drug use in that milieu was explored in a context of chronic unemployment, welfare dependency, homelessness, violence, and as part of sexual relationships. An escalation to heroin paralleled his admission to adult networks with more systematic availability. It was also less an increase in dependence in response to the pharmacological properties of the drugs than a product of changes over time in the patterns of drug use in that milieu. It was a *recreational* use, related to good times, rather than to patterns of dependency. There was an absence of urgency to obtain drugs. His more recent experiments with injection may threaten the balance he has so far maintained. He injected first (with "speed") about four years previously, with someone else injecting for him—a mode he still preferred. More regular use came with an erstwhile lover, an eighteen-year-old addicted to heroin (having a short dry spell), who was reintroduced to the drug by Phillip's drug-dealing friend.

His drug use was not a lone personal practice, but part of the activities that constituted various circles he moved in. He reported that he was heavily into drug use at certain periods, each connected with a sexual relationship, for example, a short-lived affair with a rich inner-city gay guy led to increased use of "speed" and "ecstasy"—the Oxford Street drug of preference. Heroin use was related more to his western Sydney friends. He always used a clean new needle and obtained them with friends from the widespread, government-sanctioned, needle exchange and distribution programs operating out of STD clinics and pharmacies. He reported sharing a needle once only, with two HIV antibody positive men—the drug dealer and his boyfriend—and he cleaned the needle out first. Phillip was aware of the dangers he might run, not just from HIV infection via "unsafe" injection, but in taking on the patterns of drug use he witnessed in his friends. In the previous four years he had seen quite a few friends and lovers go off the rails.

Phillip was monitoring his use, stopping when he got worried, tasting again when his guard was down or a friend propelled him in that direction. He regarded his failure to achieve self-injection as an indication that he was not yet addicted. This is a fragile marker. It was as though he sensed dependency was not too far away and knew the danger of poor judgment:

Well, I'd say I won't get infected [with HIV] unless I do something stupid. I've had my experience with needles and if I ever did get infected that's [where] it would be from. (You don't think it would be through sex?) No, no way.

It is a nice confirmation of the contingent nature of drug-use functionality and the social patterning of its practice pointed out by Rachel Sharp et al. (1991). He may be right. He is "at risk," and his continued unemployability or the dynamics of a relationship may be the destabilizing factor, rather than anything to do with the drugs per se.

When he was seven or eight (about the time his father left) Phillip started having sex with two neighborhood boys, one the same age as himself, the other slightly older. It started with games of "Spin-the-Bottle" with these two boys and Phillip's younger brother in partly built houses nearby. Each afternoon after school he would have sex with one or other of the boys, mainly "munching out [sucking] on each other's bodies." The sex continued until the age of thirteen or fourteen. His brother took part in it almost as regularly as he did, but they never had sex with each other. There are two examples he gave of these sexual interactions:

Like, I'd get home from school and one guy would ring and say: "Come over" and I'd go over there. And then we'd, sort of, play around, sort of, saying: "What do you want to do?" and he'd go: "What do you want to do?" and I'd go: "What do you want to do?" and go on for about an hour the same. And then finally we'd turn round and say: "Have sex" and then we'd suddenly get into it.

Then with the other brother:

We went for a ride on our bikes and we went to this park, sort of thing. And, um, he said he had a splinter down below, and then we stopped and he started playing around with himself. And, you know, I didn't expect him—and then the next minute I know, he had a horn [an erection]. And that's how it started from then. And then every afternoon after that I used to go over there and have sex, or he used to come over here and have sex. And there was a couple of times when my brother would come over just as we were finishing and then my brother would go in and have a bit with him.

Framing these sexual experiences was an earlier sexual relationship:

Plus I had a young guy what was—used to play around with me when I was so small . . . And I was having sex with him as well. Like, if I didn't have sex with one of the guys across the road, I had sex with the other one up the end of the road.

(What sort of sex were you having with him, the older boy?)

Um. Just sucking and sort of kissing and licking.

(So you were kissing with him, were you?)

Yeah, but I didn't—I felt funny about it, if you know what I mean. And he was the one who taught me how to do all these things. You know, when I used to go up there when I was a real young kid, he used to do things to me like jerk me off and I didn't even know what he was doing. All I know was I was getting pretty sore. And he was, sort of like, my first experience.

Phillip was six or seven, the other boy was nine or ten, and this relationship went on for six or seven years. Just how frequently these sexual activities occurred, with the older boy and the neighbors, is hard to judge. Phillip gave the impression they were almost a daily occurrence.

There were other elements of the story that lead to the conclusion that he had a fairly active sex life and one not occurring solely in private. One of the neighborhood brothers with a few mates caught Phillip and the other brother at it again, and they all decided they wanted their share:

And then they went to school and told everybody. And then it was funny how I had a lot of friends after that. . . . Like I'd, sort of, be in a classroom, sort of, sitting there and then suddenly some guy would sit next to me. And the next minute I know he'd be playing with my leg, and he'd ask if he could come home for lunch with me and I'd come over and have sex with him.

(So by the time you'd left school, how many mates at school do you think you'd had sex with?)

Oh, I can't say. I had a couple—it would have been well over ten.

Phillip's childhood and adolescent sex practices underwent a significant shift in range, meaning, and investment when he entered new sexual communities and subcultures beyond his school and region.

Roxy's is a large inner-Sydney roller-skating rink. It is a mecca for young Westies coming to town for a good time there, at the cinemas across the road, and in the many pinball parlors in that precinct. It is also a well-known drug venue and has for more than a decade been regarded as a major institution in the lives of Sydney's street kids, rent boys, and pimps. Phillip started going to Roxy's at about age eleven. Soon he discovered it contained thrills beyond skating. He found out that older youths and young men (late teens, early twenties) would offer a willing youngster money for sex in the toilets, generally a "head job" or they would ask Phillip to fuck them. Nullangardie was not alone in having a youthful masculine sexual (dis)order.

Within three years he had also found out about Oxford Street. This marked the second period in his life, and he presented the next ten years as a continuous round of lovers, drug dealers, and increasing and more serious drug use, punctuated by erratic participation in the inner-Sydney gay community. His sporadic prostitution began at age fourteen, mainly giving head jobs or fucking the punters, with only one remembered instance of allowing himself to be fucked for $130. He was raped by two men who bought his services, drugged him, and offered him to guests as dessert at a dinner party. He spent a lot of time going to many gay venues, saunas, sex shops, and fuck bars because "half the time they let me in for nothing, 'cause I was so young. They got used to me and they liked me, sort of thing."

Sex during this time became focused on two things: short-term emotional relationships and casual sexual encounters. His first relationship had occurred at age fourteen, and it was the moment of his first receptive anal intercourse. He did not like it and has rarely allowed it to happen since: "It just feels like something wants to come out that's not coming out; it's going up." From then on in anal sex he almost always did the inserting:

I don't really like fucking either. I mean I'll fuck someone, but when you do a beat and you fuck someone—I mean, you wear a condom but you still get it on you, you know. And I just get turned off because I have to go with that on my thing and then go home with it. And then, you know, it's really yuk. So now when guys say to me: "I want to fuck you," I just go down. Because I hate coming out with a disappointment, and not being able to wash it off. (Right, so you suck them off?) Yeah. I'll get into it. I love sucking and I love being sucked.

He was not into esoteric sex but can participate if asked:

I don't like fisting, but I like using dildos on guys. . . . I just love munching out while I'm using a dildo on them. . . . I love having sex. I don't get enough of what I like.

The source of most casual sex was the beats. Phillip discovered glory holes (but he did not know that phrase) in a carpark toilet, while working in the reformatory-arranged retail job. He started to spend his lunch hours in the beat. Beats have remained important. He listed off the local ones and described what sounded like the heyday of the shopping-center beat:

That is the best beat I've ever seen in my whole life. Because you find guys, like, in the stairways getting off, you know, a bunch of guys getting off. And you'd go up the top of the whole building, sort of thing, and there'd be guys getting off in cars. There'd be guys sitting there in the nude. And then you'd go downstairs again back to the beat [toilet] and guys in there getting off.

These beats operated all day, he reported, but each has its time and moments — some of them unpleasant. The police once busted him and a casual partner in a toilet with his pants around his ankles and charged him with offensive behavior. He was bashed at a nearby beat four or five months before the interview. In a scene reminiscent of Neil Davidson's experience, one guy approached Phillip who demurred. The guy's mate came over and they beat him up.

He had a standard pattern of beat use: he left home late at night, caught the train to a suburb a few stops down the line and visited the local beat near the station. He timed it so that he could also visit a friend nearby and still get the last train home. Perhaps the extent of his beat use was best revealed when I asked him what was the best sex he'd ever had: "It's hard to say. I really can't say, because, I mean, I've had so much sex. . . . Well, all my life I've been doing it in strange places, you know, like in creeks and pipes down at the creeks, parks, toilets, in buildings, you know, just done them everywhere. So sometimes sex is really good; sometimes it's quite boring, type of thing." There were also a number of female sexual partners but always in threesomes with other boys met at dances and parties. He was raped a second time by a carload of "poofter bashers" during these later years after being picked up walking along a road, "but that only happened twice, thank God."

Phillip had certainly been through a full but messy sexual journey, and clearly, sex was more than a mere pastime for him. It held some key to his sense of self and it formed a major bargaining chip in dealing with life. An end in itself some of the time, sex was also part of the mix of needs he brought to his relationships.

At age fourteen Phillip was living with his first same-age boyfriend in the latter's parents' home. This relationship lasted four months. The boyfriend's mother had just left the (drunken) father, and the unsupervised boyfriend liked to steal the father's car to joyride. They were caught, and Phillip went to the reformatory for a few months. After that came a relationship with a pedophile and the drug dealer. These two men were in their late twenties and became Phillip's lovers, friends, and employers on-and-off over the next few years.

Other lovers have come and gone: the pedophile's and the drug dealer's own lovers who were Phillip's lovers either before or afterward; the eighteen-year-old heroin addict; the rich inner-city "speed" freak; a short-lived affair with a worker in a gay community–based AIDS service organization, which was ending at the time of interview. He still held out the hope of finding the right person. He did not want monogamy, nor did he require a sexual relationship; he was content with closeness and with getting sex elsewhere, if necessary. This kind of relationship has occurred once for him—with a woman.

He met Vicki at the technical college, and they became very close. It was never a sexual relationship (she knew he was gay), but after she and her sister had hassles with her family, they and Phillip squatted in an empty government house around the corner from his mother. This started the last phase of his life before the interview, a period of about three years. Vicki and Phillip for a few years joined forces against the world. They fought the government over the house, and after considerable bad publicity for a government then fighting an election, they were given another Housing Commission home in a nearby suburb. But the network of friends again were the spoilers. Vicki's sister moved out. A lover of the drug dealer moved in and out and in again. Then the dealer himself moved in temporarily, seducing Phillip's newest boyfriend, who not only took to the drug dealer, and his lover, but also the drugs. They set up a threesome elsewhere, leaving Phillip alone.

Finally, a group of thugs, mates of a temporary resident, bashed Phillip. The bashers were charged—hence the criminal compensation case on whose decision Phillip pinned his future. Relations with Vicki became strained by all of this. She started some part-time prostitution to earn money and eventually moved out. An older woman and her son moved in, but after a supposed act of interference with the boy by one of Phillip's friends, Phillip finally gave up the house, his right to purchase it—the lot—and moved back home.

It is a depressing tale of intersecting woe and misery. The rapid deterioration and changeability in his relations with other people is indicative of the basic level of social instability within Phillip's milieu in western Sydney. The effects of lives like this on others is devastating. These are the homeless, the unemployable, the wounded on welfare. They are networked together in a common bond of marginality and dependency; they also collide in their attempt to help each other out. This is the other side to the "cooperative coping" (Connell, Ashenden, Kessler, and Dowsett 1982: 39) noted of working-class people—a resource they each offer and rely on—

but in this case it takes a negative and abrasive form. For Phillip it is a trap; he cannot easily leave it, bound as he is by familiarity, loyalty, and dependency. The one possible place he could go, Oxford Street and its gay community, has failed to embrace or hold him.

Phillip had a somewhat rosy view of Oxford Street. He failed to distinguish between venues and their nuances and subtleties of desire. He participated in the sex life there but failed to negotiate its political and sociocultural life. In Oxford Street, he was a loner, enjoying periodically the joie de vivre:

> I met one guy [the pedophile] and he took me into town and showed me what Oxford Street was all about and it was a real good feeling. I've never experienced a feeling like that before. . . . Just the atmosphere and the music what I liked—the music . . . Flo's—that was the first place I walked into. And when I walked in it was so small and it was flickering lighting. It was just really good. And after that I went to Caps, and I thought it was even better. Remember that song "When Our Lips were Sore" came out? . . . Well that's when I went there.

The city became a magic place, somewhere to escape to. One bar led to another. Then he was introduced to a sex shop with a back room, a fuck bar (by the pedophile), and the saunas (by a drug-dealing cop). But saunas were difficult: "Like I have this thing about taking my clothes off. I only like taking my clothes off if I—if I'm with someone. But I won't walk around, sort of, like a piece of meat, sort of thing." His sexual success in such places was attributed to: "My hair, my big dick, I don't know. My hair, I don't know. . . . Could be 'cause I give good head."

The sexual engagement did not come easily; it was threaded with doubt and uncertainty and dependent on skill. His entry and trajectory were also contingent on assistance. Casual liaisons with partners found in Oxford Street did not develop into relationships, and Phillip's sociocultural involvement there never developed into full friendship circles and social networks. The AIDS service organization worker, a likely introduction to gay activism, politics, and culture, was "too well educated. . . . That's what he kept saying to me: he was 'very well educated.'" That putdown symbolizes the difference between Oxford Street and so many of the more working-class men in this study. The cultural divide it represents, the inequality in access to and appropriation of social resources it exposes, says more about class struggle than is recognized in traditional class analysis.

Oxford Street continued to hold out hope of something better, but he did not feel able to live there: "Well, it's really nice down there. I like it, but I don't—I couldn't—it's nice to visit, but I'd like to live in a house like this, sort of thing, with a backyard. . . . In town it seems like everything's is on top of each other and it's just so fast, and it's more polluted down there than what it is up here." Gay life in western Sydney was not fulfilling either. The only gay venue, Zodiacs, was "somewhere to go. It was a place I never got hassled." At least it offered other people like himself. But neither it nor Oxford Street could offer the haven he sought, and he continued to move between the two communities seeking bits of each at times, leaving one for the other, usually dissatisfied.

Phillip is homosexual, possibly drug-dependent, a convicted criminal, unemployable, and alone. His injuries from the bashing look like they are sufficient for a disability pension, and if so, his social marginalization will be almost complete. If anyone ever doubted that gender is about damage to men too, the hurt Phillip has experienced at the hands of other men should convince them that patriarchy is not in the interests of many men either.

What is remarkable about Phillip was his resilience: his persistent attempt to shift ground from one gay arena to another, from drug user to drug-free; his undaunted pursuit of sex and relationships; his enjoyment of the present, his planning for the future. The main danger (when it comes to avoiding HIV infection) lies in his injecting drug use. He is at risk because his patterns of gay community attachment are not stable or uniformly supportive and his injecting drug user network is unpredictable. He has access to few social mechanisms sufficiently reliable to protect him; and if tested, his own resources will probably be found wanting.

I have spent some considerable time laying out this life history for two reasons. First, Phillip illustrates the intricate and elaborate interconnectedness of a life. Concentration on any individual aspect—his employment situation, for example—yields only part of the dynamic within which he lives. His experience of government instrumentalities illuminates only partly the class limitations involved in the direction his life has taken. His homosexuality alone does not explain the parlous state of his psyche or his fragile grip on social relationships. Indeed, no single factor holds the key to understanding the twists and turns of his life.

This must reinforce the need for any adequate social analysis to integrate analytical concepts, such as class, gender, race, sexuality, age and generation, history, ideology, and discourse. One cannot deny the buffeting Phillip has received, or fail to recognize its origins in larger forces that shape the terms of his struggle. Nor can one deny the struggle itself, the determined efforts to make sense of the experiences, of the contradictions between discourse and experience (particularly in sex), and of the unaccountable propensity for collapse in his relations with family, friends, milieu.

Phillip offers a contrast to Barney, for whom sex is a discrete aspect of life, a delightfully wicked and pleasurable diversion from the day-to-day. The lack of distinction between sex and everything else in Phillip's case raises a question: has there been a shift within one generation, that is, about forty years, in the meaning and significance of sex and sexuality? Phillip's undifferentiated desire lacks Barney's compartmentalization or Harriet's energetically constructed four-part identity, which offer manageable ways of living gay lives. Phillip's sexual subjectivity is not disaggregated, but he has no vantage point from which to understand it. His is also different from that of a gay liberationist like Pip Bowles, who cut his teeth in the inner-London gay community and managed the transition to Australian gay life easily. In contrast, the west of Sydney did not prepare Phillip for Oxford Street.

Phillip has no framework for understanding his sexuality within a larger sexual order, as does Ren Pinch. He struggles from within a far more dispersed and less specified discourse on sexuality, with meaning derived from embodied experience, in pleasures practiced, and through snippets of understanding garnered from a baffling din around him in western Sydney. On leaving this behind when he encounters the more systematic framework of relations offered by gay community life, he finds its appropriation difficult. His accumulation of meaning through practice is too clumsy for these more nuanced accounts of sexuality propounded and pervasive within the modern gay communities. He has no aesthetic. But, in contrast to Barney's increasing marginalization, Phillip remains attached to the idea of gay community life, in its possibilities for salvation. Phillip is caught on the horns of a dilemma; he has yet to find a place in which he can resolve his homosexual desire comfortably in the context of the other conflictual and uncertain parts of his life.

Phillip's lack of resolution might also be simply a product of immaturity. Currently an unfashionable concept, immaturity may yet have explanatory power; another young man in this study, the youngest, offers some evidence to support this possibility.

## Simon Little

Simon Little comes from an inner-city working-class family, his stepfather is a technician, his mother a "nail artist." He is twenty years old and has a twin sister, who is a lesbian, and one heterosexual younger brother. The family was initially raised in an old inner-city working-class area, Newtown, before moving to western Sydney. Simon was close to his mother but not to the stepfather. The twins have become much closer since they came out to each other. His sister's lesbian identity is more definitely political, his sexual identity is more personal. His sexuality is *his* business, and he does not "run around blurting and telling everybody . . . it's what happens in your bedroom more or less. The rest of your life is like everybody else's."

Simon left school as soon as he could and, like Phillip Gibbs, his work history since has been filled with unskilled, mindless, and trivial tasks. He went from this job to that, occasionally with help from family acquaintances, a bar course, instant print work, work in a drunks' pub where he saw a bit of the seamy side of life. There were no other expectations. But it was not factory work and at least he had worked, unlike Phillip. He was trying to get some training in computers; but the idea was no more specific than that, and without qualifications he will face a difficult time.

Simon left home not long after leaving school and returned to Newtown. But the area had changed; it was now less working-class and more gay. He contrasted it with Oxford Street, indicating that his choice of Newtown was aided by this consideration and by knowing gay people from the Newtown Hotel, a major local gay venue. Simon was very anti–Oxford Street:

I hate Oxford Street [and] most people associated with it. I think they give the gay community a hard time about it. You don't have to be a "girl" to be gay, the way I see it. After what happened in this area and on the streets—gives me the shits. . . . And I look at it this way: if you're doing so much for gay rights, gay this, gay that—it pisses me off, because they are trying to get people to accept what they are. Being pro-gay this and pro-gay that is separating themselves from the rest of them. They're pushing themselves but they're not getting any closer, and that's not the way to do it.

In contrast, gay people in Newtown "don't tend to corrupt themselves." There he met other young gay people and started sharing houses with them. These group houses were mixed: lesbians and gay men, non Anglo- and Anglo-Australians. These and other arrangements with gay Aborigines and Islanders were fraught with conflict and short-lived. (It is clear that Simon moved in circles where young black and non Anglo-Australian gays are part of the network. This certainly makes for a different milieu from the Oxford Street crowd he disdained.) At the time of the interview he was sharing a house in an adjacent inner-western suburb with his lover.

Sex came to Simon at fifteen. He knew he was the only one at school who had not done "it"; only he was not sure what "it" was. The first try had ended in vain: the girl told him to "practice on someone else." Then he tried with a girl who turned out to be more sexually experienced than he was, and who twigged to his virgin state immediately. She gave him a quick lesson. This is a far cry from *Puberty Blues* (Lette and Carey 1979) and its picture of the innocent reluctance of young girls pressured by the mindless bollocks of randy boys, which has dominated the discourse on suburban Australian teenage sexuality for far too long. Simon's experience offers a contrasting picture of eager and compliant young boys *and* girls, owning their sexuality and engaging in it in a more resourceful and egalitarian mode than the previous generation.

Simon still considered his part in these explorations "shameful." These attempts were not simply those of a gay boy trying to find or resist his real sexual orientation; he was simply a boy trying to get laid for the first time, just like everybody else. There were a few more attempts, but Simon engaged the heterosexual fray with little success. His early adolescent years were profoundly painful and he reports having spent a lot of time breaking into tears at the drop of a hat. This led to difficulties with schoolmates, but also signaled something about the process of his struggle with his sexuality.

Simon linked this period to an increasing realization that he was attracted to men and that he might be a homosexual. Although deeply troubled by that, he started to find his feet among friends, including young gay people, back in his old suburb. A visit to the Newtown Hotel with a supportive female friend was an eye-opener: "I found myself kind of in seventh heaven. Ah, people like me, all guys, all of that."

Sex with a man came not long after starting work. An older workmate, recognizing the hassling Simon was receiving from other straight employees, became a bit of a protector and eventually they had sex. The older man led Simon gently through the first encounter, using a video as a stimulus. But it was not a grand revelation: "I certainly didn't want to touch him, I was far too scared. I didn't know what I wanted to do. I felt like something—I mean, he didn't pick [up on the fact] that I really didn't quite know what to do." The man clearly desired Simon, but Simon offered no account of what actually occurred. But it was not a discovery of pleasure, a clarification of his interests, a new possibility opening up, a resolution to doubt and uncertainty:

I went home and I spent an hour scrubbing in the shower, scrubbing and scrubbing. I really felt dirty. I couldn't touch myself. It was kind of like I didn't really know what happened. I kind of understand [now] how I felt. I didn't want to touch myself. I hated the thought of it. I didn't want to go downstairs to my family because I felt like everybody was staring at me, even though everybody was behaving as normal except for me.

The anguish was physical. It centered on his body. He thought he was somehow physically, *visibly* changed.

This alerts us to two aspects of early sexual experience. First, Simon's disgust had as much to do with shame at a homosexual act, as with being a "poof." It was a public shame drawn from a discursive realm; he had done something homosexual (not a term he used), something he believed others had long accused him of doing. Everything he was frightened of about himself had been confirmed. This is reminiscent of Ralph Coles after his second beat encounter.

Second, Simon found the physicality of the sex acts themselves repulsive. He could not touch the other man during, or himself after, the event. He "scrubbed and scrubbed," hoping to remove the discursive and physical evidence. It was all in vain; no matter how clean he became and no matter how invisible his shame was to others, he was stained for life. He feared his body would betray his public shame in some way. Unlike Phillip's headlong pursuit of such pleasure, Simon found gay sex profoundly hurtful and damaging. Further, the isolation in which some young men deal with such events contrasts with the experiences of Harriet and his mate doing the beats on their bikes, or with Harry Wight's easy recognition (and subsequent exploitation) of toilets on the way to class. The sexual (dis)order is not easily accessed by all.

The Newtown Hotel and a small "queens corner" at a pub where he worked began to provide partners for further homosexual encounters, some of them in groups. His interest in men began to focus on their physicality. He found that "muscles turned me on instead of [women's] figures. The physique of a guy, the way he looks, the muscle toning. . . . I like the whole lot. I like their legs . . . the face . . . the whole lot. . . . I like big balls." This experimentation, this beginning of a sex life was occurring at the same time as he was trying to find work and moving jobs, and trying to leave home. His new sexual interests and opportunities were an added impetus to leave western Sydney and return to the inner city.

Having a sex life is not the same thing as having sex; Simon found getting fucked was painful right from the earliest experiences, and eventually he stopped doing it. However, he was often the insertive partner if sex did include anal intercourse; it just as often might not, and that was okay too. It is clear that Simon had gained more confidence in sex by age twenty, and part of that confidence came from being in a relationship.

Simon's ambivalence as a teenager about being gay was alleviated in part by his growing group of inner-city gay friends, but a real change occurred as a result of finally having a relationship. Like many young men in this study, Simon was wedded to the idea of a relationship, the right partner, some other person to solve his emotional plight. Simon's first sexual-emotional relationship occurred with a gay Aboriginal Australian. He regarded this relationship in hindsight more as a symbol of attainment of an adult life than as a real, intense engagement between the men themselves. The partner's early infidelity ended the affair quickly and not too painfully. Simon's subsequent and few short stop-start affairs followed a similar path. These were interspersed with a number of one-night stands, about which he felt some guilt, shame, and misgiving.

When Simon referred to his current relationship, the interview took on a lighter almost demure quality. It was a relatively new affair, and Simon was certainly watchful of those "drooling" over his lover, particularly as he was one of the most adored in gay life—a barman at a gay pub. The lover was also HIV-infected, and this meant a sudden immersion in the epidemic for Simon. They practice "safe" sex and since Simon does not engage in receptive anal intercourse anyway, negotiating sex was that much easier. There was the underlying threat of possible progression of the lover's as yet asymptomatic infection. This was one threat to the bliss Simon reported both were experiencing.

Simon first participated in the Sydney Gay and Lesbian Mardi Gras in 1989, dancing on the back of a float wearing nothing but a G-string, accompanying drag queen friends who were, in contrast, frocked to the eyeballs. The float had been entered in the parade by a gay social group from western Sydney. This might be construed as a newly found rapport with the gay community. Yet at this point of the interview Simon immediately returned to the critical theme outlined earlier:

I looked at the newspaper clipping and there was one shot [of the Mardi Gras parade] in it I didn't like—just ridiculous. . . . I look at the way it's publicized on the news and things like that and that's—Mardi Gras I think was originally supposed to be set up for gay people, you know, it's just to let people know that we're here. But the whole idea it's presenting now is just a bunch of queens who love getting round in fancy dress and partying on, and have no ideas of reality, like, there's work the next day and, you know, things like that. They just seem to party all the time.

Simon also referred to the problem of having relationships among Oxford Street gays:

Oh, it's a meat market out there. . . . If you're after a relationship, it's hard to get one. And if you do get one, you got to hang on like all death to keep it, because if you break up, believe me, there's somebody willing and able to jump right in there without even giving you and the person you split up with any chance of kind of making up and working it out, because they're all in like Flynn,[2] either trying to pick you or the other person.

Part of the reason for this bitter response to Oxford Street men is Simon's own unresolved sexual identity:

I think people have got the attitude that gays are always having fun and being happy, and that's bullshit! . . . It's much like everybody else at times, only it can be more depressing.

Simon regarded being gay as more difficult than being straight, and he stated that if he had the choice he'd be straight because it was "easier."

A third stinging attack on gay community–based AIDS service organizations revealed a further aspect of his anxiety: "They're singling themselves out and saying: 'We want this, we want to do this.' *We* all the time, never— why don't [they talk about *all* of] *us*—you know it's just *we*." He went on to argue that gay activists merely push themselves down other people's throats, not giving others a chance to understand and, maybe, accept gays. Those being accosted by gays are then forced to "come back" and will "aggress," as he termed it. Activism, he argued, is actually self-promotion.

His distance from and disgust with the gay community has three elements. First, there is the legacy of a painful adolescence with its experience of isolation and oppression at the hands of peers, the fear of being homosexual, and the fear of self-discovery. These doubts about being gay are yet to be resolved. Second, there is a pervasive disappointment with the gay community as he discovered it: the sexual permissiveness, the lack of concern for the sanctity of relationships, the fickleness of sex/love encounters, the objectification of himself and others, and a failure to offer a resolution

---

[2] "In like Flynn" is a colloquial expression recalling the somewhat legendary sexual exploits of Australian actor Errol Flynn, famous in Hollywood films from the 1930's to the 1950's.

to his pain, that is, his need for love, protection, and safety within a relationship. Third, there is a class-related, milieu-reinforced concept of proper behavior, manners, keeping oneself to oneself, minding one's own business, keeping one's backyard in order and leaving others alone: " 'Cause not everybody has to like it [homosexuality]. People are entitled to their own opinions, right, and they don't have to like homosexuals. They don't have to do anything, so long as they don't aggress or hurt you. They're entitled to their own opinion. So, that's that way I see it."

The stridency of gay politics and the provocative presence of gay community threaten the security of gay men living in working-class milieus. Others interviewed for the study also criticized the inner-Sydney gay community, not for its outward and declared political organizations and activities, such as the Gay and Lesbian Rights Lobby, but instead for the blatancy of Oxford Street gay men, the salacity of Mardi Gras costumes, the offensiveness of the Gay Nuns, and the insistent challenge to "come out," all of which endangers carefully managed lives in less-supportive environments.

These carefully managed lives are not necessarily isolated or closeted. Simon spent most of his socializing time within two distinct homosexual milieus: the first, a group of young mixed-race working-class gays and lesbians in the inner city, whose social activities centered on the Newtown Hotel; the second, a clutch of drag queens and western Sydney gays in social groups like the Castaways (itself an evocative choice of name for a suburban social group). In these milieus, unlike Oxford Street men, people were "not pretentious, they're themselves. They don't have to put on a girlie act"—always a giveaway, an act of exposure threatening to others who are less prepared or able to reveal their sexuality in any way.

These milieus have problematic relationships to the hard-edged, more masculinist, gay community in inner Sydney, with its dance clubs, its finely honed gay aesthetic, and its connections with international gay culture. Young gays regularly ridicule older gay men from the clone-prone gay community of the 1970's as "fisties"—an extraordinary conflation. Older gay men often regard young ones as reaping the benefits of past struggles without due recognition. Drag queens still attract flak from some gay (and especially lesbian) activists and intellectuals despite their astonishing contributions to the origins of gay liberation, to the gay community fundraising programs for HIV/AIDS, and to other parts of gay life. Gay men unattached to gay communities such as Barney Sherman, Jack Sayers, and Neil Davidson are excluded by their age, among other things, and their histories. Geoff Harris and Simon Little find post-clone gay life unacceptable, unapproachable, inaccessible, and often unattainable. Martin Ridgeway has not even tried to approach Oxford Street, apart from the odd visit for a drink in a bar with friends. Of all the young men only Dennis Partridge and Pip Bowles succeeded in joining in Oxford Street gay life.

The process of exclusion described here makes the negotiation of Oxford Street difficult and possibly unachievable. Like Barney Sherman, Simon was not able to fathom the semiotics of modern gay life; it threatened his fragile, still-forming gay identity and exacerbated the quite unsteady grasp he had on his life in terms of relationships, employment and economic security, a sense of direction, and emotional safety. In other words, gayness was still for Simon not so much a resolution to a sexual crisis, but a resignation to a less than welcome state. Unlike Barney, the young, good-looking Simon was sexually sought after (although he experienced this as exploitation); but he was unable to jump in feet first (as Barney would have gladly done) and fuck like a bunny for the hell of it. Emotionally he was not (yet) prepared to appropriate that version of gay life. Sex neither provided the solution (as it did for Richard Cochrane), nor did it compensate for the downside of being gay (as it does for Phillip Gibbs).

Simon's popularity at least means he is no longer pursuing his homosexuality alone. Mardi Gras and the shows at Castaways have convinced him that others see him as a good-looking young man. Confirmation of his attractiveness also comes from friends' complaints that likely sex partners often seek help from them in approaching him. Yet, like Phillip, he does not rate himself as "anything special." Simon is convinced that he is not attractive enough to keep his lover's interest. The lover is taller, more solidly built, and a barman! This contrasts with Simon's "skinny body," although he rates his face as his best feature.

These doubts exist in the face of ritualized validation of his sexual attractiveness. His involvement with drag shows has developed through friends. He performs every few weeks as a dancer to an audience of western Sydney gay men and lesbians, who are "straight-acting, thank God." This involves lip-synching songs, dancing, and generally acting the subordinate cute "boy" to the drag queens' superordinate presentations. Although untrained, he regards his performance as passable and he works at it, practicing seriously at home. He refuses to appear in G-strings there though, or take his clothes off: "No way! They'd run out the door. They want to keep their customers [laughter]." Even in this culturally validated position of the beautiful "boy" Simon still doubts his attractiveness. For Simon, there is no easy alignment between sexual pleasure, his body, his history, his emotional-relational needs, and a gay identity. Much of his unresolved sense of difference as a gay man is still being assessed *against* other gay men rather than *with* them.

Compared with Phillip, however, there is at least a sense of resolution in Simon. He has found gay milieus to join and he has a lover. His economic situation is fragile but he has work. He lives in a very small rented house, sparsely furnished, lacking anything gay apart from Madonna posters; yet he and his lover are living together and he has been looking after himself adequately since he left home. It was a struggle, but he is managing to survive and make a life.

Simon offers yet another example of the process of coming out, dealing with being gay, and of the very paradoxical position the modern gay community occupies in that process. But it is clear that gay community, particularly its current inner-city version, has not as yet presented Simon an approachable option; gay community has yet to develop a workable entry point for either Simon or Phillip.

## Dennis Partridge

Dennis Partridge was Ralph Coles's lover. Dennis is an amusing and interesting person, with a wry sense of humor, and seemed a touch world-weary in manner at the time of the interview. His was a life undergoing great change, and central to the process was his relationship with Ralph. Dennis offered a contrast to Phillip Gibbs and Simon Little—one of total integration in the Oxford Street area. Perhaps gay community can perform after all?

Dennis came from a classic nuclear family: Mum, Dad, and two kids, an older girl and himself. His father, Sydney-born, worked as an auditor in the same company for many years. His mother worked in a shop. They were respectable, white-collar people just one step removed from the Anglo-Australian working class. Their comfortable life was barely secure; an attempted business venture, for which Dennis's father was ill equipped, failed. The mother went to work to support the family and has worked ever since, slowly asserting her rights with increasing confidence and control—a nice example of "contested patriarchy" (Kessler et al. 1982) in the petite bourgeoisie. Dennis's relationship with his parents was difficult. Of his father he said: "My father, I had never really been all that close to. . . . I wasn't the kind of son he would have wanted. He wanted the really, I suppose, the really straight type." Of his mother little was said except that during his late teens, after her ascendancy, she regarded Dennis as wayward and difficult. He resisted her increased pressure about getting a job, too much going out, and so on, and finally left home. Relations were abrasive and distant for years, but had improved recently.

Dennis was educated at the local state schools. He was not a top student, but the consensus was that it was better to finish school. There was some pressure for Dennis to follow his father's path, and obviously some tension in picking school subjects that facilitated or barred entry into that job. There was no evidence that Dennis resisted his father's pressure strongly; rather, he followed his nose and his peers. He was part of a group, not a loner like Phillip, but not one of the sports or academic stars either. He does not regard himself as a sissy, nor was he regarded as such by his peers. He was quite effeminate though; hence my question about being a "sissy":

> I wouldn't exactly say sissy, I don't think, what the straight community think [of] as a "wrist flapper." I don't know, I think it all depends on what your definition of masculinity is. I don't think that all gay boys who turn into gay men are sissies. I have to admit that when I was seventeen, eighteen, I use to think, never having met any gays, well, obviously there are only two types: there's ones like me—there would be ones, like, who are gay, but not really bitch; and then there are the wrist flappers, the real girlie ones.

Dennis is a trainee community worker. He took on the job because it was a way of "helping other people" and because, as he said wryly, his previous work as a prostitute revealed an interest in people. He wants eventually to work in an AIDS agency to help others "of his own sexuality" because "you can't help thinking: there but for the grace of God go I."

He was living with his parents at the time of the interview. This arrangement developed as a way of renewing his relationship with them, and as support during his training. He moved in with Ralph sometime after the interview. There was a sense of some enculturation occurring, with Ralph teaching him about classical music and introducing him to friends and colleagues in the more intellectual milieu Ralph inhabited.

ᕬ

> at first
> a feeling like
> silk, then
> a slight motion
> of lip on lip
> and breathing.
> I take your
> lower lip
> into my mouth,
> delight
> in its blood-round
> softness, re-

lease it. we kiss.
your tongue
explores; for
the first time
it touches mine:
tip and surface,
root and vein.
our eyes open.
—Robert Peters,
*The First Kiss*, 1973

Dennis considered Ralph "attractive . . . nice-looking . . . attractive personality . . . warm . . . thoughtful. . . . I just don't know how to explain it. It is just when I am with him I get that sort of feeling that nothing bad can happen. Nothing bad can happen to me." When Ralph is not there, "I don't feel complete," Dennis said. He used to believe that relationships were not going to happen for him:

> I'd tried having other relationships before. But, I mean, it was either one
> thing or another. It was usually they found out what I had been doing
> before I met them. I'd meet them and a week later I would think, well
> I can't keep working as a prostitute. I have to, you know, because I am
> with them and I am beginning to like them. . . . And at times I felt I
> should be honest and I said it: "You know I use to be a prostitute, but I
> haven't worked since I met you." Some said: "That's okay, that doesn't
> worry me." And a couple of months later they would really freak out
> about it.

Dennis met Ralph in a backroom fuck bar off Oxford Street. One night after "working," Dennis, somewhat drunk, headed there for some sex of his own. A stranger in a dark passage way kissed him and they went home together. It was more than your average kiss on both their accounts. Dennis contrasted his relationship with Ralph to the experiences he had with other lovers. To Ralph he revealed he was a prostitute immediately, and Ralph "didn't bat an eyelid." Sex with Ralph was "very intense . . . we became one." Kissing formed a major part of intimacy. Oral sex offered less on this count, but they went to great lengths to ensure that they kissed a lot when having anal intercourse. In this, the act became definitional with reference to their relationship, in symbolic and real terms.

Ralph was HIV positive; Dennis had been tested six weeks before their first night together and was (very probably) uninfected when they met. Their first night together Ralph fucked Dennis without a condom and ejaculated inside him. They argued that they were both drunk that first

night and had unprotected anal intercourse in a "moment of lust." Dennis
was not sure that he had not had unprotected anal intercourse in the interim since his last test, and so did not blame Ralph for his infection. He
was sure that he was now infected, having had the symptoms of acute HIV
infection a few weeks after they met. He had not been retested to check.

Anal intercourse not only began their sexual relationship, but cemented
it symbolically. In the name of love (and Dennis's undoubted seroposi-
tivity), from that moment on they fucked regularly without condoms. Even
if he was not infected on that first night he undoubtedly was so by now.
This is reminiscent of *Tristan und Isolde*—a bond that grows ever stronger
in the face of exacerbating circumstances, in this case probable illness and
possible early death. Treichler (1988) was only scratching the surface of her
own thought in her "epidemic of signification."

Dennis's first-ever sexual encounter was a homosexual one. On the way
home from school one afternoon, at age seventeen, he had to walk past
a well-known (though not to him) beat. A drunkard walking toward the
toilet offered him $20. Dennis was not entirely clear for what reason. He
refused and walked off home, thinking all the way about the difference between his $2 weekly pocket money and the $20 offer. Even though he was
unsure of what he was to do, he headed back to the toilet again. There were
now many parked cars. The drunkard was not there, but there were others
in various states of undress having sex, and Dennis went into a cubicle with
one of them and did likewise.

He started to go more regularly to the beat and soon learned that being
in school uniform meant much more sex. That suited him because he was
always attracted to older men:

It did not really amaze me that I would get off with a guy, because even
though I was naive in a lot of respects, I think I had known since I was
seven or eight or nine that I was attracted to men. But not until then
was [it] in a sexual sense. It was a feeling of wanting to be really close,
but wanting to be next to or close to a certain boy. . . . Not all boys,
but certain boys. And then after my first sexual experience I thought,
well, I put that [sex] on top of wanting to be really close to them.

The sexual experience distilled a gnawing sense of difference into a dramatic reassessment. Dennis had already experienced the pain of having a
crush on another boy at school, always wanting to be near him, but this
attraction was not simply a sexual urge. He had tried having a girlfriend
like all the other boys; it led to much kissing but little attraction. The crush
remained. He kept thinking it was "wrong," "not natural." So there were

already discourses of perversion in operation in the daily life of the school. But the point here is that Dennis had already physically and emotionally responded to sensations from his body and suggestions from his psyche *before* the realization dawned that these feelings and sensations could also be defined and encapsulated in the homophobic phrases being expressed around him (probably by him, too) in the schoolyard.

I asked Dennis why he thought he was gay:

> Well, if I wanted to analyze myself, which I wouldn't because I don't know enough about it. But I don't know. I don't think—a lot of people say it's because you've got a dominant mother and a weak father. Well, I suppose in my situation, yes, I suppose that is true, *now*. But I started to realize, as I said when I was seven or eight or nine that I was attracted to guys *then*. And you know, I had the kind of family that everybody else has, you know, the strong father and mother who stayed at home. . . . But I do not know, I tend to think that I am gay because I am gay—because I was born that way. Maybe a genetic defect or something.

I quote this in full because it is luxuriant with interpretative offerings. Here we have the process of struggle revealed. He grasps for simplistic renderings of a complex professional discourse, from psychoanalysis, without knowing where the ideas come from. But he rejects it on *experience* because his family relations changed *after* Dennis had already experienced his attraction to other boys/men. A more dangerous appropriation of discourse comes from the "born that way" offering. Here we see a classic use of the one axis of the nature/perversion explanation, but emphasized by the reference to genetics. Or so it would seem. For what is noticeable in listening to the tape at this point and not available from the typescript is the intonation of that last sentence; it was said as a throwaway line, with a somewhat humorous inflection—a joke with a serious underside. This struggle to explain confirms the vital part played by essentialist discourse for these men in their examination and explication of their sexuality. Yet they are not merely absorbers of discourse; Dennis's rejection of the parenting theory shows how these men work to make sense of such ideas.

It is clear that the discursive formulation of homosexuality pervasive in Dennis's immediate milieu was largely that of the schoolyard, plus the general pejorative comments made (probably) by family and friends. These were not the powerful formulations of modern discourses, discussed by Foucault, although they were perhaps influenced by them. Not only should the elite or master discourses not be regarded as dominant in the shaping of Dennis's sexuality, but the earliest of his experiences—his attraction to men, the beat encounter—were not dealt with directly in either the elite or lay discourses. He experienced these events and sensations, and made sense as best he could *after the event*—just as he did with the lay explanations of homosexuality he continually pondered. Even for someone who came to sexual activity as late as Dennis, he did so with the discursive silence about homosexuality only beginning to fill.

In the midst of these sexual experiences on the beats, Dennis came upon an old copy of *Campaign*, Australia's oldest continuous gay magazine. He found an excuse to travel to the city to buy a more recent copy, then went home and read about the bars, venues, and events in the Oxford Street precinct. Three months later he made his first furtive trip to Oxford Street. He was by then out of school, and was working at Burger King at the time. He got dressed up in his best clothes and headed to Patches, the major young gays venue at the time, for his first foray into gay life. There he realized that he was in the wrong clothes, "very suburban, very straight." Everyone else was in tight jeans and short shorts. So he went all the way home, changed into a T-shirt, a pair of shorts "one size too small," footy socks, and runners. He headed back to Patches and

> Took one really deep breath and thought, well it's now or never. And walking into Patches—I don't know, because I realized that everybody in this place, at least I thought there might have been straight people there too. I don't know. But the feeling that everybody in this place felt the same way as I did. . . . But I had known like before I had gone up to Patches that being gay [was] the way I was meant to be.

What is fascinating about this account is the agency. He was decisive, determined, and clever. And he did it all on his own, no going hidden among a bunch of sightseeing friends or with a girlfriend for cover. The quick recognition of the unsuitability of his image and style and his resourceful handling of that was another element in a pragmatic response. His determination contrasts with the incidental accumulation of experience in Harry, the fear-ridden stifling experienced by Neil, or the disjointed excursions into inner-city gay life by Phillip.

This may be partly due to being of a younger generation; *Campaign* existed, bars were advertised in it, the word "gay" was used prominently to describe the growing movement/community represented in the media. A somewhere existed that might offer an explanation, a somewhere not available to older men in the study like Jack Sayers, who only joined a gay organization after he had retired. For Dennis there was already a subculture, its politics and practices — its own discursive practices[3] — calling to his experiences and his dilemma. Its essentialist identity function cannot be clearer. Dennis now knew what he was: "I just thought to myself, if you're gay, you're gay."

But it was clear to Dennis right from the start that what you are and how you do it were different things. He had already heard stories from men on the beats, married men who cheated on their wives and hid their sexuality. He argued in a moment of retrospective reconstruction that he was determined not to be like that. But a positive way to be gay was not that easy to find. He had already learnt enough to know about school uniforms and shorts, however:

I think the biggest shock was when I walked into the disco area looking at the dance floor, and I could still see these two guys, who looked like truck drivers: really big-muscly, short hair, moustached, tattoos down one arm, dancing together, and kissing. I just could not believe it. Like I said before, I thought guys were either sort of straight-acting sort of thing like me, or really girlie. But I didn't think that there were these really butch-looking types; that just knocked me for six!

He started going to Patches regularly. Life became a big party — such a big party that he stopped going for job interviews and eventually left Burger King. He went on the dole and stayed over frequently with new friends in town. Eventually he decided to leave an increasingly troubled home. Two friends, met through gay venues, had a flat in the Oxford Street quarter. They said they were shift workers and that he could move in. Dennis had finally made it to the "ghetto."

This is a nice example of what the Gay Liberation Movement would regard as liberation: a resolution, a satisfactory *inclusion* and positioning for the way forward toward a gay life. However, Dennis reported this resolution on a number of occasions in terms of getting "sidetracked"; an idea given extra weight by his determination to leave prostitution behind. It suggests something more of the contingent nature of the process of gay community attachment itself.

Dennis was unemployed and on the dole when he moved into the inner-

---

[3] I like Dollimore's definition of *discursive practices* here: "a term used to indicate the inseparability of cultural formations and the language used within them; specifically, to denote the interrelationship of (1) representation of the social, (2) interpretation of the social and (3) praxis within the social" (1991: 65).

Sydney area. He went for a number of unsuccessful job interviews, aware that his expenses were now larger than they had been at his parents' home, and money became a problem. As it turned out, his two new flatmates were prostitutes. Dennis's first reaction was to be "confused" and "disgusted." After hanging around the Rex Hotel (long known for its rent boys) with the flatmates and hearing their tales about "cracking it," the negotiation, the techniques, Dennis decided that it might be "exciting" and even "glamorous." His flatmates had said in response to a critic: "I get off with about as many guys as you do. The only difference is I get paid for it."

Concerning the issue of sexual choice—of *desirable* sexual partners—Dennis rationalized that beat sex often led to sexual compromise. One could not always get off with hunks; one often took second best because one wanted sex. He was getting some sex with men, but as a shy person (his words) he usually did not initiate. All of this formed a part of his thinking as he worked his way toward his first night on the game. Business was slow, but he was picked up on the second night, driven to a secluded spot and there he sucked the guy off. He was embarrassed to tell me this. I had to ask a second time about what they actually did. His whole account of working as a prostitute was covered with a kind of thin veil, either because he did not trust me or because he was embarrassed or ashamed.

He put paid to the idea that prostitution is all easy money; most of the time, he insisted, was spent standing around, waiting. The transactions were not always easy. He did not make a lot of money, though "more than what I would if I had been working in a shop." Punters, often married men, or businessmen needing to be discreet, were a varied lot: some were attractive, others were not; some wanted straightforward sex, others wanted to be punished, or fisted. Dennis would comply, although he took a while to get used to some of this. He never allowed himself to be mistreated or put into a dangerous situation, for example, being tied up. He specialized in working a particular park, the Rex Hotel and around Kings Cross. He thought about brothel work but decided against it because they take 50 percent of the money earned. Dennis wanted to remain in control of the action. Like Harriet, he was running his own show.

Dennis presented himself as an athlete, a jogger—very tight short shorts, T-shirt, footy socks, and runners. This was his masquerade in Harriet's taxonomy of desire. He has very athletic legs and knows it. And so winter or summer he strutted his stuff bare-legged on and off for nearly ten years, supplemented at times by the dole. By adopting this masquerade he became desirable, not merely attractive, and "desired." Dennis became a sex *object* in the clearest socially scripted way.

Prostitutes are discursively formed as objects of desire. They are compleat sexual objects, not simply objectified others. They promise and guarantee the satisfaction of desire. They embody sex in a way different from that of women for men or gay men for each other. And they are attainable. There are no encumbrances on their desirability—no pregnancy, no responsibility, no need to reciprocate or provide pleasure (unless one wants to). Sex worker activists emphasize the fact that sex is *sold*, that prostitution has its "industrial aspects," and neglect the fact that more than a service is being traded, that desire is being distilled not in an exchange, but in a transaction in which only the client is satisfied. Or so it would appear in theory; actual prostitution appears to be more complex and human in practice, at least some of the time.

Most of the theoretical work on masculine desire and sexuality is concerned with the subjectivity of sexuality. The life histories in this study have concentrated on the experiential pursuit of homosexuality, the discursive formation of the desiring self, the learning of practices, the construction of homosexually defined lives. In contrast, the discursive formation of Dennis's sexuality was reactive; it was built on being objectified by others. He has experienced his sexuality as *being desired* more than *desiring*: the first offer of money as a schoolboy; the recognition of the school uniform's capacity for attraction; his "dressing up" for Patches; his athletic persona as a prostitute: these were all geared to being desired.

What is it like to embody/inhabit desire, and actualize it rather than hold it at bay? What must it be like to have one's sexuality formed objectively? Most of us do experience or have experienced being desired, but not in so powerfully constructed a way as a prostitute is positioned as the desired, the gazed-at, the longed-for, the enactment of, the source of, the embodiment of sexuality, that is, everyone else's. There is a decidedly masculine character to this desirability; male prostitutes do not transgress masculine sexual desire in the same way that female prostitutes are generally regarded as having transgressed feminine desire.

One resonant account of this subjectivity as object is found in an interview by the late George Stambolian in *Male Fantasies/Gay Realities*, with his "Handsome Man" (1984: 74ff.). The man's flat was full of mirrors and he videotaped the interview for his own purposes; except the videocamera was focused on a mirror reflecting his image as he was being interviewed. The handsome man undressed during the interview because he wanted to watch Stambolian desire him, and he wanted to exhibit his desirability in order to capture a response to it. His desire was shaped around being desired and gazed at and exercised itself in being exhibited.

There is definite incongruity embodied in being an object of desire as a prostitute. Often prostitutes, once hired and chosen for a promise of satisfaction or a special something—remember Dennis's naked legs, come rain, hail, or shine—are then asked to act out some other fantasy, to repeat a sequence, to reenact a previous experience, or be another real or imagined person, one beyond their own masquerade. They may cease to be objects of desire in their own right, and their sexual skills become their most important contribution. It is then the technician who reigns.

How can one regard prostitution simply as work and discount the impact such work must have at the deepest level of the self? Often a sex worker activist argues for prostitution to be seen as work, seeking to connect it with other trades such as clerical work or car servicing; thereby removing from consideration elements of more problematic discourse about the damage such work does to souls, psyches, minds, bodies, and lives. There is good reason to be skeptical about the simple characterization of prostitution as sex work. This skepticism does not dispute the importance of industrial issues and struggles about working conditions and legal status for sex workers, but draws more on the neglected emotional and psychic underpinnings of prostitution in the current political position prostitutes take.

Dennis indicated how he worked at gearing himself up for the emotional challenge of sex with clients: "I work myself up into the mentality of saying to myself when I was out on the street: this is a business deal, that is all as far as I am concerned. They want something and I want something. They want sex and I want money. And it is just like a business merger." This steeling of nerve must have an impact on the sexuality of the prostitute. Dennis's refusal to work when in love is very similar to another proscription common in prostitution. He never let the clients kiss him: "Some tried and I just turned my face away, and they ended up kissing me on the cheek." Similarly, "safe" sex is practiced with clients and unprotected sex is reserved for the lovers, boyfriends, or spouses. In discussing his sexual repertoire Dennis refused some practices because he "could never get that relaxed with clients," indicating the part played by trust in these interactions. No wonder—one client slashed him with a razor blade saying that he had paid for Dennis and so he could do what he wanted with him, and he wanted to leave his initial in Dennis's leg! Whatever else this says about being the object of desire, it is clear that the negotiation in prostitution goes far beyond the financial and the sexual repertoire; there are other, more contingent relational, emotional, and psychic dimensions, and these have a deeper impact.

Dennis talked of fantasizing to produce an erection when necessary, mobilizing his own desire as a functional technique. This is a particular problem for male prostitutes; a non-erection is a very visible absence. It is not surprising if his own sexual capacity was affected in a more serious way than the binary of work/private sex allows. The sex was rarely good or erotic, and it was clear that prostitution had exhausted him. There was none of Harriet's enthusiasm and glee here. In contrast, Dennis experienced long hours on the game, the sensations deadened by drugs ("speed" and "dope," no hard stuff) and displaced by bouts of recreational sex later in gay sex venues, in an attempt to reclaim a diminishing private sexual self. This was still playing itself out in problems in sex with Ralph: "I had a lot of hangups about actually cumming."

Some questions remain. Why ten years on the game? That period was one of increasing intensity about HIV/AIDS, marked by the development of considerable gay community–based services. Although there were fewer sex-on-premises venues of the sort popular in the 1970's, the overall scope of gay life in Sydney had increased markedly. This was also the decade of the remarkable growth of the Mardi Gras, gay newspapers, and legitimate gay businesses. The Oxford Street precinct had many gay bars, video shops, restaurants, and other businesses that usually employed openly gay men. Even Phillip Gibbs gave its black economy a try for a while. Why did Dennis not move to this kind of work?

It seems that Dennis was not sponsored either—no older gay man took him in, introduced him around, or found him work. He remained tangential to the burgeoning gay community, "sidetracked" by aimlessness, unemployability (perhaps), rather than trapped in prostitution by drug addiction or some other reason. Gay community did not reach out to Dennis during these years in prostitution. The key may lie in his failure to develop relationships with other gay men. Perhaps gay community is not as accepting of prostitutes as it pretends to be. Although the prostitute might appear validated by the fantastic photographic images used to advertise their services in gay newspapers, as Harriet noted, *gay* men do not pay for it.

Dennis expressed the need for two correctives to the dilemmas produced by this period of his life: "a job I can at least talk about" and "someone to care about me." Through Ralph and his community work training he seems to have found both. Dennis has now finally embarked on a new gay life of his own—facing an uncertain future in terms of his own health, and a few short years after his interview, Ralph's death.

## Understanding the Sexuality of Boys and Young Men

His feelings, thoughts, etc., were the work of people around him.
Men particularly. The first made a weirdly detached person out of
his body and mind when he was thirteen or something. The next
man corrected his predecessor's mistakes. The next changed some
stuff. The last few had only tinkered because Henry was perfect,
aside from a few bad habits.

—Dennis Cooper, *Frisk*, 1991

A series of themes emerges from the case studies of Phillip, Simon, and
Dennis which elaborate aspects of homoerotic desire revealed in the analysis of Barney, Harriet, Harry, Ralph, and Neil. These themes concern the
process of resolving the dilemma facing men who develop early awareness
of homoerotic interests; namely, the development of homoerotic desire in
early childhood and adolescence through the experience of homosexual
activity; early ambivalence concerning the sex acts themselves; the negotiation of a sexual repertoire; dealing with the character and meaning of
adult homosexual relationships in the context of various sexual communities; and the appropriation of a gay identity and attachment to a particular
gay community.

A striking feature of these life histories is the pre-adult sexual experience. Is Freud's notion of *sexual precocity* sufficient, even in its essentialism, to explain the downright permissive perversity of these youngsters? Is
a *capacity* for sexual expression an adequate basis for understanding the
subsequent sexual explorations among these boys? Does it help us understand the struggle made by these men to resolve the dilemmas of dealing
with homoerotic desire and its embodied sensations? We need a social account of construction beyond that capacity; precocity is a concept awaiting
content.

The circumstances of many of these childhood and youthful sexual
events should not surprise us: sex play with brothers, neighborhood playmates, and school friends is reasonably common. Some cultures regard
such sexual activity as a "natural" part of growing up. Whether couched in
naturalistic terms such as "phases," "stages," "sex play," gesturing toward
a universal human propensity to investigate, to be inquisitive, or configured
as experimentation linked to the "drive" to reproduce, to select partners,
to test physical capacities as part of experiential learning, there are many
ways to conceptualize childhood and adolescent sexual activity, but most
of them ignore the agency of the youngsters themselves.

This is particularly common in the orthodoxies about pedophilia in the
West, despite considerable empirical work on the younger persons' actual

contribution toward, and comprehension of, intergenerational sexual re-
lations (e.g., Tsang 1981; Virkkunen 1981; Wilson 1981; O'Carroll 1982;
Sandfort 1982, 1987; Sandfort, Brongersma, and van Naerssen 1990; Li,
West, and Woodhouse 1990).

Through its intensive cross-cultural analysis anthropological work has
been very important in challenging the universality of the Western version
of sexuality in general, and childhood sexuality and homosexuality in particular (Blackwood 1986; Feierman 1990). However, its scientific approach
has a tendency to categorize and classify, to ritualize and incorporate sexual
activity into a perfectly acceptable, all-encompassing comprehensibility. It
too robs us of glimpses of other, sometimes paradoxical, sides of sexual
interest and contributes to the sanitizing of discourse about childhood and
adolescent sexuality. This sanitizing has not been without some benefit.
There is now a more open recognition of the sexual experimentation of
children. Women's magazines (not men's) and popular-science coffee table
books often contain quite clear messages that "sexual activity is as natural
among children as any other sort of activity" (Diamond 1984: 100).

There are three frameworks commonly used to grapple with this issue.
The most readily recognized is *sex research* or *sexology*, the so-called scientific study of sex. The second relies on *social* scientific accounts and most
often deals with sexuality within the framework of *gender*. The third and
the least often recognized (but more regularly used by gay activists and
theorists) is a more *cultural* and *historical* account. These will be dealt with
briefly in turn.

Some might regard the precocious sexual activities of men such as
Phillip Gibbs or Harriet as unusual, perhaps unfortunate. A few might
even regard them as dangerous. But such sex play is not uncommon among
boys. The scientific literature on childhood sexuality is large and not the
subject of intensive review here. It is sufficient to note that commentators report *without alarm* sexual interests in young children, exploratory
genital activity among children, to include mounting and presenting behavior, masturbation, and so on (see Kinsey, Pomeroy, and Martin 1948;
Schofield 1965).

The loosening of sexual constraints on children has also been reported.
Thore Langfeldt (1981) notes that the incidence of nocturnal emissions (*wet
dreams* is a far more evocative term) among boys in Norway has decreased
considerably due, he asserts, to the increase in masturbation in that more
sexually relaxed society. He also notes that the visibility of boys' sexual
arousal and ejaculation, the development of a sexual language (formal and
informal) among boys earlier than girls, and the cultural expectations for
male sexuality offer the ingredients for a more open and public sexual

arena of discourse and practice. In asserting the easier time boys have of it, Langfeldt notes, for example, that a boy could readily use the word *penis* in certain situations—family discussions, jokes—whereas a girl could not as easily say *clitoris*.

A. C. Kinsey, W. D. Pomeroy, and C. E. Martin (1948) reported that 70 percent of the preadolescent boys in that study admitted to childhood sexual activity with peers (more often with boys than girls) and a third of the sexually active boys continued the activity over a period of five years (p. 167). Forty-eight percent of older males and 60 percent of the pre-adolescent boys in the study reported that such sex play included homosexual activities. Seventeen percent of those engaging in homosexual sex reported anal intercourse, 16 percent reported "oral manipulation," 67 percent reported "mutual manipulation of the genitals" (pp. 170-71). Kinsey, Pomeroy, and Martin went on to say that the chances were greater (one in two) among those with lower educational levels that such play continued into adolescence.

Their data on adolescence is similarly informative. They reported that the sexual activities of boys experiencing an earlier capacity to ejaculate "are far from incidental" (p. 303). Twice as many of the early-maturing boys experienced homosexual activities than the later maturing boys (p. 315). Of those who reach college level, 45 percent have had some homosexual experience. They note in passing that "as a factor in the development of the homosexual, age of onset of adolescence (which probably means the metabolic drive of the individual) may prove to be more significant than the much discussed Oedipal relation of Freudian philosophy" (p. 315). Leaving aside the obvious biologistic thrust of the comment in parenthesis, these data point to a frequency and patterning of homosexual experience far more widespread than many would prefer to acknowledge, much less applaud. Indeed, their report was greeted with incredulity and outrage. It appears, then, using Kinsey, Pomeroy, and Martin as a rough guide (on the datedness and cultural specificity of their data, see Fay et al. 1989), that the early homosexual activity reported by the men in this present study is far from unusual. What is notable is the open, collective, and almost *systematic* nature of that sexual activity.

There is another neglected theme that runs through Kinsey, Pomeroy, and Martin's analysis: the issue of social class. They reported that homosexual relations "occur most often in the group that goes to high school *but not beyond*, and least often in the group that goes to college" (p. 357). The incidence of homosexual activity for single males educated to the "high-school only" level began at 32 percent in early adolescence and rose to 46 percent among those who remain unmarried by age thirty. The accumulated incidence for these unmarried high-school educated men was 54 percent by age thirty. Just short of 50 percent of this category of men experienced homosexual activity between the onset of adolescence and marriage (p. 357).[4] A breakdown by occupational categories was less conclusive, but it reveals a higher incidence of such activity among men in lower-status occupations.

The Australian surveys of sexual behavior among homosexually active men undertaken since the onset of the HIV epidemic—similar in their findings to overseas studies—indicate that over 40 percent of the respondents have university degrees or their equivalent (Connell et al. 1988: 18). A little education is clearly a dangerous thing! Connell et al. note the familiarity of such sampling biases in similar surveys abroad, but also argue the possibility that homosexuality may not be expressed in the same way among men from lower-class backgrounds as it is among the better-educated (p. 24), among whom the gains of (largely university-educated) gay liberation activists have significantly reformulated contemporary homosexual lifestyles as gay. Undoubtedly, there are working-class gay men who identify as gay. The point here concerns not their sexual identity but the structuring of sex taking place among such men in their early years, during youth and young adulthood, and as mature adults pursuing active sex lives before, during, and after marriage. It is this structuring of collective sexual activity, its meanings and relations, that sexology and conventional sex research fail to investigate and understand.

In order to capture a sense of the structuring of this sexual activity, social science has often incorporated sexual experience within the framework of gender, thereby picking up on the male (or female) potential of bodies, and assessing the contribution of sexual experience to the production of men and women. Gender is an attractive concept, since it allows sexual adventuring to be investigated with an eye on the sociocultural resolution of sexual difference. There would appear to be something definitively "male" about the sexual adventuring of boys and youths and something immediately "masculine" about the ease and freedom with which it is explored. But as Harriet has already shown us, gender can be a trap when applied to the actuality of the lives of these men, in particular through its privileging, by definition, of the male/female binary as the fundamental social relation.

The most structural account of gender using this model offered in re-

---

[4] Kinsey et al. (1948) do note the large number of men in this educational category in the armed forces, and in a number of places in their report they note the contribution of such institutional settings to homosexual activity.

cent years is that of Connell (1987), who dealt with sexuality by configuring a substructure of cathexis within gender. This configuration relies on two central concepts: "gender order" and "gender regime." The term "gender order" captures the state of play in historically produced relations within and between the sexes operating in society at a given moment (however incoherent and contested they may be) and includes the creation and contestation of definitions of sexuality and sexual character; the term "gender regime" refers to the state of play in gender relations in any institution at a given time, for example, in a school. There is a sense that regimes contribute in complex ways to the overall gender order and that sexuality is one axis upon which gender regimes and the gender order expend considerable energy, thereby contributing to the overall structure of gender relations in a given society. Can we locate the sexual exploration of the youngsters in this study within this kind of framework?

Harriet's school and Phillip's lunchtime trysts were definitely not part of school policy; nor were they pursued in conscious defiance of it. These experiences do not qualify as part of its gender regime. There is no institutional quality to these explorations, as there is in boarding schools or among boy scouts. Barney's boarding-school experiences were hardly products of school policy either, and even in the reformatory Phillip experienced no homosexual activity. The only example he reported concerned a warder who had sex with a few boys in the showers. If there are consequences for the deployment of power between the boys and the warder in this instance, it is one that could lead to an increase in the warder's vulnerability to exposure.

The contribution of the school's gender regime, if any, lies in its lack of discursive framing of the sex play among boys. For Phillip Gibbs, sex with high-school mates finished in the ninth grade:

(What caused it to finish?)

Um, well, they just started hanging around all their mates and all that. . . .
    They started to, sort of, come out into the straight image and started getting into the drugs and all that sort of stuff, started hanging round rough people. And I, sort of, thought I don't want to do that type of crap, you know, because they're all covered with tatts and big beards.

Although the gender regime of a school is directly concerned with sexual activity among its charges, it concentrates on the suppression and parameters of *heterosexual* relations and activities almost entirely. What amounts to undifferentiated sex play among the boys becomes progressively *homosexual* by default. Those doing it become *poofters*, that is, not real men (with their tatts, their beards, their straight image, their rough behavior), and Phillip was well placed to become the local poofter: "Everybody knew what I was." In this way, the collision of this sex play with the unwitting gender regime of a school does squeeze out homosexual activity, and participants must seek gratification elsewhere when the sexual horseplay in that milieu comes to an end. But to attribute to unwitting gender regimes in their heterosexual parameter development a structural power over boyhood sex play and the body itself is too heavy-handed; this merely shifts the conceptual "weight" from the formative capacity of the sex play itself to something easier to pinpoint.

If the notion of a gender regime cannot serve to conceptualize the systematic and publicized homosexual activity of boys, can we use Connell's overarching term "gender order"? The answer is no. It would be a mistake to configure these collective sexual transgressions as part of a clearly recognized gender order, for they are not part of a hegemonic discourse about masculinity, nor are they simple manifestations of opposition or resistance to it.

On first view it appears that such sexual exploration is situated within the relations between boys and forms part of their masculinizing process. Boys hang around together, they swap toys, cards, stories, and male gossip, they beat each other up, and they have sex with each other. There is a constant interplay of pleasure and power. Each boy negotiates this in his own way.

Kessler et al. (1982) used the term "hegemonic masculinity" to define a culturally dominant, though not necessarily common (or majority) construction, within which boys assess and produce themselves. For example, a school's First Eleven cricket team may represent all that is demanded of, and dreamed about, in being a "real" man; yet most boys never make the First Eleven and are set up for failure by the very process. Other boys are severely marginalized by the process, for example, those nonsporty types, and children like Harriet. In this sense the gender regime of a school (and indeed of a family), in its preoccupation with heterosexual bodies, establishes an ongoing process of defining masculinity as an internal process within masculinity itself, as well as defining it against femininity. Undoubtedly, homosexually desiring boys respond to this process, and there is certainly some evidence that hegemonic masculinity is implicated in the production of objects of desire. Ren Pinch is the clearest example of this, and it is the bodies of men, the muscles, the feel, that Simon Little finds attractive and which he (like Phillip Gibbs and Pip Bowles) contrasts to his own body.

But Ren Pinch's sexual tastes developed beyond this early shaping to very diverse attractions. Other men noted no such connection with heterosexual masculinity as the primary determining object of desire. The younger men speak more of the relational character of sex than its external or fantastic shaping. There are just as many, if not more, gay men indifferent to macho gay as there are interested in it.

To use the idea of a gender order would require the incorporation of these homosexual activities and desire into the general order of sexual things, an acceptable part of being/growing up male. Or it would demand of the concept a capacity to embrace and contain ever-widening resistances, discontinuities, and oppositions. Such an incorporation of homosexuality is definitely not the case either now or ever in this culture (in contrast, see Herdt 1981). Even in its marginalization or resistance, homosexual activity between men is not a tolerated aberration, but an oppressed representation of a not-to-be-spoken-of possibility or history.

To position sexuality within gender, in order to take into account the contribution of sexuality to the formation of sexed and gendered beings and their relations, would seem logical if it is true that "two principles of organization are very obvious in our culture. Objects of desire are generally defined by the dichotomy and opposition of feminine and masculine; and sexual practice is mainly organised in couple relationships" (Connell 1987: 112). These two principles may hold a hegemonic position discursively, and may indeed shanghai heterosexual relations and practices. It is inaccurate to use either of these principles to describe the experiences of the men in this study. In the discursive silence within which these boys/ youths pursue homosex these principles play little or no part. The sexual construction of these men's lives has already moved on apace, before any such heterosexual incursion achieves a formative weight. Beyond this early sex play, these adult homosexual men in their sexual-emotional relations and practices derived little from these two principles. The sexual lineage that produced the intense sexual explorations of Ren Pinch, Robert Cusack, and Richard Cochrane in the gay community displayed little impact from these heterosexual principles either.

Gender fails to accommodate these men, for its preoccupation with the male/female binary relegates homosexuality to marginality or resistance. To investigate the social lives of homosexual men we must leave aside notions of gender order and regime and claim sexuality, with its powerful structuring capacity, as a conceptual tool in its own right.

ᔍ

> man to
> Man. admit
>     it. There's
> Something clean about a well-kissed
> Boy.
>
> —Jim Eggeling, *Aphorism*, 1973

The third discursive field brings to the debate a conceptualization of childhood and youthful sexuality in terms far more erotic than those of the more scientific approaches. It reclaims the body and its sensations for the debate on sexuality and foregrounds the physical experiences of sex. I would like to spend a little time outlining this field of inquiry because, first, it is less well known than the two fields outlined above and, second, it has in recent times become the source of much new work on homosexuality and sexuality theory. I am referring to art, literature, cultural studies, history, and literary theory.

In *Articulate Flesh*, Gregory Woods's analysis of male homoeroticism and modern poetry (1987), the opening chapter, "The Male Body," offers a typology of men, or rather a sexual taxonomy that, he argues, captures the key elements of homoerotic attraction through the ages. Using classical mythology, he outlines the "adolescent pliancy of Narcissus," "the potency of Heracles," and "Apollo's firm but graceful maturity" (p. 9) as three components of a single male body. This tripartite body offers not only a template for configuring aspects of masculinity, but corresponds to three physical attributes of the sexualized male: the adolescent Narcissus "chiefly admired for the delightful promise of his backside," the "unequivocal" phallic talents of Heracles, and finally the ideal of Apollo encompassing all male beauty and sexual possibilities in one being. Woods explores these themes in poetry from a number of angles, but here I chiefly concentrate on the formulation of the sexual attractions of boys and young men.

One of the major discourses on boyhood sexuality Woods offers is a view from an adult man (nowadays firmly, but incorrectly, labeled by many as pedophilic). In addition to the three mythical figures/paradigms already mentioned, he outlines a clear genealogy from a firm conviction about the "ages" of youth to the Ganymede myth, and on to other iconographical figures—Saint Sebastian, Orpheus, and Christ. It is a stunning analysis of the historical formulation of male sexuality within the discourse of poetry; a discourse that underpins the very language and concepts used to create today's images. This framework helps situate the careful positioning of pederasty in John Addington Symonds's *Male Love: A Problem in Greek Ethics and Other Writing* (1983) in which he removes any sense of lust from desire. It is a highly rarefied, ennobling sexuality with (as Robert Peters's "Foreword" points out) more than a keen eye to the debates about homosexuality in late-nineteenth-century England.

With a similar view to the politics of the late twentieth century, David Halperin's work (1990) echoes that of Foucault (1985) in redrawing the terms of our understanding of ancient male-to-male sexual activity and man-boy love (as it is often called today). There is a marked continuity between Symonds, Foucault, and Halperin in presenting a view of the younger partners' place in homosexual relations in terms relevant only to the adult partners, as in the issues of "Ethics" and the "Use of Pleasure." These writers offer a remarkably filleted picture of homoeroticism and sexual activity itself. There are no "bodily fluids"; no one gets "sore" or has love bites on his neck; no one loses an erection or gags when a partner ejaculates in his mouth.

James Saslow's analysis (1986) of the myth of Ganymede in European painting does note the sanitizing of the sexual elements of the rape and abduction of the youth by Zeus. He traces the transformation of Ganymede from the beautiful adolescent youth, through a period of gender confusion from androgyne to hermaphrodite, to the squalling infant of Rembrandt.[5] He reveals a cleansing of the storyline paralleling the historical twists and turns in European sexual politics, but confirms the pervasive discursive position of the Ganymede myth in the development of Western ideas about (male) youthful sexuality.

Another exploration of youthful erotics occurs in work on Herman Melville's book and Benjamin Britten's opera, *Billy Budd* (see Sedgwick 1990). While passion has clearly returned to artistic works such as these, Sedgwick's rereading of them again robs us of sex. In what is otherwise a remarkable structural analysis of the discursive underpinnings of sexuality, her intellectual/academic reading neglects the powerful tensions available to the novelist and the performer, a tension observable in a sensational reading of Thomas Mann's *Death in Venice* by the Sydney Dance Company in their full-length ballet *After Venice*.

In this re-creation the sexual tensions in the original novel are rendered irrefutably homoerotic in a scene set in a Turkish bath where the naked

---

[5] The late John Boswell would have been pleased to note, as evidence of a more continuous gay aesthetic and a relatedness between homoerotic forms throughout history, that Michelangelo's drawing clearly features Ganymede, a beautiful, fully grown youth, about to be mounted from behind, his legs being firmly forced apart by the sharp talons of the transformed Zeus. And to give Rembrandt his due, his nasty infant Ganymede at least registers a displaced sexual response to his plight—he pisses himself!

Tadzio struts his stuff before the voracious eyes of the other naked male dancers. Aschenbach's incapacity to pursue his love sexually is conspicuous; his character remains fully dressed in the scene. Britten, in his last opera, *Death in Venice*, struggled with the same issue of erotic representation and tension and also solved the problem by making Tadzio a dancer. Britten thereby presented directly a sexually embodied youth and enhanced his sexual mystery by making him mute in an opera! As a consequence, Tadzio's own sexual quest remains silenced.

These representations all rely on adult views of youthful sexuality, sexual interests, and sexual urges. Collectively, they form a powerful genealogy from which gay theory and politics have drawn remarkable insights into human sexuality. These discourses have also been deployed with less political and intellectual success in some discussions of pedophilia, an issue still dogging all gay politics and receiving an undeserved thrashing in the current bedlam that marks the sexual abuse debate. This in itself should warn us of the historically contingent nature of any discursive endeavor.

· · ·

> At the country picnic the 12 year old boy
>     wanders off by himself in the woods,
>     he knows the perfect spot.
> On his study-hall break to the library
>     the 13 year old stops in the empty john,
>     just enough time for a quickie,
>
> · · ·
>
> The voluptuous 19 year old youth knows
>     he's got the whole beach to himself today,
> He basks naked in the sun till baked,
>     then floating on the bosom of the lake
>     gives himself the best handjob of his life.
>
> · · ·
>
> He just smiles remembering the first time
>     he jacked off from a cliff,
> The ecstatic boyhood semen spurting and spurting,
>     tumbling thousands of feet
>     into the valley below.
>
> · · ·
>
> (Antler, *What Every Boy Knows*, 1983)

This poem exemplifies a second reading of boyish/youthful sexual interest, presenting a view of an authentic sexuality from within a continuum of masculine sexuality. Antler's poem offers an alternative to the previous almost unerotic readings of boys'/youths' sexuality by adults; but it too is concerned with a natural and autonomous sexuality. Antler's boys masturbate whenever and wherever they can. They are sexual and lusty. He presents a picture of an insatiable drive, a perverse will to orgasm, an opportunistic exploitation of possibilities for sexual activity. Similarly, William Burroughs's *The Wild Boys* (1982), with its hallucinogenic undercurrent of transgression and subversion, posits a *collective* will to sex among boys: "Five snake boys release cobras above a police post. As the snakes glide down the boys move their heads from side to side. Phalluses sway and stiffen. The boys snap their heads forward mouths open and ejaculate. Strangled cries from the police box. Faces impassive the boys wait until their erections subside" (p. 229).

In the visual arts from Greek pottery, through von Gloeden's *Taormina* photographs to William Higgins's video pornography, similar encoding of boyhood and youthful sexual interests occurs. Whichever of these two points of view we take—Halperin's or Foucault's discussions of the intergenerational homosexual lives of the Greeks, or J. D. Cardinot's pornography with youths fucking each other in schools, reformatories, scout camps, or seaside resorts (the *sanitized* or the *authentic*)—there is a clear discursive continuity underlying these formulations. There is a certain acceptance that childhood (itself a problematic term) has its sexual side. There is no argument with Freud. Nevertheless, a kind of legitimacy is sought and imposed by most analysts through the employment of concepts such as ritual (Herdt) or culture (Halperin), or historicity (Foucault), nature (von Gloeden) or perversity (Cardinot), and so on.

There is an almost unacknowledged acceptance that these discursive configurations represent the sexuality of actual boys. Take, for example, von Gloeden's photographs of Sicilian boys and youths (1984). In these we have a German aristocrat rendering the local youngsters as forever desirable, sexual but in a very "natural" way (their nude bodies readily positioned in innocent proximity to one another). They are also presented in another "naturalistic" dimension (rocky coves, Mediterranean beaches, trees, wild landscapes), yet culturally inscribed too (Greek allusions, large pots, trailing cloth, garlands, Arcadia). The occasional unequivocal sexual signifiers (touch, particular stances, a naked adult male caning a naked boy's buttocks, a certain positioning of genitals in the photographs) betray another interest/fantasy.[6] These photographs were originally regarded as collectors' items for the classically educated aristocrats of Europe, winning prizes. Today, they are again major works in the collections of famous

---

[6] The difference between "nude" and "naked" is a debated one in art, particularly when the sexual explicitness of representation is in question. If the subject is male then the issue is further confused (Saunders 1989).

art galleries, though their homoerotic element is much more explicitly recognized (Cooper 1984). They are also sold to tourists as postcards by the villagers of Taormina (Leslie 1978), raising the question of how the young men of Taormina today see their sexuality and how they are seen by visitors to the village.

These few examples reveal the often deterministic accounts of sexuality that dominate the social constructionist *versus* essentialist debate by introducing other countervailing, historically specific, yet rarely subversive discourses that inform conceptions of male homoeroticism. There is much work to be done here reformulating and redirecting our post-Foucauldian thinking, to recognize a more fragmented and multifaceted discursive formulation of male homoeroticism (a larger frame than homosexuality), as a context within which all young men come to their early sexual experiences and feelings, and some seek deliberately to define themselves.

The few contributory fields of inquiry sketched here reveal a still largely deductive and text-preoccupied technique; yet most come from a distinctly post–gay liberation era. The rise of international gay communities has offered an enlarged range of possible ways to capture and reformulate much of the discursive territory of homoeroticism. Many of the works mentioned above were defiantly gay-produced. The two poems come from *The Male Muse: A Gay Anthology* (Young 1973) and *The Son of the Male Muse: New Gay Poetry* (Young 1983). The references on von Gloeden (1984) come from, in order, a book published by Gay Men's Press and a lightly informative and softly pornographic gay magazine *Blueboy* (Leslie 1978).

These represent two of many publications, organizations, media outlets, and cultural producers responsible for the ongoing seizure and reformulation of homoeroticism through cultural discourse among gay men internationally. They add to a collectivist project of manufacturing gayness through such clearly identifiable codification, burgeoning political activity, and increasing theoretical work among a gay intelligentsia. These activities occur concurrently with an ongoing organization of gay men's lives into recognizable gay communities. This politico-cultural seizure is deeply implicated in the production of modern gay communities socially, sexually, and culturally.

It is this discursive complexity which informs many gay activists and theorists and underlies our prevailing understandings of the lives of Phillip, Simon, and Dennis. This formulation of boyish/youthful sexuality comes largely from the adult point of view, with its concurrent strand of libertarian autonomy presented in poetry, literature, opera, sifted through in theory production, cultural representation, and political activism. These affect how we understand homoeroticism as much as, if not more today than, the structuralist frameworks prevailing in gay theory a few years ago. It is no longer adequate to render to Caesar, Jehovah, or Hippocrates only; we are responsible for our own homosexuality.

Yet these remarkable and challenging conceptualizations fail us; or more accurately, fail Simon, Barney, Phillip, Harriet, and many others who took part in this study. Theorists and activists alike remain ignorant of how these men live, love, loathe, and leave each other; how they deal with oppression, with bashers, with the state; how they are handling HIV/AIDS, safe sex, death, and dying. These men offer a quite different narrative from that of our discursively informed, powerfully deduced, but ultimately theoretical account of homosexuality.

A simple example of this failure is found in dealings with the body. Phillip Gibbs gave no account of the physical sensations of his first sexual experiences, except to say that he got "sore." Simon Little readily acknowledged difficulties in the first experiences of anal intercourse and gave it up fairly quickly. The taste of semen in oral sex, the smell of bodies (again, Simon's first encounter comes to mind) provide further evidence sufficient to acknowledge that the process of sexual skilling is difficult and none too straightforward in practice. There is a startling contrast between the experiences of these boys and those discourses which inform gay communities about (homo)sex. Compare the following:

> I don't really like fucking either. I mean I'll fuck someone . . . but you still get it on you, you know. And I just get turned off because I have to go with that on my thing and then go home with it . . . it's really yuk . . . I just go down. Because I hate coming out with a disappointment, and not being able to wash it off. (Phillip Gibbs)

with:

> . . .
>
> At my penetration
> he quivers like oceans cupped among continents.
> But we contain each other, and he is safe.
> . . .
>
> From the anus of the earth
> perfumes of sensibility and learned blossoms ascend;
> we sweat casual beauty.
>
> From the remorseless cabins of his body
> love reeks; and I exult that from seeds of excrement
> I breed poems.
>
> (Laurence Collinson, *Himn*, 1977)

## Toward a Structure of Sexuality

In order to grasp fully the constitutive nature of sex and sexual relations in the lives of homosexually active men such as those in this study, we must establish a framework for understanding sexuality that stretches beyond these existing paradigms toward a *structure* of sexuality. As a start to outlining a more systematic understanding of this structure, I have employed the idea of a *sexual milieu* to describe the early sexual activities of these boys and youths, their collective nature and their ritualistic character occurring within a *discursive silence*. A second field of practice is that of the *sexual community*, a terrain covering more diverse and (dis)orderly sexual possibilities, with often conflictual and competing discursive formulations informing its action, seeking to fill the silence. A third domain is that of *gay community*, now a self-sustaining and generating sociocultural field of practice, sexually constructed/ive and shaped by a rapidly evolving reformulation of homosexual practice and sexual subjectivity.

Phillip's explorations with his boyhood mates took place behind a veil of secrecy. Although Phillip encountered no direct injunctions from parents and other authorities, the transgressive connotations of sex were carried beyond the circumstances of the activity and into the choreography of sex itself. What is clear from Phillip's story was the central importance of such activity to him. Sex became the medium of exchange between him and other boys in a small, localized sexual economy. It was a major source of bodily pleasure for them all, a fact not to be disregarded or played down. Above all, it was an integrated component of their play, their explorations of the local area, and of each other.

Phillip was not the lone masturbating child. The two sets of brothers in his story were fairly open about their sex lives with each other—these were not furtive foursomes—and the high school paramours were alarmingly forthright about trading information on and accepting Phillip's services. This corresponds with similar activity talked of by other men in this study. There is an acknowledged collective homoerotic practice wherein boys pursue pleasure with each other.

The formative nature of such early sexual experiences is difficult to estimate, but there are some standard elements in the story. Both Barney Sherman and Jack Sayers experienced childhood sex play on farms with male cousins. Jack continued the play throughout his childhood and early adolescence unnoticed, but Barney's early idyllic play gave way temporarily to a clear injunction from the mother. From that moment on Barney's sexual activity became unnatural, naughty, clandestine; it became transgressive.

But the risk attached to further exploration was outweighed for Barney by what? the physical pleasure? the naughty delight? willful disobedience? Whatever it was, the clearest legacy of these injunctions, though, was that sexual pleasure must be hidden.

In a similar vein, whatever the kudos obtained from his childhood sex tales by Harriet today, the sexual badgering he attracted as a child was a powerful counterpoint to his experience of a daunting injunction against sex. The public betrayal by his parents, a confusing police car ride and the humiliating rectal examination did not lead to abstinence. It did not prevent an even more open exploration of sex from age six or seven, again on a neighborhood scale and across generations for "ten cents a poke. No, hang on, a shillin'," with boys banging on his door demanding sex, particularly older boys, and as well as one of his father's mates.

The attempted suppression of sexual interest—Barney's knife-wielding mother, Harriet's humiliating encounter with the police—cements in place not only the need for secrecy but also notions of an (often unspecified) wrongness of sex. These incidents structure sexuality at a physical and psychic level. They are part of systematic, yet strangely incoherent antisexual discourses informing and shaping these boys' practices, which render homosexuality as a silent domain of pleasure and transgression. I say incoherent because it is not at all clearly spelled out; and, anyway, beyond the post hoc injunctions lay tempting pleasures already tasted and priapic peers stalking sexually engaged/aroused boys, offering an insistent counterpoint in permissive practice to the discourse of continence and constraint.

What I call a *discursive silence* is the unspecified and confusing structuring of sexual interest; a silence which in its very embarrassment and disregard for childhood sexuality offers little or no detail on the nature of sexual wrongdoing. The men in this study as boys were left largely to their own devices within this silence to follow the pleasures of their own bodies. Its single victory was secrecy not celibacy.

A sexual milieu must remain a small local and periodic phenomenon, existing in moments such as in Phillip's neighborhood, Harriet's street of beaus, or particular conjunctions in Barney's boarding school. These milieus are contingent on a number of factors: a certain tolerance (turning a "blind eye"), a facilitating change in previous social conditions (a new shopping center or recreational facility), a change in personnel (new boy in town), physical conditions that create opportunities (the beach pavilion, changing sheds, the housing estate construction site), and so on.

Individual entry into sexual milieus is clearly not *individual*, as such. These are moments of entry into existing milieus, collectively, historically, and experientially formed, yet anarchic in character, in that they rely on the pursuit of the body's unclassified possibilities in the face of inapt (and inept) generalized prohibitions about sex. It is important to remember also that the sensations of the body have often been explored already by individual boys alone (as Ren Pinch revealed) and then are brought to sexual milieus and engage each other in this discursive silence.

There is instability and contingency in these milieus, derived from within the history of the local area by its participants, old hands and newcomers, through the passing interests and fads or fashions among its young, often tangential to its masculinizing practices. As well, the sexual activities are influenced by external deployments of power: the local toughs, the rapes, the tyranny of kids over each other; the sexual politics of families; the actions of police, teachers, welfare workers, and local government.

There is an absence of discursive formation of the preponderant character required by such concepts as "sexuality," "gender," "drive," and "libido." The determinative nature of much of this discursive paraphernalia, and also of the psychoanalytic account of sexual interest, renders the experiences of these youngsters as functionalist end products of preset configurations of desire. In fact, the sex play of many of the boys is an exploration of bodies and sensations wildly oblivious to more serious and oppressive (sexually repressive) frameworks within which these men may, later, reformulate their comprehension of these acts.

In contrast, the highly elaborate, explicit discourse relating to "homosexual" activity of Herdt's Sambian male youths fully *informs* the sensations of the sex act (1981). The acts themselves are deeply embedded in supportive cultural elaboration and explication. The childhood and youthful explorations illustrated by Barney, Phillip, and others in this study rely far too much on happenstance and opportunity to be considered manifestations of larger structuring or discursive formations or deeply etched libidinous enactments. It would be a mistake to ask that such collective practice carry the weight of perversion, a refusal to conform, a desire to retain wayward possibilities, a denial of constraint.

However, sexual milieus are capable of structuring practice and meaning, of clustering and encoding possibilities, and are formative in that sense. The conceptual dilemma is to render these pleasurable sexual explorations and transgressions in terms that suggest the systematic, formative, and deeply social nature of the pursuits, but avoid a deterministic account. There is order here. There is even predictability. But Foucault's "deployment of sexuality," while existing largely in the operation of the state and the elite discourses, has made little incursion into these sexual milieus.

The youthful sexual experiences of some of these men takes us from the local sexual milieus to more institutional settings. Homoeroticism among schoolboys in single-sex schools is well known, and Barney's experience was only remarkable in his passivity. It would be tempting to cast the incidents with the school teacher, for example, as sexual abuse; an interpretation favored at present as the *only* way to understand intergenerational sex (see Maasen 1990). But there is a strong element of voluntarism in Barney's account; he was willing and he was able. What's more, he did not remain passive for long. He sought similar contact after school. The readily available sex between men and youths reveals a glimpse of a sexual (dis)order that quite frequently and systematically provided boys and men with opportunities for significant "sexual outlet" (to use a term from Kinsey, Pomeroy, and Martin [1948] which seems strangely appropriate in this instance).

Barney's era of adolescent sexual exploration occurred at the same moment in history as the Kinsey data were being collected. The 1940's was a period when a large number of men were in uniform, and Australian cities were responding to the war with a not inconsiderable, unofficially sanctioned easing of morality. Sydney's Kings Cross was then (and remains) the center for prostitution synonymous with the fast lanes of sex and corruption. The homosexual subcultures of that era intersected with this seamy side of Sydney life (Wotherspoon 1991). Barney's twenties also coincided with an era in Australia of high economic growth, plenty of money, and a significant easing in sexual morality. The wowsers were no longer in control.

Barney's is not a classic example of a passive young man being "done" by exploitative adults. Although there is no evidence in these tales of his initiating anything sexual, it all seemed to occur without much effort on his part. And, as he indicated, he went looking for it. It is an age-old ritual really, recognized by all protagonists: the boys present themselves and seek out contact; the men know how to read the signs and take advantage of the curiosity. Both know the sites and circumstances where such activity can occur.

One of the astonishing (and frightening for the press and police) aspects of the infamous Clarrie Osborne case in Brisbane in the 1970's was the ease with which boys, approximately 2500 of them, sought and engaged repeatedly in sex with the unprepossessing, aging, balding parliamentary reporter and, moreover, were prepared to be photographed and documented for his extensive records. Osborne argued he could always tell a boy was interested in sex just by looking at him (Wilson 1981). Osborne's accounts to Wilson are full of detailed "scripts" wherein Clarrie could encourage the boys to have sex with him by utilizing a very sympathetic and detailed understanding of the sexual urges and experiences of the youths. The boys themselves reported:

He seemed a nice guy and he could talk about anything and I knew he wanted to do something with me even though he wasn't being heavy about it. And when he was talking he put his hand on my cock and just gently rubbed it and it seemed nice. I can't honestly remember whether he told me to take my pants off or whether I just took them off so he could get his hand around my cock more easily, but it didn't really matter because I wanted to do it. . . . I enjoyed talking to him and I enjoyed the sex as well. . . . All I know is that I wanted to have some sex then and I got it. (Wilson 1981: 39)

Had the anthropologists who had investigated male sexual behavior in Melanesia (see Herdt 1984) observed the sexual adventuring of youthful Barney Sherman, or the adult Clarrie Osborne for that matter, they would have classified these practices as rituals in the following manner:

There are many designated places where men and boys meet in order to engage in sex, such as parks, large cinemas, and seaside pavilions. Here, boys go when they are looking for sexual activity; men await the boys and instigate various sexual acts once contact has been established. This usually occurs in silence in the back section of these cinemas and sometimes in automobiles, public toilets, or changing rooms. This male-to-male sexual activity is markedly more hidden and unspoken than in countries to the north of Australia, where boys fellate their elders as an acknowledged part of the manhood initiation rites. However, many of these Australian boys engaging in sex with men also experiment sexually with peers, male and female, and some do so with older women. Most would appear to transfer all or most of their sexual energies to the opposite sex later in life, as also happens to the north, partly for the purposes of reproduction. However, a small proportion retain a sexual interest in their own sex and become a specific subculture known as "gays." A larger but unspecifiable number marry, yet continue to meet with men for sex in such venues.

The point need not be pushed any further. Anthropologists debate their proclivity in analyzing cultures in such ways. It serves to highlight the contrary approach wherein most sex researchers looking at our own societies usually constitute male-to-male sexual activity among boys and between boys and men as deviant, marginal, *ab*normal.

From this study a different picture emerges; one where a considerable number of adolescent (and occasionally younger) boys would seem to engage in sexual encounters of various kinds with other boys and, to a lesser degree, with men, in and outside family life. This homosexual activity is more commonplace and *normal*, even worthy of being thought of as ritu-alistic. Such a proposition would not require all males to engage in male-to-male sex; rituals can be constituted by significant minorities. Barney's experiences may represent those of a significant minority of men and boys, most of whom do not become or remain homosexual.

In contrast to any notions of repression, these youths embarked on fully fledged sex lives, experiencing bodily, not just fantastically, the demands of desire. They found a range of sexual possibilities, from beats to localized clutches of queens, dragons, and peers.

The sexual communities of Nullangardie, the beats, the networks of the western suburbs of Sydney, the secondary gay community around New-town opened up broader opportunities for sex with men. Martin Ridge-way's is a clear example of this process. He had his first sex at a beat in western Sydney at age twelve. After more random events, he went with various partners in their cars to parks or secluded places for sex, even-tually being asked home by one partner. While visiting homes of other sexual partners he met their friends. Return visits constituted relationships of sorts, often in the context of outings with such partners to local gay venues. There he met others his own age and recognized a culture beyond sex. Eventually he fell in love, and by age twenty was living in a gay couple, complete with house, garden, swimming pool, and room for a pony.

The beats were central to many of these men. Beyond the freely avail-able and wanton sexual activity itself, they offered possibilities of explor-ing relations beyond sex. For Harriet they also provided entry to social and sexual networks of men in Nullangardie. These sexual communities were quite diverse, providing discursive possibilities for shaping and fram-ing sexual identities. Harriet emerged from the process a fully fledged "dragon," Martin became a "couple," and Simon became a "non-scene" gay man.

For others, these were confusing moments. Dennis Partridge struggled to interpret his crushes on other boys until his quite delayed sexual initia-tion in the beats. Even then, the physical sensation of the experiences (in a manner similar to eighteen-year-old Harry in the toilets on the way to college) provided a powerful counterpoint to the patchy incursion of pro-hibitive discourse. Dennis Partridge's determined first trip to Oxford Street quickly led to further trips, new friends, and sex partners, and the space created by the discursive silence began to fill quickly.

These sexual communities provided relational bases for explorations of homosex and preliminary discursive practices in which to refine a sexual identity and consolidate other aspects of an emerging sexual subjectivity.

The men brought with them to these sexual communities a number of resources: bodily experiences of physical pleasure; a recognition of collective transgression; an inchoate discursive framework for understanding sex (the practice) and desire (the sensate yearning) in the process of being encoded in various, often contradictory ways; and established patterns of practice in pursuing these sexual pleasures. These resources offered a more than adequate position from which to bypass, override, or ignore (rather than refuse or resist) their slowly intensifying definition as deviant, as homosexual.

The young men in this chapter had in common a pursuit of the social and sexual possibilities of the inner-Sydney gay community; a community where the dilemmas of their sexual interests might find some resolution. Yet each was less than successful in attaching himself to it. An important component of this was the framing and shaping of homosexual desire itself, a confusing aspect of which was their experience of being desired.

The idea of being objectified and desired rather than (or as well as) desiring is quite important in the structuring of a sexual subjectivity. Phillip did experience being desired, and understood it in terms of the attractiveness of his hair and, less surely, his big cock. In spite of this, he remained uncertain about his sex appeal, and he pursued sex in beats rather than in the more socially demanding clubs, bars, and cultural events.

Simon experienced his desirability as less welcome. Although he was a popular "boy" for the drag queens, he still experienced sexual advances as predatory, as a manifestation of a "meat rack" sensibility. For all the bravado of the G-string on the Mardi Gras float, Simon insisted that gay men, the *desiring*, were spoiling it all for him, threatening his security, undermining his coming-out process, invalidating his friendships, and threatening to steal his lover at the drop of a pair of 501s.

Dennis, his desirability confirmed already within the adult sexual sphere of the beats and his legs clearly acknowledged as a sexual attraction, launched himself into the new sexual world of Oxford Street. Yet within a short time he was a prostitute, and that desirability encompassed a quite different range of meanings and was mobilized for purposes at odds with his own sexual pleasure. He experienced diminished satisfaction in his private sexual domain, and a series of damaging relationships revealed a gay community rather intolerant of his prostitution; he was desired only on certain terms. Being desirable/desired is a mixed blessing.

Discourses on men as the desired, and particularly the desired of other men, are not generally available. Certainly they are in short supply for homosexually active youth. Those so desired may borrow from heterosexual discourses on women's desirability to explain others' responses to them and to shape their reaction and self-formation. The increasing influence of gay male representations of the homoerotically desiring and desired, and the exercise and embodiment of such desirability in homosexual praxis undoubtedly contributes to a more general formulation and development of a desired/desirable male. The dilemma is that the passivity of being desired is at odds with hegemonic masculinity. It is not surprising that these desired young men experience some confusion about their sexual subjectivity in the process of moving from a more carefree sexual milieu to a more complex sexual community, and beyond to a problematic gay community.

In their transition from suburban life to inner city, from sexual milieus to gay communities, these men confronted other constitutive aspects of sexual subjectivity: its cultural and representational manifestations within gay community. Simon got closest in his G-string. Dennis played out its fantasies bare-legged on the game. Phillip gained temporary success in free entry to sex clubs. Yet, faced with the prevailing discourses of male homoerotic desire in the Sydney gay community, none of these men has yet begun to succeed as Robert Cusack, Ren Pinch, or Richard Cochrane did in their time.

Along with the poetry, theater, and art, which offer a discursive framing of youngsters' sexuality and of the experience of sex, new discursive formations and visual representations of homosexuality and the images and practices of gayness in modern gay communities are shaping sexual life. Here I briefly examine two fields of practice and representation that dominate the ongoing recalibration of gayness and gay community: the Sydney Gay and Lesbian Mardi Gras, and pornography.

One of the wonders of the annual Mardi Gras is the representation of male homosexuality as living works of art. The celebration of gayness; the exhibition of sexual interests in a semiotics of desire and their actual exploration; the barest of bodies; the drugs, dancing, and daring: the Mardi Gras must be acknowledged as presenting all with a dilemma. The desiring, the desired, and the desiring-to-be-desired are all encoded and on display. The event becomes a collective representational festival of sexual subjectivity. This blatant act of public representation has its major moment in the Mardi Gras parade, but for the Australian and, increasingly, the world's gay communities the month-long cultural and sporting festival and the all-night dance party offer a more community-specific focus.

At all the Mardi Gras events, dress (or the lack of it) offers one clear code. Where did the minuscule lycra dance shorts as a signal of gay desirability come from? And before them, where did the gym/bicycle shorts come from? Before that, cut-off jeans? Before that, the strategic holes cut in the jeans? Before that, the jeans themselves, the 501s? Right the way back to, twenty years ago, black bell-bottomed trousers with three-button waist bands and gold pendants? The external shape of desire has been changing before our eyes.

The increasing presence of naked flesh, particularly muscled flesh, in gay community culture is a little less difficult to document, for physique photography was catering to a wide homosexual audience and formed a major discourse on sexual freedom in the 1950's and earlier. But even in physique photos of the 1950's pectorals were not anywhere near as present or lauded then as they are today. The body has become less a biological given and more a sculpted and transformable possibility, with specific attributes—chests, penises, buttocks—assuming iconographic status.

The early days of gay liberation lauded the androgyne and eroticized smooth, lithe, hairless bodies and long hair. Today it is nuggetty little muscles and ponytails. Hairless chests and shaved legs are features of approved beauty. Yet ten years ago moustaches, hairy chests, and dark features were lusted after. There is a new relationship between youthful beauty and its androgynous yet narcissistic masculine promise; "macho" has been replaced by "machette."

If we look at images used in gay community advertising about HIV/AIDS for example, we can see some familiar sights: the use of erotic imagery predominates, nudity is frequent, youthfulness always a factor. There are familiar items present; subcultural icons of a gay life to which all gay men are assumed to have access and in which all might participate. It is argued by gay community–based AIDS service organizations that it is important to attract gay men's attention and that such images are what gay men want to look at. What exactly do those images promise: practicing safe sex will net a gorgeous guy like the one in this ad? If you practice safe sex, you will be gorgeous too? If you keep safe sex up, there's a promise of erotic experiences beyond your current repertoire? There's an intimacy to be had through safe sex that you may not have had in your life until now? There is a sense of belonging to a community to be found through safe sex? Do these images really say that? In this study some of the working-class participants indicated that although not averse to nudity and homoeroticism, they prefer different images.

Gay communities are constantly manufacturing gayness, and this process has expanded, with HIV/AIDS educational materials adding to other forms of cultural production. These meet in the middle in publications such as *Ecstatic Antibodies* (Boffin and Gupta 1990), *AIDS DEMO GRAPHICS* (Crimp with Rolston 1990), the HIV/AIDS issue of *Art and Text* (1991), and

*Don't Leave Me This Way: Art in the Age of AIDS* (Gott 1994), which, in their commentary on the process of representation, actually produce further encodings.

How do the old, the ugly, the physically different, the black, feel when faced with these evolving representations of gay sexuality? Could it be that these representations *exclude* as much as they *include*; that they *invalidate* as much as they *validate*; that they *distance* some expressions of homosexual desire as they seek to *incorporate* and *colonize* others?

These images build on a larger existing culture of representational and discursive manufacturing of gay community and gayness. The burgeoning gay publishing industry offers a steady stream of new novels, poetry, short stories, glossy news/info monthly magazines, imprints of old "classics," unending glossy photographic essays on the male nude, and refulgent theory development. Gay film festivals reveal a surging interest in any and every film with even a hint of the "celluloid closet" (Russo 1981). These all have an impact on gay sexual subjectivity and enhance gay identity by situating it not just in a collectivity, in a local "scene," but also within an international and historical framework. It is a powerful sociocultural transformation.

There are further challenges in homosexual practices themselves. Some of this influence can also be understood by examining the nature of the emerging international gay culture. An English AIDS activist recently told me that among other types of men, he really likes having sex with Castro clones, that is, the classic macho gay men from San Francisco. The reason: when he has sex with a Castro clone he knows exactly what is going to happen, how it will start, the sequence of moves, the sounds, smells, and drugs. The choreography of sex is perfectly familiar right down to the dirty talk and the buttock slapping accompanied by all those phrases that pass for dialogue in pornographic movies: "Yeah, do it, do it! Fuck me, fuck me! Suck that big cock! [Slap]." Sex is predictable; the men become almost interchangeable and you can be sure that you will cum every time.

Now while this account is a none too subtle British dig at the North Americans, it does point to something about the sex gay men engage in: that it is also shaped to a great extent outside the actual sexual moments themselves. Sex is actually a collectively structured pursuit rather than a private act. Gay men may constantly learn from experience, but also learn from the meanings given those experiences by others. Attention is drawn to the particular activities, body parts, sequences of events, images, and language, and these help mold the experience of sex in ways often transparent. And nothing draws attention in the sexual domain of gay life more than pornography.

My first visit to the huge supermarkets in Canberra from where pornography is distributed by post all over Australia was disappointing. It was astonishing how "vanilla" the gay pornography was. It was porn as art rather than lust; beauty featured more than action, and the closest it came to exploring the perverse was a little bit of highly predictable leather. While one is not so weary of sex that these expensive images of youths disporting themselves in and on each other has no effect, one must ask: Have gay men finally become respectable? Are gay men no longer "sexual outlaws"? It is not my intention here to discuss pornography in terms of the fruitless pro-porn/anti-porn debates seen over the last few years. One hopes the work of Lynne Segal and Mary McIntosh (1992) might at long last counter the destructive, antisex stridency of feminist antipornography crusaders, or the largely guilt-ridden pleadings of the Men's Movement (e.g., Kimmel 1990).

Let us consider instead pornography as a lecture in technique, a fantastic adventure out of the mundane, a visitation to a pleasure dome, an exploration of the self, that is, as an erotic practice. Essentially, gay porn is a bit like watching television when there are only two channels: a North American channel, and a French channel. The West Coast of North America seems preoccupied with size—size of penises, chests, thighs—with white teeth and unblemished protein-fed, currently hairless (though previously hairy), prime hunkettes, who mumble their monosyllables and bravely take or give it like a man. The French are preoccupied more with youth, with androgynous beauty, and with extending the perversity of gay sex by exploring setting, context, the frisson that comes with transgressive sex—sex where, by some other standard, it ought not to be. Asian and South American pornography is taking off but offers no challenge in imagery or plot. A neophyte Australian porn industry capitalizes on a similarity to North Americans; if there is a local authenticity, it comes, I suspect, from small budgets and the absence of body doubles.

Irrespective of the source, the viewer is offered a particular cultural vision of gay sex, a hegemonic image that subordinates other representations of gay sex. It is also exemplary sex; they always fuck, they always come, they are always beautiful, they are always desired, and they will forever be so. It is consciously pursued sex; these are directly embodied pleasures. Nothing deeper is offered. The viewer seeks and sees skin, sweat, semen, and for some inexplicable reason, socks (usually white ones). Those fucking lack darker or more complex motives, even if the "plot" pretends to sketch out such possibilities. They will—damn them—never, never step out of the TV set and walk toward you. In the meantime the porn user is left spent, satisfied for the time being, perusing the catalog for a new image, a new fantasy, another sexual exemplar, another orgasm.

I do not consider it dangerous to watch or read pornography. Most gay men have a quite functional relationship to it. It may be obsessive for some; but then so is romance. The question I pose concerns the lack among theorists of a critical relationship to pornography at the level of sexual practice, and beyond that to the discourses that shape desire. (An exception is Randall 1989.) Pornography is a major discourse that contributes to shaping images of homosexual beings in its constant reflection and re-alignment of the pleasurable, its redefinition of the erotic. This continual remaking of desire in gay pornography, over and above the actual experiences of sex itself, is transparent to the user. In this way it contributes to the daily manufacture of homosexuality.

Pornography has been another player in the first decade of HIV/AIDS, and it will continue to be a major player for the foreseeable future. Its contribution to living with the sexual constraints of the epidemic, to representing gay men's struggles in homosex itself, and to gay men's sense of ourselves as sexual beings in the face of an ongoing health threat is yet to be determined.

Pornography and the Gay and Lesbian Mardi Gras are bright, larger-than-life representations of gay sexuality, but as they assume iconographic status their power to disturb grows. It is this power, this hegemony, that Simon rails against in relation to the photographs of the Mardi Gras parade. It is this pressure for a certain kind of gayness that Harriet resists in his frocking up for an HIV/AIDS fundraiser, ignoring the calls for male strippers coming from the younger gay men now used to tours of Australia by West Coast American porn stars like Jeff Stryker and Blade Thompson.

Yet Mardi Gras and pornography are not the only images of homosexual desire. Other images are appropriated from a number of sources, much of it the North American discourse, which dominates international gay culture. It is not that the incorporation of imagery, the translation of homoerotic desires into codes is inauthentic at all, or to be rejected. They are vital to the reorganization of gay men's lives, and each man's appropriation is real; they do signify the self-in-community. In this, they are further elements in the overall production of a collective sexual subjectivity. These responses to homoerotic representations and their ongoing transformations should not obscure from view the social character of the process. What these men reveal is the struggle involved in that appropriation and the difficulty they experience in keeping up with an explosion of hegemonic gayness that marks the contemporary gay community. Moreover, the "pace" with which this transformation of gay life has occurred, especially in the last twenty years, is remarkable, as is the "distance" covered in that time. It is precisely that distance which Phillip, Simon, and Dennis try to cover. It is the pace from which Barney and Harriet have increasingly slowed and so fallen behind. It is a transformation in which Neil Davidson and Jack Sayers have been bypassed.

Each has learned to deal, to some extent, with the subordinate and oppressed condition of homosexuality; though pertinent, this is not the main source of their difficulties. In response, Phillip, for example, seeks a sanctuary for gay people; Simon wants a quiet stable acceptance; Dennis seeks a "respectable" place of worth. For all three, the resolution to the dilemma of their desire for other men is only partly resolved by their attempts to appropriate gayness.

The young men's dilemma—how to deal with homosexual desire and extensive sexual practice in sexual milieus and other sexual communities—left them seeking a resolution in the discursive frameworks and practices on homosexuality and gayness in the gay community. Although all three are sexually attractive to other men, this newer sexual community did not answer their needs, nor do they find it satisfactory.

Of none of them can it be confidently said that they have resolved their dilemmas of desire. For none is sex with men the problem. Phillip is no longer "sore," and Simon no longer needs to "scrub and scrub"; Dennis no longer needs to press his "private" sexual desires into service. But these men found (homo)sex far from ideal in assisting them in gaining for themselves a place in the sexual firmament. All have experienced difficulty in forming and sustaining relationships with men.

Phillip, Simon, Dennis, Harriet, Barney, Martin, Geoff, and others offer a quite important picture of the structuring of sexual experience. Not only are the elite discourses and their practices—medicine, law, science, the church—startlingly absent from the lives of these men when boys or youths, but so are these more cultural/literary/political configurations of homosexuality. The latter appear highly romantic, fictional, and absurdly artificial in comparison with the sexual milieus in Phillip's neighborhood and the toilets of Nullangardie.

By the time these youths/men approached the gay community of inner Sydney, the impact of its cultural and political seizure had been transforming understandings of homoeroticism well beyond a sexual identity as gay. The homoeroticism of modern gay communities now offers, and is continually building on, a sophisticated political and sociocultural architecture of reorganized sexual practice within a powerful discursive framework and a highly elaborated and choreographed sexual cultivation. The edifice created has to be breached by those trying to gain entry; this is obviously much harder for some than others.

Neither Phillip nor Simon has managed to find or experience a fit with the prevailing forms of contemporary gay life. Each has tried and, like Barney, has experienced partial success. Their rejection of/by Oxford Street came about not because they had aged (as Barney has) but because (like Barney) they brought to the task of appropriation a limited set of tools.

Gay community reveals itself now as far more complex than a range of practices, a code for understanding the immersion of homosexual men into the newly configured and ever-growing development of gayness, as a resolution for sexual desires for men, or a collection of like-minded persons into a group. These three men reveal much about the process of trying to attach oneself to a gay community. They offer examples of earnest explorations and of the traps and pitfalls of the process. They exemplify the partial appropriation of a gay sexual identity and offer the beginnings of an explanation to the dilemmas gay communities face in building that social sanctuary men like Phillip (still) imagine. *Being* gay is simply not enough.

These lives also point to a definite structure of sexuality; one based firmly in sexual experience and contextualized within overlapping patterns of social relations. The trajectory—the sensations of individual bodies engaging a collective abandon in the discursive silence of sexual milieus; the slow discursive definition in the (dis)orderly practices of various sexual communities; the negotiation and appropriation of gay community as a sexual, political, and sociocultural sexual subjectivity—is neither fixed, sequential, nor universally experienced, nor is each part necessary. Although the gay communities are building an ever more attractive proposition, there is no definite or single outcome. Yet. But there is no doubt that these experiences are neither random nor accidental; there is too much order for that. These are not simply aberrant experiences of individuals or of a tiny minority; rather they are historically formed, quite widely experienced patterns of sexual relations between boys, youths, and men that offer quite systematic possibilities for the resolution of desire.

# 8

# Reflections

⸜

It seems trite to say sexuality is complex, but it is important to say that homosexuality is what makes sexuality complex. But further, I should think that it is beyond doubt nowadays that it is homosexuality that constitutes sexuality, at least as it is understood in modern industrial societies and, increasingly, in the developing world. By this I mean that the very core or heart of our understandings about, and our theoretical and empirical work on, sexuality to date has relied, a priori, on that discursive construction known as the homosexual. This we know from the work of those theoreticians famous in sexuality, many of whom have already been cited in this book.

In the same vein as these insights, it is important to note that from this moment on, the deployment of sexuality will rely increasingly on the discursive construction of the pedophile, who for the coming century will perform the task that the homosexual performed for the century nearly past. In the same way, gender will have to contend with/rely on the discursive construction of the transsexual.

This complexity of sexuality, however, relies largely for its sense-making on individuated formulations, in particular, the *identities* of which we are so fond in theory and politics, and on the binaries of male/female, masculine/feminine, homosexual/heterosexual, as the starting points for demarking the differences that fascinate us. These individuated formulations and the binaries that support them then allow us to comprehend desire, fetish, object choice, pleasure, pain, even power, in sexual activity, as either a socially constructed event or process, or as a coming to the self, a finding of truths, a redemptive moment of human progress.

There is one trap in all aspects of these formulations: they leave out what is difficult to fit into the picture. They delete the ambiguities we experience in relation to object choice and in the emotional-sexual relationships we make. They omit the ambivalence we experience toward our own and others' bodies. The contextual disaggregation of desire, captured better by our poets and fiction writers, seems strangely absent in the sexuality we theorists represent.

As the men in this study were interviewed, as they revealed their proclivities and trajectories, as they revealed the seeming incongruities that constitute their sexual subjectivity, the complexity of sexuality, the disaggregated nature of desire, the impossibility of identity, became clearer and clearer. The misgivings I experienced so strongly in relation to the two Amsterdam conferences were consolidated. The dangers in the formulations of sexual activity I saw dominating HIV/AIDS behavioral research were convincingly confirmed. Both rendered gay men as passive and subjugated, if in very different ways. Both boxed (homo)sexuality into a marginalized compartment within and from which little movement was possible. The theoreticians, burrowing their way toward the textuality of desire, lost the texture of sex; the behavioral researchers, counting the contacts, marginalized the meaning and numbed the sensation. Sexuality is rendered self-ish.

The dangers of these formulations are clear in a number of pressing concerns for gay and homosexually active men, and it is to these this study now turns. As the men in this study show us, being gay (or homosexually active) in the era of AIDS is a complex ongoing struggle, a struggle with the self at each moment of sexual engagement, a struggle with other men similarly engaged, a struggle framed powerfully by homosexuality itself, both as discourse and as practice.

## HIV/AIDS

It is no wonder that in the face of the exigencies of the HIV epidemic, gay community–based educators are struggling with a never-ending list of prevention and care/support issues and to sustain their efforts and compliance with safe sex guidelines in gay communities, increasingly in the absence of applicable theory and usable research findings. The practice of HIV/AIDS education, its pedagogy and curriculum, have been left to chance. Little research has ever been undertaken on the *educational* processes that guided the mammoth change in sexual behavior achieved over the last decade in gay communities in response to the epidemic. (Davis, Klemmer, and Dowsett 1991 and Davis et al. 1993 are exceptions.)

None of the men in this study is unaffected by the epidemic, whose full impact in the Sydney gay community will be seen in the next few years. The gay community newspapers in Sydney are often full of obituaries; the rate of loss is increasing; the burden of care is nearing its height. The survival of a number of these men, such as Ren Pinch, depends on state-of-the-art antiviral therapies and awaits further scientific breakthroughs. For those on these various drugs, or awaiting trials of new ones, their health is fair. But Richard Cochrane and Ralph Coles will not be the only men in this study to die of AIDS-related conditions. That fate is ever present for Ren Pinch, Geoff Harris, Dennis Partridge, Barney Sherman, and Dan Berger, all of whom are caring or have cared for other HIV seropositive men.

None of the uninfected men finds the HIV epidemic distant or unimportant. Many are activists, care givers, friends, fundraisers, lovers, and ex-lovers of men infected with HIV. HIV/AIDS suffuses their lives. Even for Alex Lawes. His status as a married, bisexually active man enables him to regard HIV/AIDS as someone else's problem. Yet, HIV/AIDS has a nagging presence. He donates blood regularly and, since the Blood Bank tests every donation for HIV antibodies, he uses this as a periodic indicator that he is still uninfected. He has reason to be concerned. Morrie Layton is also a married, bisexually active man. However, he is dying of AIDS, cared for by an uninfected wife. These two men remind us that not all homosexually active men register a connection with gay community, gayness, or even being gay, and this is still an obstacle in dealing adequately with the epidemic.

There are other effects of the epidemic that these men exemplify. Most men told of a close shave with "unsafe" sex—events that are useful to investigate, since they reflect on the always vexing issue of sustaining safe sex among the gay communities in the second decade of the epidemic.

Peter Standard reported being HIV-seronegative in the SAPA survey in 1986, but at the time of his interview for this study (one year later) he declined to discuss his antibody status. It had been some time since his regular partnership of many years ended and the sex practices he allowed with casual partners in his safe sex regime definitely ensured that he would not come in contact with HIV: he restricted his activity to mutual masturbation, kissing, and some body rubbing and massage. His sexual frustration was evident in diatribes against the local gay community–based AIDS service organization for continually failing to clarify the safety of oral sex. Having given up anal intercourse completely, Peter argued that if only some clarification were offered on oral sex he might at least obtain some satisfaction in that practice. His very strict regime even went as far as masturbating side by side so that no precum or semen could land on his body. The tension in this regime was palpable, and its restrictiveness had proven unsustainable on three occasions in the previous year. On each occasion Peter allowed the partners to fellate him and he ejaculated in their mouths.

Dan Berger has broken his safe sex rules on the odd occasion in casual encounters. It is unlikely that he put his partners at risk: in fellating a few men and swallowing their semen, he may have actually put himself (given his compromised immune system) at risk of STD infection or, possibly, HIV reinfection.[1] It is in these *lapses* we see something of the difficulty some men have in keeping to their safe sex decisions.[2] It reminds us of the fact that safe sex is not simply achieved; it is an ongoing struggle.

For Ralph Coles, the development of gay community safe sex guidelines occurred at the same time as he was infected. He knew all the right answers to questions about what is "safe" and what is "unsafe." In spite of this, Ralph decided that if a casual partner suggested an "unsafe" practice, either verbally or by body movement, it meant that the partner was probably infected too; otherwise, why would anyone take such as a risk? Ralph did not believe in HIV reinfection, so he thought that he was neither running a risk of endangering his own health nor endangering the other "infected" man.

As we know, this was a delusion. Dennis Partridge had been tested a few times and was HIV-seronegative when he met Ralph:

Ralph kept saying to me all the time, it is "unsafe." What we are going to do is "unsafe." And, I don't know, I just thought, this is just a one-off . . . it's hard to express. I think at the back of my mind I still had that same mentality. I'm careful most of the time, so if I slip up once, maybe I will get lucky and not get it.

It was a moment when two imperfect safe sex strategies collided and went badly awry.

The examples of safe sex rule breakage involving oral sex, which many regard as of "small risk" of HIV transmission, indicate something of the ongoing process of *doing* safe sex. Dan Berger and Peter Standard went (in their terms) all the way; their "unsafe" lapses represent an enormous jump from no oral sex to full ejaculation in the mouth. Peter, the man who called anal intercourse "double the pleasure," currently allows no anal

---

[1] There is dispute over the possibility or the likely effects of HIV I reinfection.

[2] "Lapse," though markedly inadequate to the task, has become a common term to distinguish single events of "unsafe" sex from a return to a persistent pattern of "unsafe" behavior, namely, "relapse" (Kippax et al., "Relapse," 1992; Adib, Ostrow, and Joseph 1992).

intercourse. Is he likely to go "all the way" if and when he lapses? It would appear from the example of Ralph Coles and Dennis Partridge that this is distinctly possible, even among well-informed men and when the risk of HIV transmission is very high. If a man has made the adjustment to using condoms for anal intercourse, a slip to unprotected anal intercourse is a small (but no less dangerous) leap. However, a move to engage in unprotected anal intercourse from a safe sex regime that bans all anal contact is a much more complex posture for HIV/AIDS educators.[3]

This points to a need not just to concentrate on getting the message about the riskiness of unprotected anal intercourse across to gay and homosexually active men, but also to offer a graduated list of sexual activities that explains more about safe sex than protected intercourse. For example, a message about not sharing sex toys can be expanded to include clear statements about the "safe" use of dildos and fingerfucking, as well as the usual step-by-step instructions about lubricated condom use. Programs that eroticize safe sex need to focus on the internal contents of specific sex practices. Attempting to shift the emphasis toward "safe" activities, particularly those not focused on oral or anal contact, can have only limited appeal among men for whom such contact is both the most important emotional and physical source of sexual pleasure.

Even Robert Cusack, who has seen so much death, can make a mistake:

> I'd gone for a very, a very attractive man at the sauna, and [we] just sort of [got] carried away and I probably said: "Oh hell, forget the condoms" or things like that, you know. We had, I, I, we had anal or [pause] he screwed me and er, we sort of said afterwards [that] it was very foolish, but he knew that he was negative and I knew I was negative at that stage but—
>
> (Did you talk about that at the time?)
>
> We, we discussed it afterward.
>
> (Afterward?)
>
> Yes, we knew how stupid we were sort of thing, but he had more to lose than I did 'cause he had a lover.

Beyond the practices of safe sex, the men in this study exemplify great diversity in their sexual activity, relations, and meanings. In particular they

---

[3] In the Netherlands for a long time the safe sex message for gay men advocated no anal intercourse at all. This has proved unsustainable, and the Netherlands in the 1990's began to report the highest levels of unprotected anal intercourse and the lowest level of condom use among gay men in the European Community (Pollak et al. 1992).

reveal the need in HIV/AIDS work to take into account various components of homoeroticism. The significance of certain practices comes not only from their physical pleasures, but also from the skill associated with their enactment, from memories of experience, and from a recognition of the body's capacities. The choreography of sexual encounters and the great diversity of sites and circumstances for homosex in gay communities and in the wider sexual (dis)order point to a cacophony of meanings, fantasies, and representations in which to encode "safe" sexual practice and with which to tease out its attractions. In preventive education, variations on the theme of one particular practice or another need to be offered in detail, and the promise of satisfactions encompassed by those variations must be assessed realistically. I have yet to see a safe sex pamphlet (written in clear simple language for a high-school dropout) address Phillip Gibbs's favorite practice: "munching out" while he fucks his partner with a dildo. And there is an urgent need to address Barney Sherman's inventive use of condoms: "I always find that a bit of cream over your penis first before you put your condom on—that's where I find success. Because the condom will grip . . . the anus, and your prick slides in and out of the condom."

Each sex practice, which in its unprotected form is capable of transmitting HIV, has a "safe" counterpart: condoms for anal sex, gloves for fisting, dental dams for cunnilingus and rimming. But it was not Ralph Coles's lack of knowledge about condoms that allowed him to fabricate his negotiated "unsafe" incidents and to lay the groundwork for infecting Dennis. It is the relationality of these acts which contextualizes the action and invokes and creates meaning. The continued reification of sex practices in most of the current research on gay men's responses to the epidemic will never explain, beyond their frequency, the *construction* of sexual moments, particularly the "unsafe" ones, in any terms leading to either a comprehension of the phenomenon or the development of adequate prevention pedagogy. The concentration on convergence in such research, namely, finding the majoritarian experience, neglects the immense diversity of meaning associated with each man's sexual intentions.

Beyond practice-focused educational strategies, the question of intimacy and sexual negotiation within relationships is vital. The contrast between Harry Wight's successful strategy in threesomes and Dennis Partridge's unrolling the condom from Ralph's penis in that highly charged *Liebesbeweis* could not be stronger. Intimacy in anal sex is a central motif for most of the men in this study who practice it. Education about safe sex must move beyond its concern with abstracted practice to assess these relational contexts of sex, its symbolic dimensions, the process of negotiating safe sex, and the (mis)use of HIV-antibody test status involved in that negotiation.

This last issue emerges in many forms: HIV-seropositive men choosing only to have sex with other already infected men; HIV-seroconcordant men assuming that trust is enough and the condom is not needed. These pressing problems of prevention emerge *because* of the complexity of sexual meaning and context for gay and homosexually active men. It is precisely the ingenuity that led to the invention of safe sex which is leading to these ever more complex reinventions of how to have (homo)sex in the epidemic.

This dispersal of concerns, problems, and issues in prevention raises the question about the representation of gay sexuality offered to gay and homosexually active men by their various communities, their AIDS service organizations, their sex services, pornography, magazines, travel promises, images of gayness, and so on. How safe sex is represented is vital to achieving compliance with its ideals. The men in this study exemplify a more fractured homoeroticism than our gay community–focused and -situated AIDS educators often recognize. Therefore, any representations of, or metaphors from, Robert Cusack's and Ren Pinch's sexual adventures within the gay community will have little resonance for Simon Little or Neil Davidson. Yet these representations dominate, and their dominance in safe sex education obscures the fact that the particular medley of sexual experience reflected was achieved by only some men.

There is no doubting the loss to gay men that safe sex constitutes; in particular the multiplicity of meanings and pleasures associated with anal intercourse detailed by the men in this study. There is a disturbing possibility that the long-term effects on gay sexual culture are more serious than yet imagined. Where once male homosexual abandon was premised on a fearless exploration of flesh, fluids, and numerous and fantastic permissions to transgress, now wariness is ever present. Gay men's bodies have become untrustworthy. Pleasures are forgone and that is a real loss. The once-shared meanings have altered: there is a cautiousness about and distrust of sex; nagging doubts about safety persist; concerns about partner choice linger; the need to negotiate, the need to protect oneself and the other, bedevil sex itself. These are changing the intrinsic character of homosex, gay life, and being gay. The impact of the epidemic on gay communities and their sexual culture is profound, and the impact of this transformation of gay sex is yet to be fully witnessed or assessed.

Yet there is extraordinary resilience among gay men if those in this study are any guide. Their resourcefulness in dealing with HIV/AIDS and safe sex highlights their individual contributions to stemming the epidemic.

Harriet received a lecture from a friend early in the AIDS scare, after a particularly messy group encounter where he was the receptive partner. Since then he has used condoms for oral and anal sex, lots of lubricant, lots of relaxation, especially for the "big" men. And he has developed a style all his own in insertive intercourse:

> With any guy that I let fuck me these days—if I do, I've got to be really, really, greased before I let anything up me. And then even when I'm fucking someone now I'll pull it out after a couple of pushes, right, to get it—pull out to see if the rubber is okay. Then after I go for about five minutes I pull it out again and just to have a look. And I make it part of the root, like, pull it all the way out and check and get back in. And even before I blow I'll still pull out to see if I'm okay with the rubber.

This is not paranoia but carefulness. Would that all gay and homosexually active men were so consciously responsible for both pleasure and protection.

### Safe Sex and Beats

Given the central place of beats in the lives of these men, particularly in their sexual explorations as youngsters, it is important to consider the consequences of the epidemic on beat sex. There is still "unsafe" sex occurring at beats (Bennett, Chapman, and Bray 1989). But Harriet, a barefoot educator if ever there was one, has one solution:

> Well, if I was a beat worker and I walked in, I'd stand there, I'd put my hand on my hip and I'd say: "Look you pair, do youse know what youse are into? Have you got a rubber on? No. Well, do you know what diseases you can get from fuckin' like that without a rubber. If youse want to do anything, for fuck's sake put rubbers on because youse are only—if youse are sick, youse are spreadin' it. And if you're sick you've just given it to him and vice versa. Youse have gotta do something, you know. Youse can't go on infectin' each other. But youse are 'okay'? How can you know he's not sick?" I'd have a go at 'em, definitely, but I'd also hand 'em a rubber and say: "Look, if youse are gonna do anything, please wear this. So I don't have to worry and people don't have to worry about you."

Yet this "known homosexual" is not allowed to contribute his obvious skill to fighting the epidemic this way. The Nullangardie gay community foolishly disowns Harriet as a gay man, and by choosing the approved (Sydney) model of a beats worker invalidates him further. It is a terrible loss to HIV/AIDS prevention education.

The experiences of the men in this study offer little doubt that "beat sex" is everywhere—in Sydney's parks, at truck stops in the Midwest of the United States, in the public toilets of London, on the beaches of Spain, in railway stations in Bombay, or knee-deep in the snow in Copenhagen. The masculine sexual (dis)order that beats represent so clearly must disturb any pretense that the homosexual/heterosexual binary has any status at all; rather, the conditions for venturing across the binary become the substantive concern for HIV prevention.

## The Issue of HIV Positivity

Ralph Coles remembered vividly his moment of infection with HIV, as did a number of men in the study. At a beat one afternoon Ralph was fucked *seriatim* by three men. He regarded this as a matchless sexual moment: "But even though I know that's when I got it, I still look back on that as a fantasy—being fucked by three different people." He experienced acute HIV infection symptoms two weeks later.

At his interview for this study, Ralph had resigned himself to an early death, probably between five and ten years hence; it was exactly five. Dennis Partridge is roughly three years behind him by their reckoning. Ralph was involved in AIDS care, education, and politics. He saw many die, including clients he had cared for as a volunteer. It was difficult to face his own future so frequently and so determinedly, but he did so courageously. Geoff Harris, in contrast, has refused to be involved in HIV/AIDS support groups for this very reason. In his own efforts looking after sick friends and lovers, he strongly resists becoming part of the gay community volunteer programs that offer support to those caring for people with HIV. For Geoff, it is his normality within/as gay that sustains him; he fears its loss inside his HIV serostatus would cripple him.

In a similar way, Dennis Partridge does not want to know of his ongoing health status. He regards the ordeal Ralph went through of regular T-cell tests, his angst about their levels, as far too worrisome. Dennis regarded AIDS as "an unreal illness until you get full-blown AIDS. Because you can go on your merry way maybe for five years with this thing inside you and still feel one hundred percent." He refrained from thinking about AIDS as much as possible (even if he worried about Ralph). But with Ralph's death, the focus of the infection has shifted to Dennis.

In interviewing the men who were HIV-infected, I tried to ascertain their interest in, and access to, therapies and support programs available through the gay community–based AIDS service organizations. Findings that access to such treatments and programs of support is related to social inequality would not be unusual in any study of healthcare systems in advanced industrial societies, including Australia (Sharp 1991). But things get more complicated when it comes to gay men.

One consequence of the second interview with Barney Sherman was the recognition of just how much my understanding of HIV/AIDS treatment issues is determined by my access to inside information from government, health professionals, other researchers and gay community activists. My words—"treatment regimes," "trials," "PCP," "access"—were gobbledygook to Barney. He talked of "tablets," "trying out this new drug," "this chest thing." He had no synonym in his vocabulary for "access."

This was not simply a case of the usual researcher-subject mismatch in language or education level. The cluster of issues around therapies and treatment politics is an area I know something of through my professional involvement with HIV/AIDS. My conceptual categories come from gay community forums and scientific conferences and are useful in my research; but they do not relate to Barney's experience of the epidemic at all. The day after I saw Barney the second time, a survey appeared in all Australian gay magazines and community newspapers. Among the questions it asked was the following: "Please circle any of the following drugs you currently take." Here are the answers listed exactly as they appear on the questionnaire: "AZT, ddI, ddC, Prophylaxis for PCP (Bactrim etc.)." I thought of Barney's "chest thing" and wondered how the proposed education program to encourage early use of treatments, to be developed from the findings of this survey, would be able to make sense of, or even reach, Barney and others like him. Except that they need not do so, for few of Barney's class participate in such surveys anyway and gaining an understanding of Barney's situation would not emerge in that kind of survey as a result.

The importance of this mismatch goes beyond research methodologies or treatment interventions to the heart of the gay community response to PLWHAs. The formation of an HIV-positive identity is a phenomenon commented on often as if walking on eggshells, and is an issue where researchers, in particular gay researchers, should take a strong interest. The phrase, "I am HIV," stands in stark contrast to "I have cancer." This identification of the self with a virus is reasonably unique: one doesn't hear "I am CMV" or "I am spirochete." We should be cautious, however, and not overinterpret what might simply be idiomatic shorthand.

The development of an "HIV identity," or an "HIV career"—and some would argue also an "HIV community" — is something worth investigating, if only because its consequences for the fight against the epidemic are difficult to estimate (Ariss, Carrigan, and Dowsett 1992). There are cultural and political determinants of this development, much again coming from North American experiences of the epidemic and shaped by the particular configuration of gay minority-style politics that predominates in the United States. The suggestion made in Chapter 2 that one could bowdlerize Dennis Altman's early book title and speak of the "Americanization" of the PLWHA seems less cheeky.

Since the early days of the epidemic there have been warnings about the peculiar nexus between HIV/AIDS and homosexuality, particularly those kinds of homosexual desire which form gay communities. In 1986 Christopher Spence, the director of London Lighthouse, warned of the possibility that issues of being homosexual, particularly deep and unresolved emotional issues, may collapse in on gay men as they grapple with the far more uncertain consequences of being HIV-infected.

The transference of terms — "coming out" as seropositive, the very notion of there being an HIV "identity" — borrows heavily from gay liberation tropes and political tactics. The notion of certain "rights" pertaining to PLWHAs, for example, to treatments, drug trials, and so on, derives much of its character from civil liberties struggles by gay men and lesbians over the last twenty-five years. The collectivity of interest in HIV borrows heavily from gay "community."

Various commentators have noted the development and use of the phrases "positive" and "negative" and the wider ramifications of those terms on the condition of being infected or uninfected with HIV. These terms have now become another binary, growing beyond the original medical test result terminology, with its often complete blindness to the social consequences of its work, to have far more meaning. There is an increasing danger of a polarized identity and a social process and politics growing out of that binary, which, inter alia, threatens to constitute uninfected gay men as the "other." Whereas, as any uninfected man knows, he is merely the "proximate" (to borrow again from Dollimore [1991]), uninfected due more to luck and circumstance than by design and decision, and always but one slip away from becoming infected.

This discursive formation of an HIV identity and its consequences are of concern. There are infected men in this study, such as Richard Cochrane, who have gained considerable social support and personal resources in programs run by local gay community–based AIDS service organizations and, inter alia, from their collective approach to being HIV-infected. Equally, there are others, such as Geoff Harris, who resent separation from other gay men implicit in certain configurations of HIV-identity politics. Yet others, like Barney Sherman, socially excluded from gay communities, reject the need for support groups and are confused by those particular definitions of their situation.

The marginalization from these conceptualizations of being HIV-infected represents yet another mechanism whereby gay community is found wanting. It rehearses a broader dynamic in gay community seen in the cases of Barney, Phillip, Harriet, Simon, and Richard. It points to a larger consequence for the whole gay liberation project: its need to come to grips with the structuring of social and sexual inequality.

## Gay Community and Class

A pervasive theme in this study has been that of men from working-class backgrounds dealing with their homosexuality. Any attempt to comprehend the process of coming to a (homo)sexual subjectivity that ignores the larger social and economic relations within which these men live is doomed to failure. The working-class men in this study have tense relations with the gay communities, relations that are enacted in sociocultural terms and in processes of inclusion and exclusion. Even where a successful transition to gay community life has occurred, there are costs.

These men offer fascinating accounts of the construction of working-class homosexual lives. Harry Wight has remained close to his families, not only geographically but also in his daily activities. This active engagement with family is far less common among modern inner-Sydney gay men. This extended beyond biological families to his and his partner's social network, to their heterosexual friends, workmates, neighbors, clubs. This is a fleshing out of the finding in Connell et al. (1991) that working-class men experience less separation from a broader heterosexual matrix than other, middle-class, gay community–identifying men.

Another example is the use of sexual language. Harry offered insight into working-class life in other ways, for example, in the use of expressions such as "goin' birko" (derived from the whistling "Birko" electric kettle popular in the 1950's), "youse" for "you," and camp language such as "bitch" and "butch." Yet he was quite well spoken and expressive; there was none of the hesitation and slips of the tongue or syntax evident in, say, Robert Cusack.

There was a lovely moment where Harry's expressiveness and directness came through in describing looking after a sick "queen" at a dance:

The first dance, fuckin' drama everywhere. Right. Got to about twelve
o'clock after the show and he was paralytic. We said to Hazel [the drag
queen who organizes the dances], we'll take him home and put him to
bed in the spare room. Because he'd already put the hard word on us
anyway, and we'd said yes. Someone's off their dial, there's no point,
ya know. So: "Come on, we'll take you home." So we bought [*sic*] him
home, took his clothes off. I washed him down because he was all,
blaaah, put a bucket next to the bed. I said: "If you spew on that car-
pet, I'll rub your fuckin' nose in it when I get back."

This is the Harry who did not seduce the excited rookie in his bed in the
armed forces. This is the Harry who pulled a friend's teenage nephew out
of a beat and lectured him about safe sex, gave him condoms, and drove
him back!

Yet the interview with Harry also contained poignant reminders of the
subordination of Harry and his concerns. At one point he wanted to describe the older boy who initiated him into insertive anal intercourse as
"bitch" (receptive in anal intercourse) or as "passive." He asked for my
approval for his terminology. I assented to whichever he preferred and he
chose "bitch." But it was clear that I represented a modern fag, a Sydney
queen, a gay liberationist, an activist connected with a gay community
AIDS service organization, a middle-class academic, or some unnamable
combination of authenticity, expertise, and deference. He was also aware
that some gay men nowadays eschew "girlie" terms and, if nothing else,
he wanted to check whether I was from that milieu. One way or another it
represented a moment in hegemony.

Barney used some strange expressions: "what for have you" instead
of "what have you," "debenture" for "dementia," and "Baclin" for "Bactrim." But Barney's approximation of knowledge, his experiential learning
style, ought to be regarded as a resource for prevention and care education, not a barrier—something to be worked *with*, not *against*. For all the
semantic differences, here is a potential available to HIV/AIDS work. In
the examples of Barney working as a volunteer for Neighbourhood Watch
and various gay social groups; in Harriet's tireless fundraising; in Robert
Cusack's giving years of his life to building up the gay leather bikie club;
in Neil Davidson's contributing through his activities in a group for gay
men leaving married life: these men exemplify the positive side of the "cooperative coping" (Connell, Ashenden, Kessler, and Dowsett 1982) aspect
of working-class life.

Where is the recognition of this work? The gay community, while so dependent on the collective contribution of its members, barely notices them (as Barney bitterly recalled) and unwittingly contributes to their exclusion from its ranks. This is a remarkable but untapped resource for HIV/AIDS work and for the building of gay community. Phillip Gibbs experienced this lack of recognition, this marginalization, as cultural dissonance: his active rejection by the "too well-educated" HIV/AIDS worker paralleled his complaint that the leaders in his young gay men's HIV/AIDS peer education group always talked of films, plays, and inner-city life, the very lifestyle he had failed to appropriate.

Social inequality and marginalization are not simply about these dissonances in style and custom, language and manners; they are also related to the effects of significant limitation in opportunity. Robert Cusack and Richard Cochrane lived all their lives on meager incomes. Their work prospects, already limited by working-class backgrounds, were foreshortened by a dedication to pleasure, although they derived from their gay lives some respite from the daily grind. Ren Pinch, who did not need to work, was the only one of the three community-attached men to construct a "career" for himself as an HIV/AIDS activist, and a good one, too. But the cost in social and economic terms for others cannot be understated.

Robert lived in a very small two-room flat, the single living space crammed with a "laminex" kitchen table, a television set and shelves of memorabilia, treasures, and tack. Mass-produced postcards of male beauty in plastic frames competed with sideshow prizes, family mementos, and leather bike club trophies for attention from a single viewing point in a lone vinyl armchair. This was not a smart loft in New York City, a cozy flat in Camden Town, London, or a neat Victorian terrace in Darlinghurst, Sydney.

Harriet lived in a granny flat. Jack Sayers lived on the suburban fringes of western Sydney, the only place where he could afford his own home on a retirement income. Richard Cochrane's wages were insufficient to provide savings to sustain him in his illness; he went home. Simon Little lives in a tiny rented run-down inner-city terrace house with minimal furniture and only his much-loved Madonna posters to decorate the bare walls.

For many working-class men in this study, living with the realities of low incomes and a shrinking labor market for unskilled workers (and particularly for young people) means a life of limited options. Here "choices" is an absurd middle-class notion. Some do decide to forgo a more reliable salary in, say, a factory in Nullangardie (Alan Cunningham's job) for low wages flogging their bodies behind gay bars (Richard Cochrane). For all its glamour, gay bar work is hard and uncertain and has no future. How many middle-aged gay barmen are there?

Gay work is certainly safe work, in the sense of being in a place where being gay in itself does not lead to harassment or strained workplace relations. Where else could Harriet survive? Richard certainly had no regrets about his working life, for it enhanced his sexual possibilities, but it is certain that Richard's sexual exertions cost him dearly in more ways than one.

Robert suggested that discrimination against him as a (presumed) gay man was partly responsible for his lack of advancement. Undoubtedly discrimination against gay people in the workforce is real (see Anti-Discrimination Board [NSW] 1982), even though it is illegal in New South Wales. Yet there is also a hint of something lacking in Robert—a certain ambition, or determination to strive for a "career," to fulfill the promise of postwar social mobility he embarked on. Similarly, Barney Sherman never really succeeded as a small businessman; he remained a self-employed tradesman. Alan Cunningham reported that being gay never entirely disappeared from others' sense of him; he has to be ever watchful in the factory. Jack Sayers always refused promotion above foreman, leaving jobs if the pressure to move to middle management became too great.

For working-class gay men like these, life is profoundly shaped by their experience of training, work, and the labor market. They experience considerable constraint in their capacity to shape their lives in ways that many other gay men like Ren Pinch can. There is no sense of achievement like that Neil Davidson experienced. Rather, they have a sense of cultural limitation, only sometimes self-imposed, which underscores their confusion in the face of something large and unfathomable.

Just as gay liberation utilized the concept of *internalized oppression* to analyze the limiting effects of social marginalization and stigmatization, so too working-class men like these carry within them a sense of personal limitation: a record of failure in school and work; a sense of helplessness in the face of an ever tighter labor market; a perplexing acquiescence to restrictions through low earnings, reliance on the welfare system, and poor prospects of mobility. This adds up to considerable social vulnerability and directly shapes their homosexuality.

There is a relationship between work and sexuality, not just an accidental one, but one where sexuality and work are interlinked structurally. Pringle (1988) has pointed out that sexuality does not simply enter into workplace relations, but that sexuality actually constitutes workplace relationships and the labor process itself, even when no actual sex occurs.

A case in point would be the hospitality industry Richard worked in. His entry to this industry came about through a familiar process among working-class people—a friend got him the job. The industry is commonly thought of as a place for gay people. But why? The work attracts inadequate pay, has poor working conditions even compared with lowly paid public-sector work, and has little career structure. Some gay men may simply choose this industry because it offers a chance to travel, as Richard did, or to gain work and be able to move on at will, or to meet other gay men by working in gay-positive venues. In other words, there are trade-offs.

But neither Richard nor Harriet were doing bar work while they completed a degree or as a second job to save for the house or the overseas trip. The hospitality industry[4] is a major source of employment for the unskilled, or for those on the fringes of the skilled labor market. It is one of the few places, outside the ever-decreasing jobs in factory work and blue-collar public-sector work, where men like Richard and Harriet can go. While some of the men in this study were boilermakers, like Alan Cunningham, others, like Barney Sherman, have a trade. Many found the hospitality industry the only other place to gain work. In a tight labor market the hotels, restaurants, and shops are not just choices for temporary work until something better comes along; they *are* the available jobs for many working-class gay men.

In Richard's case something else occurred; these jobs provided him with entry into a particular kind of gay life. Bar work opened the doors to a fully fledged, modern gay life and he lived it to the limit. Harriet told a related but different story. He became a "dragon" and a popular one at that, working clubs as both an entertainer and bar worker; yet Harriet made more money as a prostitute (in drag) working the street. When "working" eventually became too difficult, Harriet reverted to sandwich making.

These two men live their gayness in very different ways. Is their gayness the reason why these men live permanently on the unstable fringe of the labor market, with poverty never too far away? Is it possible that the work helped shape their gayness? It seems plausible that Richard's limited work options landed him in a situation where certain forms of gayness became available for appropriation. Had Harriet not started in drag work, he might have gone down a different track. And what of the directly sexual character of much of Phillip Gibbs's experiences of the black economy?

The relationship between work and sexuality is not simple. It is not that

---

[4] The hospitality industry encompasses such employment possibilities as hotel and bar work, restaurant service work, and other such personal services.

work determines sexuality, or that sexuality determines work. But there is a relationship between homosexuality and the construction of one's own version of it that is definitely related to issues of class, in this case represented by job opportunities, labor market exigencies and economic circumstances. In the common thread of friends' getting the men these jobs, the collectivity in these gay men's lives shines through again.

The sexualized nature of the workplaces these men inhabit cannot be omitted from the mix. Jack Sayers specialized in seducing younger men at work (not that much younger than he, but this may account for why he refused promotion). He retained a number of friendships with these youths long after they left and got married, and there are a few who bring their wives and kids to visit him in his retirement. Alan Cunningham reported initiation practices in his factory that were definitely sexual in character. And his workmates delighted in getting details of Alan's weekend trysts, even if these were often met with feigned repugnance. Harriet more than anyone experienced the sexual nature of work; being a drag queen and bar "girl" in a gay pub is hard work, but definitively sexual, as Simon Little's boyfriend also exemplifies.

In this sense, sexual expression and sexual meaning-making for these men as gay men is deeply involved in the day-to-day practice of their work, its opportunities (or lack of them), the character of the workplace relationships, and in the case of the hospitality industry a fair chance that workmates will be gay as well. It is no wonder then, as gay communities grow in infrastructure and commerce that these precincts become small labor markets of their own. Yet even here Dennis Partridge's and Phillip Gibbs's experiences indicate that *being* gay is simply not enough.

The construction of homosexual lives, their components, meanings, and experiences are, for these men, profoundly affected by the limitations of their backgrounds and by the constraints of an unequal social order. There are undoubtedly powerful structures that shape gay men's lives and the labor market is one of these, not just by limiting economic opportunity, but also as an element implicated in the project of becoming gay. It is implicated in the whole process of trying to be a part of a gay community, of learning to live a gay life. This is most clearly exemplified in the examples of Phillip Gibbs, Harriet, and Simon Little. Their working-class style (values, attitudes, expectations, manners) is inappropriate in Sydney's gay community; they just do not "fit." This is not a social wrinkle that simply gets ironed out after the "status and culture"–dependent "arrival point" is passed by each man as he enters a gay community (Herdt and Boxer 1992: 6); these social costs and inequalities pervade gay community life.

## Sexual Subjectivity

The stories these men told served quite clearly to link seamlessly an often sexually active childhood to a sexual adulthood. These explanations should be understood not so much as a claim to essentialism but as an *essential* part of the sense-making activities of gay and homosexually active men. On this issue, these men answer the challenge of Dianne Fuss (1991) with reference to the performative aspects of sexual identity. When faced with the ongoing daily struggles of these men, it is rhetorical to debate the correctness of their interpretations of homosexuality and its purpose, or the delusions contained within the frameworks they utilize.

Harriet's four-part identity is my construction; for Harriet terms such as "gay," "camp," or "homosexual" are interchangeable. Barney hardly relies on a sexual identity at all. It may be that the nineteenth-century emergence of the homosexual as a species (and eventually an identity) left out as much as it put in. The discursive formulation of the homosexual bypassed the commonplace and dispersed sexual relations involved in homoeroticism as a whole. The pathologized individual, which emerged to trouble elite discourse and its deployment, was in the main bourgeois. Only some sodomites became homosexual; the discursive silence left offered transgressive disorderly space able to be exploited by the men of Nullangardie over time and reproduced by the likes of Barney, Harriet, and friends in their daily sexual practice.

These men display the components of a homosexual subjectivity for us with detail and clarity. Beyond the performativity of what is often termed identity, the contribution of the body itself to the formation of sexual subjectivity is vital. The body, its experiences, sensations, and the processes whereby we come to judge our sexual capacities, pleasures, preferences, and so on, cannot simply be regarded as *tabula rasa*, upon which discourse etches its historical product. The input from embodied practice, from the sensate experiences of men in sexual milieus and other sexual communities gives prominence to a kind of social constructionism concerned with the agentive and collective exploration of bodies' capacities in a discursive silence. In this, the pursuit of transgressive pleasure in the sexual (dis)order is by definition neither revolt nor resistance; rather, it only sometimes and later becomes an increasingly strident counterpoint, historically structured and reproduced in collective practice of gay community.

The meanings encountered and made in the sexual (dis)order cannot be simply regarded as local narratives or crude extracts of powerful discourses;

they have lives of their own, derived from an historically produced collective experience of embodied sexual activity. And in the choreography of sex between men, these meanings make a mockery of the terms that comfort theory: that which gender purports to enclose in fact disaggregates in this sexual (dis)order, offering new ingredients for pleasure, recasting its elements into sexuality. If we utilize sexuality as the structural category of equivalent weight to gender, a new vision emerges of the organization of social life, one that does not by definition subordinate gay men and lesbians to heterosexuality. Yet a warning must be sounded here: the purpose of this study was not to develop a new structuralist frame—Foucault already did that in a vision that lacks content: there is no sex in its sexuality.

The role of social theory is to explicate contributions to the production of history. To be working in social theory development in sexuality would be an irrelevant act if it neglected the lives of men like Barney, Harriet, Phillip, and Simon and relegated them to the ranks of the deluded or cast them as supporting actors in the playing of history. The real question to ask might more appropriately be: whose (gay) history, whose sexuality, has been written and understood to date?

Gayness remains emergent in social action, and may never quite become internalised, so that each night we seek to rediscover that identity by performing those rights of hyper-exchange based on rituals of endless, byzantine moves whose purpose is definitional at least as much as it is the trading off of sperm (an objective which in homosexuality itself is largely symbolic in its transformation of natural to cultural purposes). (Michaels 1990: 99)

Eric Michaels puts his finger on a permanent tension in homosexuality in our society, but individualizes it and thereby fails to recognize the tremendous collective effort in performing those "rituals." And even Michaels is still convinced by "gay." The sexual trajectories of the men in this study offer dramatic evidence of another profoundly social and collective character to homoerotic activity.

It is through this investigation of men's lives, largely though not all working-class, that a fuller content of sexuality starts to emerge. These men should convince us that gay life, homosexuality, gay community, constitute a far less certain and defined field of inquiry than underpinned the Amsterdam conferences. In discomforting "gay," these men offer the possibility of evaluating the quarter-century-old gay liberation experiment.

## Gay Community

The undoubted success of the gay communities in dealing with HIV/ AIDS must argue for a judgment that gay community as a social phenomenon is a remarkable accomplishment. In Australia at least (but also in some other countries), the gay community AIDS service organizations are among the largest government-funded nongovernmental organizations in the country, and they certainly must be credited with doing most of what has contributed to the reduction in HIV infection among gay men. Whatever other evidence might be offered, the epidemiology of HIV in Australia confirms that these gay communities have done a mighty job.

For some men, the gay communities remain a safe space in an unsafe world, one where ungrateful elements still attack the "gay lobby" and its "hijacking" of HIV/AIDS. This attack has generated little widespread public acceptance as yet, despite its having been made a number of times during the epidemic. But it signals the ongoing need for a protective place from which to defend homosexual desire and the gains made in gay community. The deconstructionism of the early 1980's, which gestured toward the end of homosexuality, has yet to attract those men in gay communities to its somewhat uncertain prospects.

Gay community is not simply an aggregation of individuals; nor is it any longer just a sexual subculture linked by sex practices or an historically formed sexual community accumulating common interests. Rather, gay community is an interactive construction and

May be reconceptualized as social and cultural forms in their own right, albeit emergent ones and thus still fuzzily defined, undercoded, or discursively dependent on more established forms . . . [which] acts as an agency of social process whose mode of functioning is both interactive and yet resistant, both participatory and yet distinct, claiming at once equality and difference, demanding political representation while insisting on its material and historical specificity. (de Lauretis 1991: i)

De Lauretis captures a good deal of the tension in her deconstruction of gay community in this formulation. But there is a need, however, to move beyond gay community, or communities, as emergent and dynamic within a structure/resistance binary. And where (again? still?) is sex?

The pursuit of homosexuality and the project of sexual liberation as it stands certainly do show considerable progress toward a resolution of sorts in gay community. October 1995 saw Sydney's annual Sleaze Ball celebrated by 16,500 gay men (mainly) and lesbians in an atmosphere of direct sexual revelry and a flesh-filled fanfare for homoeroticism. At Sleaze the "sexed" and "gendered" bodies display all the inversions, transformations, deconstructed and destabilized, confirming the shortcomings of gender and sexual difference as analytical concepts on their own. Sleaze demonstrates the need to establish sexuality as a worthy theoretical framework in rethinking the transformation of desires and the appropriation of gayness as culture and politics, and in the structuring of the social.

As representations of community and (homo)sexual culture, annual events such as Sleaze and Mardi Gras point also to the enormous "community" that now exists in Sydney. The "pink vote" in the Oxford Street precinct now determines the local seat in the New South Wales State Parliament. Antivilification laws were enacted in New South Wales in 1994 to restrict anti-gay incitement activity. Trade unions and employer organizations are debating the inclusion of gay households and relationships in industrial awards, so that provisions for family leave apply equally. There have been great gains for many gay men and lesbians drawn from civil rights activism within the Sydney gay community. These reveal a particular participation, a certain form of attachment. For the likes of Ren Pinch, gay community has been the "making of the modern homosexual" (Plummer 1981). Yet Barney does not like the noise and drugs at parties; Harriet's drag acts attract less support at community fundraisers; Martin Ridgeway and Neil Davidson rarely visit Oxford Street; Simon Little resents the "political" gays. So, whose community is it?

Gay community is still in process and has a long way to go before it fully encompasses its constituency, if it ever can—or should for that matter. It remains to be seen whether the edifice being erected in Oxford Street can accommodate all gay and homosexually active men, the young and the old, the beautiful and the plain, the ill and the well, the poor and the well-off, the ill-educated and the highly cultured, Anglo-Australians and the mixed races and ethnicities of Australia, the desired and the desiring; and do so without creating merely a marginalized inner-city minority on the political and social fringes of Australian culture.

## Postscript

In early 1995, I attended yet another HIV/AIDS conference, the IUVDT World STD/AIDS Congress. This time it was in Singapore, revealing just how far the locus of the HIV epidemic has shifted since those Amsterdam conferences. There were few Europeans there. Almost all of the Australians attending, many of whom had been involved in HIV/AIDS work nationally and internationally for quite some time, had strong links with the gay communities' efforts back home. A particular scientific STD research model dominated papers at the congress, with notions of "core groups," particularly sex workers (always assumed to be female), blocking the vision.

HIV/AIDS has made a major incursion in the STD field over the last ten years, yet only two sessions featured gay men and gay communities specifically, partly in an attempt by some of the congress organizers to unsettle this narrow venereological vision. In the first I presented an overview of the prevention efforts of gay communities in Australia in a session titled "Successful Prevention Efforts," based on the work discussed here in Chapter 2. This was the fifth time I had done this kind of presentation in such a forum, hoping yet again that audiences could see beyond the gayness of these prevention successes to the real possibilities for HIV prevention *everywhere*.

The second session was convened by Australian gay academic Dennis Altman as a panel discussion of delegates from HIV/AIDS organizations in five Southeast Asian countries with emerging HIV epidemics, where gay men were struggling for recognition. These delegates argued strongly for diverse configurations of homoeroticism lodged firmly within the cultural specificities of an emerging "Asian" identity—not dissimilar to the contemporary "construction" of Europe. They were engaged in a struggle, for postcolonial morality still dogs sexuality in this part of the world—homosexual sex is illegal in Singapore, for example. So in seeking to convince the audience of the varied legitimacies of same-sex sexual desire, various modes of organic (homo)sexual expression were detailed, for example, the transsexual *waria* of Surabaya, and the effeminate *bakla* of Manila (see Altman 1995).

Simultaneously, the nascent gay communities of these regions, whose extraordinary work in HIV/AIDS is finally being recognized, embody the assertion that homosexual expression finds new legitimacy in the concepts "gay" and "gay community." The wielding of gay identity by these proudly gay men was worthy of all that gay liberation hoped for, in the sense of its liberationist tropes, its internationalism, and the accompanying and empowering commitment to fighting HIV/AIDS. It was moving and galvanizing. Yet this sat uneasily with the claims to preexisting, culturally specific forms of male homoeroticism. When questioned on this apparent contradiction, delegates invoked social constructionist frameworks to camouflage what is actually a paradox: if these varied cultural configurations of homoeroticism serve well the claim to age-old sexual possibilities, why is "gay" needed?

Yet the attractions of gay identities in the Westernizing cities of these rapidly industrializing economies are obvious, and the strategy of gay community as a resolution to sexual dilemmas of postcolonial cultures such as these would seem definite. This is particularly the case where the emerging Asian-ness eschews Western concepts of individualized rights for the more collective and conformist responsibilites of the citizen. Struggles around sexuality take on this politics squarely, if unevenly. Yet it was a salutary moment in the making of sexuality and a revealing moment in hegemony to see the prospect of gay community emerge in this context.

As I sat and listened to these men, I reflected that in my own country the promise of gay community—to reveal something of the magnificence of human sexual expression, to lust lovingly and to love lustfully one's own sex—still awaits fulfillment. As a gay man living in the heart of Sydney's gay community, as a gay man who came out after Stonewall, for all the surety I am surrounded with in this gay community, I am still unclear about the extent of the resolution to be found in gay. If gay community is to achieve its promise then, when it happens, it must do this in a manner that ensures that our Barney Shermans die surrounded by gay friends and lovers, that our Harriets' wonderful creations are validated, and our Phillip Gibbses practice their desire in safety.

# Reference Matter

# References Cited

Adib, S. M., D. G. Ostrow, and J. G. Joseph. 1992. "Longitudinal Patterns of Sexual Behavior Change and Relapse in the Chicago MACS/CCS Cohort." Poster presented at the Eighth International Conference on AIDS, Amsterdam, July.

AIDS Council of New South Wales. 1994. *Annual Report for 1993-94*. Sydney: AIDS Council of New South Wales.

Allen, Judith. 1992. "Frameworks and Questions in Australian Sexuality Research." In R. W. Connell and G. W. Dowsett, eds., *Rethinking Sex: Social Theory and Sexuality Research*, pp. 5-31. Melbourne: Melbourne University Press.

Altman, Dennis. 1979. *Coming Out in the Seventies*. Sydney: Wild & Wooley.

———. 1982. *The Homosexualization of America: The Americanization of the Homosexual*. New York: St. Martin's Press.

———. 1986. *AIDS and the New Puritanism*. London: Pluto Press.

———. 1987. "The Creation of Sexual Politics in Australia." *Journal of Australian Studies* 20: 76-82.

———. 1989. "AIDS and the Reconceptualisation of Homosexuality." In Dennis Altman et al., *Homosexuality, Which Homosexuality? Essays from the International Scientific Conference on Gay and Lesbian Studies*, pp. 35-48. London: GMP Publishers; Amsterdam: Uitgeverij An Dekker/Schorer.

———. 1992. "AIDS and the Discourses of Sexuality." In R. W. Connell and G. W. Dowsett, eds., *Rethinking Sex: Social Theory and Sexuality Research*, pp. 32-48. Melbourne: Melbourne University Press.

———. 1995. "The New World of 'Gay Asia.'" In S. Perera, ed., *Asian and Pacific Inscriptions*, pp. 121-38. Melbourne: Meridien.

Altman, Dennis, and Kim Humphery. 1989. "Breaking Boundaries: AIDS and Social Justice in Australia." *Social Justice* 16, no. 3: 158-66.

Altman, Dennis, et al. 1989. *Homosexuality, Which Homosexuality? Essays from the International Scientific Conference on Gay and Lesbian Studies*. London: GMP Publishers; Amsterdam: Uitgeverij An Dekker/Schorer.

Andros, Phil [Samuel M. Steward]. 1983. *My Brother, My Self*. San Francisco: Perineum Press.

Anti-Discrimination Board [NSW]. 1982. *Discrimination and Homosexuality* (A Report of the Anti-Discrimination Board in Accordance with Section 119(a) of the Anti-Discrimination Act, 1977). Sydney: New South Wales Government Printer.

Antler. 1983. "What Every Boy Knows." In Ian Young, ed., *The Son of the Male Muse: New Gay Poetry*, pp. 19–21. Trumansburg, N.Y.: Crossing Press.

Ariss, Robert. 1990. "The Community and Clinical Trials." In Paul van Reyk, ed., *The Frontline View of the National HIV/AIDS Strategy: Selected Papers from the Fourth National Conference on HIV/AIDS, Canberra, August 1990*, pp. 15–20. Sydney: AIDS Council of New South Wales.

————. 1991. "Social Science Research and People Living with HIV/AIDS." *National AIDS Bulletin* 5, no. 3: 14–16.

Ariss, Robert, Tim Carrigan, and Gary Dowsett. 1992. "Sexual Identities of HIV Positive Men: Some Implications for AIDS Service Organisations." *National AIDS Bulletin* 6, no. 7: 20–24.

*Art and Text* 38, January 1991.

Australian Gonococcal Surveillance Program. 1988. "Changing Patterns of Gonococcal Infections in Australia, 1981–1987." *Medical Journal of Australia* 149: 609–12.

Australian Market Research. Unpublished. Preliminary Report: Benchmark Information on Awareness, Knowledge, Attitudes, and Behaviour in Australia Prior to the Launch of an Educational Campaign (Prepared for the National Advisory Council on AIDS and the Commonwealth Department of Health). Sydney: Australian Market Research.

Ballard, J. A. 1988. "Alternatives to the Traditional Public Health Approach." In Commonwealth of Australia, ed., *Living with AIDS: Towards the Year 2000* (Report of the Third National Conference on AIDS, Hobart, August 4–6), pp. 645–51. Canberra: Australian Government Publishing Service.

————. 1989. "The Politics of AIDS." In H. Gardner, ed., *The Politics of Health: The Australian Experience*, pp. 349–75. Melbourne: Churchill Livingstone.

————. 1990. "Social Science and HIV Policy: Mutual Failure of Response." Paper presented at the Fourth National Conference on AIDS, Canberra, August.

Bartlett, Neil. 1990. *Ready to Catch Him Should He Fall*. London: Serpent's Tail.

Bataille, Georges. 1989. *The Tears of Eros*. Trans. Peter Connor. San Francisco: City Lights Books.

Bayer, Ronald. 1981. *Homosexuality and American Psychiatry: The Politics of Diagnosis*. New York: Basic Books.

Bell, Alan P., and Martin S. Weinberg. 1978. *Homosexualities: A Study of Diversity Among Men and Women*. New York: Simon & Schuster.

Bennett, Garrett, Simon Chapman, and Fiona Bray. 1989. "Sexual Practices and 'Beats': AIDS-Related Sexual Practices in a Sample of Homosexual and Bisexual Men in the Western Area of Sydney." *Medical Journal of Australia* 151: 309–14.

Bersani, Leo. 1988. "Is the Rectum a Grave?" In Douglas Crimp, ed., *AIDS: Cultural Analysis/Cultural Activism*, pp. 197–222. Cambridge, Mass.: MIT Press.

Bhaskar, Roy. 1989. *Reclaiming Reality: A Critical Introduction to Contemporary Philosophy*. London: Verso.

Blackwood, Evelyn. 1986. *The Many Faces of Homosexuality: Anthropological Approaches to Homosexual Behavior*. New York: Harrington Park Press.

Boffin, Tessa, and Sunil Gupta. 1990. *Ecstatic Antibodies: Resisting the AIDS Mythology.* London: Rivers Oram Press.

Bolton, Ralph. 1989. "Introduction." In Ralph Bolton, ed., *The AIDS Pandemic, A Global Emergency*, pp. 1–12. New York: Gordon & Breach.

Boswell, John. 1989. "Revolutions, Universals, and Sexual Categories." In Martin Bauml Duberman, Martha Vincinus, and George Chauncey Jr., eds., *Hidden from History: Reclaiming the Gay and Lesbian Past*, pp. 17–36. New York: New American Library.

Bray, Alan. 1988. *Homosexuality in Renaissance England.* 2d ed. London: Gay Men's Press.

Bristow, Joseph. 1989. "Homophobia/Misogyny: Sexual Fears, Sexual Definitions." In Simon Shepherd and Mick Wallis, eds., *Coming On Strong: Gay Politics and Culture*, pp. 54–75. London: Unwin Hyman.

Brodsky, Joel. 1987. "A Retrospective Ethnography of the Mineshaft." Paper presented at the Homosexuality, Which Homosexuality? Conference, Amsterdam, December.

Bronski, Michael. 1989. "Death and the Erotic Imagination." In Erica Carter and Simon Watney, eds., *Taking Liberties: AIDS and Cultural Politics*, pp. 219–28. London: Serpent's Tail.

Burcham, J. L., B. Tindall, M. Marmour, D. A. Cooper, G. Berry, and R. Penny. 1989. "Incidence and Risk Factors for Human Immunodeficiency Virus Seroconversion in a Cohort of Sydney Homosexual Men." *Medical Journal of Australia* 150: 634–39.

Burgess, P. M., I. E. Goller, S. J. Finch, and J. Pead. 1990. *A Prospective Study of Factors Influencing HIV Infection in Homosexual and Bisexual Men. Interim Report of Findings: Stage II.* Melbourne: University of Melbourne, Department of Psychology.

Burgess, P. M., I. E. Goller, S. K. Palmer, and G. Dite. 1992. *A Prospective Study of Factors Influencing HIV Infection in Homosexual and Bisexual Men.* Melbourne: University of Melbourne, Department of Psychology.

Burroughs, William. 1982. *A William Burroughs Reader.* Ed. John Calder. London: Picador.

Butler, Judith. 1990. *Gender Trouble: Feminism and the Subversion of Identity.* London: Routledge & Kegan Paul.

Cain, Roy. 1991. "Disclosure and Secrecy Among Gay Men in the United States and Canada: A Shift in Views." *Journal of the History of Sexuality* 2, no. 1: 25–45.

Califia, Pat. 1987. "A Personal View of the History of the Lesbian S/M Community and Movement in San Francisco," 3d ed. Reprinted in Samois, ed., *Coming to Power.* pp. 245–83. Boston: Alyson Publications.

Callen, M. 1983. *How to Have Sex in an Epidemic.* New York: News from the Front Publications.

Campbell, I. M., P. M. Burgess, I. E. Goller, and L. Lucas. 1988. *A Prospective Study of Factors Influencing HIV Infection in Homosexual and Bisexual Men. A Report of Findings: Stage I.* Melbourne: University of Melbourne, Department of Psychology.

*Capital Q*, February 3, 1995, p. 13.

Carrigan, Timothy J. 1981. "The Theoretical Significance of the Arguments of the Gay Liberation Movement, 1969–1981." Ph.D. diss., University of Adelaide, South Australia.

Chapman, Beata E., and JoAnn C. Brannock. 1987. "Proposed Model of Lesbian Identity Development: An Empirical Examination." *Journal of Homosexuality* 14, nos. 3/4: 69–80.

Chapple, M. J., G. W. Dowsett, and G. P. Smith. 1994. "Exploring Gay Community Attachment and Negotiated Safety: New Work on Persistent Problems in HIV Prevention Among Gay and Homosexually Active Men." Paper presented at "'AIDS' Impact"—the Second International Conference on Biopsychosocial Aspects of HIV Infection, Brighton, U.K., July.

Cohen, Derek, and Richard Dyer. 1980. "The Politics of Gay Culture." In The Gay Left Collective, eds., *Homosexuality: Power and Politics*, pp. 172–86. London: Allison & Busby.

Collinson, Laurence. 1977. "Himn." In *Hovering Narcissus*, p. 18. London: Grandma Press; Melbourne: Overland.

Collyer, Fran. 1994. "Sex-Change Surgery: An 'Unacceptable' Innovation?" *Australian and New Zealand Journal of Sociology* 30, no. 1: 3–19.

Commonwealth of Australia. 1989. *National HIV/AIDS Strategy. A Policy Information Paper.* Canberra: Australian Government Publishing Service.

———. 1993. *The National HIV/AIDS Strategy, 1993-94 to 1995-96.* Canberra: Australian Government Publishing Service.

Connell, R. W. 1983. *Which Way Is Up? Essays in Class, Sex, and Culture.* Sydney: George Allen & Unwin.

———. 1985. *Teachers' Work.* Sydney: George Allen & Unwin.

———. 1987. *Gender and Power.* Sydney: George Allen & Unwin.

———. 1990. "A Whole New World: Remaking Masculinity in the Context of the Environment Movement." *Gender and Society* 4, no. 4: 452–78.

———. 1991. "Live Fast and Die Young: The Construction of Masculinity Among Young Working-Class Men on the Fringes of the Labour Market." *Australian and New Zealand Journal of Sociology* 27, no. 2: 141–71.

Connell, R. W., D. J. Ashenden, S. Kessler, and G. W. Dowsett. 1982. *Making the Difference: Schools, Families and Social Division.* Sydney: George Allen & Unwin.

Connell, R. W., J. Crawford, G. W. Dowsett, S. Kippax, V. Sinnott, P. Rodden, R. Berg, D. Baxter and L. Watson. 1990. "Danger and Context: Unsafe Anal Sexual Practice Among Homosexual and Bisexual Men in the AIDS Crisis." *The Australian and New Zealand Journal of Sociology* 26, no. 2: 187–208.

Connell, R. W., J. Crawford, S. Kippax, G. W. Dowsett, D. Baxter, L. Watson, and R. Berg. 1989. "Facing the Epidemic: Changes in the Sexual Lives of Gay and Bisexual Men in Australia and Their Implications for AIDS Prevention Strategies." *Social Problems* 36, no. 4: 384–402.

Connell, R. W., June Crawford, Susan Kippax, G. W. Dowsett, G. Bond, Don Baxter, R. Berg, and Lex Watson. 1988. *Social Aspects of the Prevention of AIDS, Study A, Report No. 1—Method and Sample.* Sydney: Macquarie University, School of Behavioural Sciences.

Connell, R. W., M. D. Davis, and G. W. Dowsett. 1993. "A Bastard of a Life: Homosexual Desire and Practice Among Men in Working-Class Milieux." *Australian and New Zealand Journal of Sociology* 29, no. 1: 112–35.

Connell, R. W., G. W. Dowsett, P. Rodden, M. D. Davis, L. Watson, and D. Baxter. 1991. "Social Class, Gay Men and AIDS Prevention." *Australian Journal of Public Health* 15, no. 3: 178–89.

Connell, R. W., and S. Kippax. 1990. "Sexuality in the AIDS Crisis: Patterns of Sexual Practice and Pleasure in a Sample of Gay and Bisexual Men." *The Journal of Sex Research* 27, no. 2: 167–98.

Cooper, Dennis. 1991. *Frisk*. London: Serpent's Tail.

Cooper, Emmanuel. 1984. "Introduction." In Wilhelm von Gloeden, *Taomina*. London: GMP.

Couch, M. 1991. "Production and Reproduction of Masculinity in a Mining Community." Paper presented at the Conference on Research on Masculinity and Men in Gender Relations, Sydney, June.

Coxon, Tony. 1988. "The Numbers Game—Gay Lifestyles, Epidemiology of AIDS and Social Science." In Peter Aggleton and Hilary Homans, eds., *Social Aspects of AIDS*, pp. 126–38. London: Falmer Press.

Cozijn, John. 1982. "Sydney 1981: A Community Taking Shape." *Gay Information* 9/10: 4–10.

Crawford, J., S. Kippax, and G. W. Dowsett. 1990. "The Role of Contact with the AIDS/HIV Epidemic in Determining Behaviour Change in a Sample of Homosexual and Bisexual Men." In P. J. Solomon, C. Fazekas de St. Groth, and S. R. Wilson, eds., *Projections of Acquired Immune Deficiency Syndrome in Australia Using Data to the End of September 1989*. Canberra: Australian National University, National Centre for Epidemiology and Population Health, Working Paper No. 16.

Crawford, June, Alison Turtle and Susan Kippax. 1990. "Student-Favoured Strategies for AIDS Prevention." *Australian Journal of Psychology* 42, no. 2: 123–37.

Cribb, Tim, and Tim Herbert. 1991. "Sydney, New South Wales." In J. Bridges, ed., *Australia and Beyond: 1991 Gay Guide to Australia and New Zealand*, pp. 35–122. Sydney: Cobyork Press.

Crimp, Douglas, with Adam Rolston. 1990. *AIDS DEMO GRAPHICS*. Seattle: Bay Press.

D'Emilio, J. 1983. *Sexual Politics, Sexual Communities: The Making of a Homosexual Minority in the United States, 1940–70*. Chicago: University of Chicago Press.

Davenport-Hines, Richard. 1990. *Sex, Death and Punishment*. London: Fontana Press.

Davies, P. M. 1993. "Safer Sex Maintenance Among Gay Men: Are We Moving in the Right Direction?" *AIDS* 7, no. 2: 279–80.

Davis, Mark. 1990. "Peer Education and a Framework for Change in Queensland." *National AIDS Bulletin* 4, no. 5: 37–40.

Davis, M. D., U. Klemmer, and G. W. Dowsett. 1991. *Bisexually Active Men and Beats: Theoretical and Educational Implications* (The Report of the Bisexually Active Men's Outreach Project). Sydney: AIDS Council of NSW and Macquarie University, AIDS Research Unit (National Centre for HIV Social Research).

Davis, Mark, Gary Dowsett, Bob Connell, Robert Ariss, Tim Carrigan, and Murray Chapple. 1993. *Class, Homosexuality and AIDS Prevention: Resource Material for Use in HIV/AIDS Education.* Sydney: National Centre for HIV Social Research, Macquarie University.

De Cecco, John P., ed. 1988. *Gay Relationships.* New York: Haworth Press.

de Kuyper, Eric. 1987. "The Construction of Heterosexuality on Homosexuality. Or: What's Wrong with Us? What's Wrong with Them?" Paper presented at the Homosexuality, Which Homosexuality? Conference, Amsterdam, December.

de Lauretis, Teresa. 1991. "Queer Theory: Lesbian and Gay Studies. An Introduction." *Differences* 3, no. 2: i–xviii.

Delaney, Samuel R. 1991. "Street Talk/Straight Talk." *Differences* 3, no. 2: 21–38.

Diamond, Milton. 1984. *Sex Watching: Looking into the World of Sexual Behaviour.* London: Macdonald.

Dollimore, Jonathan. 1991. *Sexual Dissidence: Augustine to Wilde, Freud to Foucault.* Oxford: Clarendon Press.

Donaldson, Mike. 1991. *Time of Our Lives: Labour and Love in the Working Class.* Sydney: Allen & Unwin.

Donovan, B. 1988. "Social and Behavioural Components of Clinical Studies." In Commonwealth of Australia, ed., *Living with AIDS: Toward the Year 2000* (Report of the Third National Conference on AIDS, Hobart, 4–6 August), pp. 166–71. Canberra: Australian Government Publishing Service.

Donovan, B., B. Tindall, and D. Cooper. 1986. "Brachioproctic Eroticism and Transmission of Retrovirus Associated with Acquired Immune Deficiency Syndrome (AIDS)." *Genitourinary Medicine* 62, no. 6: 390–92.

Dowsett, G. W. 1986. "Interaction in the Semi-Structured Interview." In Merrelyn Emery, ed., *Research Network No. 2—Qualitative Research*, pp. 50–56. Canberra: Australian Association of Adult Education.

———. 1988. "The Place of Research in AIDS Education: A Critical Review of Survey Research Among Gay and Bisexual Men." In Commonwealth of Australia, ed., *Living with AIDS: Toward the Year 2000* (Report of the Third National Conference on AIDS, Hobart, 4–6 August), pp. 159–66. Canberra: Australian Government Publishing Service.

———. 1989. "'You'll Never Forget the Feeling of Safe Sex!' AIDS Prevention Strategies for Gay and Bisexual Men in Sydney, Australia." Paper presented at the World Health Organization Workshop on AIDS Health Promotion Activities Directed Towards Gay and Bisexual Men, Geneva, May.

———. 1990a. "Education Targets and Evaluation Mechanisms." In Paul van Reyk, ed., *The Frontline View of the National HIV/AIDS Strategy: Selected Papers from the Fourth National Conference on HIV/AIDS. August 1990, Canberra*, pp. 42–47. Sydney: AIDS Council of New South Wales.

———. 1990b. "Reaching Men Who Have Sex with Men in Australia. An Overview of AIDS Education: Community Intervention and Community Attachment Strategies." *Australian Journal of Social Issues* 25, no. 3: 186–98.

———. 1992. "An Absence of Desire . . . and Other Related Matters: Gay Perspectives on HIV/AIDS Research." Paper presented at the Second European Conference on Homosexuality and HIV, Amsterdam, February.

————. 1993a. "I'll Show You Mine, If You'll Show Me Yours: Gay Men, Masculinity Research, Men's Studies, and Sex." *Theory and Society* 22, no. 5: 697–709.

————. 1993b. "Sustaining Safe Sex: Sexual Practices, HIV and Social Context." *AIDS 92/93* 7, suppl. 1: S257–62.

————. 1994a. "HIV Prevention Among Working-Class Gay and Homosexually Active Men." *Focus* 9, no. 3: 1–4.

————. 1994b. *Sexual Contexts and Homosexually Active Men in Australia* (Report to the Commonwealth Department of Human Services and Health). Canberra: Australian Government Publishing Service.

Dowsett, G. W., and M. D. Davis. 1992. *Transgression and Intervention: Homosexually Active Men and Beats. A Review of an Australian HIV/AIDS Outreach Prevention Strategy.* Sydney: National Centre for HIV Social Research (Macquarie University Unit).

Dowsett, G. W., M. D. Davis, and R. W. Connell. 1992a. "Gay Men, HIV/AIDS and Social Research: An Antipodean Perspective." In Peter Aggleton, Peter Davies, and Graham Hart, eds., *AIDS: Rights, Risk and Reason*, pp. 1–12. London: Falmer Press.

————. 1992b. "Working-Class Homosexuality and HIV/AIDS Prevention: Some Recent Research from Sydney, Australia." *Psychology and Health* 6: 313–24.

Dowsett, Gary, Sandra Kessler, Dean Ashenden, and Bob Connell. 1981. "Divisively to School: Some Evidence on Class, Sex and Education in the 1940's and 1950's." *Australia 1939–1988: A Bicentennial History Bulletin* 4 (August): 32–60.

Dowsett, G. W., P. Rodden, S. Kippax, J. Crawford, D. Baxter, R. Berg, R. W. Connell, and L. Watson. 1989. *Social Aspects of the Prevention of AIDS, Study A, Technical Report No. 7 — Region.* Sydney: Macquarie University, School of Behavioural Sciences.

Duberman, Martin Bauml, Martha Vicinus, and George Chauncey Jr. 1989. *Hidden from History: Reclaiming the Gay and Lesbian Past.* New York: New American Library.

Duffin, Ross. 1990. "Education for People Who Are HIV Positive by People Who Are HIV Positive." In Paul van Reyk, ed., *The Frontline View of the National AIDS Strategy: Selected Papers from the Fourth National Conference on HIV/AIDS, August 1990, Canberra*, pp. 64–73. Sydney: AIDS Council of New South Wales.

Dunne, Gary, ed. 1991. *Travelling on Love in a Time of Uncertainty: Contemporary Australian Gay Fiction.* Sydney: Blackwattle Press.

————, ed. 1994. *Fruit: A New Anthology of Contemporary Australian Gay Writing.* Sydney: Blackwattle Press.

Eggeling, Jim. 1973. "Aphorism." In Ian Young, ed., *The Male Muse: A Gay Anthology*, p. 30. Trumansburg, N.Y.: The Crossing Press.

Ekstrand, M., R. Stall, S. Kegeles, R. Hays, M. DeMayo, and T. Coates. 1993. "Safer Sex Among Gay Men: What Is the Ultimate Goal?" *AIDS* 7, no. 2: 281–82.

Fay, Robert E., Charles F. Turner, Albert D. Klassen, and John H. Gagnon. 1989. "Prevalence and Patterns of Same-Gender Sexual Contact Among Men." *Science* 243: 338–48.

Feachem, R.G.A. 1995. *Valuing the Past . . . Investing in the Future* (Evaluation of the National HIV/AIDS Strategy 1993–94 to 1995–96). Canberra: Australian Government Publishing Service.

Feierman, Jay R., ed. 1990. *Pedophilia: Biosocial Dimensions*. New York: Springer-Verlag.

Fernbach, David. 1981. *The Spiral Path*. Boston: Alyson Publications; London: Gay Men's Press.

Fielding, Nigel. 1993. "Qualitative Interviewing." In Nigel Gilbert, ed., *Researching Social Life*, pp. 135–53. London: Sage.

Fitzgerald, Frances. 1987. *Cities on a Hill: A Journey Through Contemporary American Cultures*. London: Picador.

Fletcher, John. 1989. "Freud and His Uses: Psychoanalysis and Gay Theory." In Simon Shepherd and Mick Wallis, eds., *Coming on Strong: Gay Politics and Culture*, pp. 90–118. London: Unwin Hyman.

Foucault, Michel. 1978. *The History of Sexuality, Volume 1 — An Introduction*. Trans. Robert Hurley. Harmondsworth: Penguin Books.

———. 1980. *Herculine Barbin*. Trans. Richard McDougall. New York: Pantheon Books.

———. 1985. *The Use of Pleasure — The History of Sexuality, Volume 2*. Trans. Robert Hurley. London: Penguin.

Frazer, I. H., M. McCamish, I. Hay, and P. North. 1988. "Influence of Human Immunodeficiency Virus Antibody Testing on Sexual Behaviour in a 'High-Risk' Population from a 'Low-Risk' City." *Medical Journal of Australia* 149: 365–68.

Freud, Sigmund. 1953[1905]. "Three Essays on the Theory of Sexuality." In J. Strachey, ed., *Complete Psychological Works*, standard ed., 7: 123–245. London: Hogarth.

———. 1955[1918]. "From the History of an Infantile Neurosis." In J. Strachey, ed., *Complete Psychological Works*, standard ed., 17: 3–123. London: Hogarth.

———. 1961[1930]. "Civilization and Its Discontents." In J. Strachey, ed., *Complete Psychological Works*, standard ed., 21: 57–145. London: Hogarth.

Fuss, Diana. 1991. "Inside/Out." In Diana Fuss, ed., *Inside/Out: Lesbian Theories, Gay Theories*. New York and London: Routledge.

Gagnon, John H., and William Simon. 1974. *Sexual Conduct: The Social Sources of Human Sexuality*. London: Hutchinson.

Gatens, Moira. 1983. "A Critique of the Sex/Gender Distinction." In Judith Allen and Paul Patton, eds., *Beyond Marxism? Interventions After Marx*, pp. 143–60. Sydney: Intervention Publications.

Gay Left Collective, eds. 1980. *Homosexuality: Power and Politics*. London and New York: Allison & Busby.

Gerard, K., and G. Hekma, eds. 1989. *The Pursuit of Sodomy: Male Homosexuality in Renaissance and Enlightenment Europe*. New York: Harrington Park Press.

Gifford, Sandra M., Anne Mitchell, Doreen Rosenthal, and Meredith Temple-Smith. 1994. *STD and HIV/AIDS Education for People of Non-English Speaking Background* (Report for the Commonwealth Department of Human Services and Health). Canberra: Australian Government Publishing Service.

Gold, R. S., M. J. Skinner, P. J. Grant, and D. C. Plummer. 1991. "Situational Factors and Thought Processes Associated with Unprotected Intercourse in Gay Men." *Psychology and Health* 5, no. 4: 259–78.

Gott, Ted, ed. 1994. *Don't Leave Me This Way: Art in the Age of AIDS*. Canberra: National Gallery of Australia.

Green, Richard. 1987. *The "Sissy Boy Syndrome" and the Development of Homosexuality*. New Haven: Yale University Press.

Halperin, David M. 1990. *One Hundred Years of Homosexuality and Other Essays on Greek Love*. New York: Routledge.

Hammersley, Martyn. 1992. *What's Wrong with Ethnography?* London: Routledge.

Herdt, G. 1981. *Guardians of the Flutes*. New York: McGraw-Hill.

———, ed. 1984. *Ritualized Homosexuality in Melanesia*. Berkeley and Los Angeles: University of California Press.

Herdt, Gilbert, and Andrew Boxer. 1992. "Introduction: Culture, History, and Life Course of Gay Men." In Gilbert Herdt, ed., *Gay Culture in America: Essays from the Field*, pp. 1–28. Boston: Beacon Press.

Hicks, Neville. 1989. "Ethics, Social Justice and AIDS." Paper presented at the Fourth National Conference on AIDS, Canberra, August.

Hodges, Andrew, and David Hutter. 1974. *With Downcast Gays*. London: Pomegranate Press.

Horton, Meyrick, with Peter Aggleton. 1989. "Perverts, Inverts and Experts: The Cultural Production of an AIDS Research Paradigm." In Peter Aggleton, Graham Hart, and Peter Davies, eds., *AIDS: Social Representations, Social Practices*, pp. 74–100. London: Falmer Press.

Hughes, Robert. 1987. *The Fatal Shore*. London: Collins Harvill.

Hurley, Michael. 1991. "Introduction: Writing the Body Positive." In Kerry Bashford et al., comp., *Pink Ink: An Anthology of Australian Lesbian and Gay Writers*, pp. 12–42. Sydney: Wicked Women Publications.

———. 1992. "AIDS Narratives, Gay Sex and the Hygenics of Innocence." *Southern Review* 25, no. 2 (July): 141–59.

Hurley, Michael, and Jan Hutchinson. 1991. *Two Timing*. Sydney: Local Consumption Publications.

Irvine, Janice M. 1990. *Disorders of Desire: Sex and Gender in Modern American Sexology*. Philadelphia: Temple University Press.

Jay, Karla, and Allen Young, eds. 1975. *After You're Out: Personal Experiences of Gay Men and Lesbian Women*. New York: Links Books.

Johnston, Craig. 1981. "From Movement to Community." *Gay Information* 5: 6–9 and 32–33.

———. 1981/82. "Fragments of Gay America." *Gay Information* 8: 7–11.

Kaldor, J., P. Williamson, J. Gold, P. Grimm, J. Guinan, J. Learmont, B. Tindall, and D. A. Cooper. 1991. "Seroconversion in Sydney: Measuring the Cutting Edge of the HIV Epidemic." Paper presented at the Seventh International Conference on AIDS, Florence, June.

Kessler, Sandra, Dean Ashenden, Bob Connell, and Gary Dowsett. 1982. *Ockers and Disco-maniacs: A Discussion of Sex, Gender and Secondary Schooling.* 2d ed. Sydney: Inner City Education Centre.

Kimmel, Michael S., ed. 1990. *Men Confront Pornography.* New York: Crown Publishers.

Kinsey, A. C., W. D. Pomeroy, and C. E. Martin. 1948. *Sexual Behavior in the Human Male.* Philadelphia: W. B. Saunders.

Kippax, Susan, G. Bond, V. Sinnott, June Crawford, G. W. Dowsett, Don Baxter, R. Berg, R. W. Connell, and L. Watson. 1989. *Social Aspects of the Prevention of AIDS, Study A, Report No. 4—Regional Differences in the Responses of Gay and Bisexual Men to AIDS: The Australian Capital Territory.* Sydney: Macquarie University, School of Behavioural Sciences.

Kippax, Susan, R. W. Connell, G. W. Dowsett, and June Crawford. 1993. *Sustaining Safe Sex: Gay Communities Respond to AIDS.* London: Falmer Press.

Kippax, Susan, and June Crawford. 1991. "HIV Transmission Issues—Heterosexuals." Paper presented at the Third New South Wales HIV/AIDS Educators Conference, Sydney, May.

Kippax, Susan, June Crawford, R. W. Connell, G. W. Dowsett, and Cathy Waldby. 1990. "Establishing Safe Sex Norms in the Heterosexual Community." Paper presented at the Fourth National Conference on AIDS, Canberra, August.

Kippax, Susan, June Crawford, Bob Connell, Gary Dowsett, Lex Watson, Pam Rodden, Don Baxter, and Rigmor Berg. 1992. "The Importance of Gay Community in the Prevention of HIV Transmission: A Study of Australian Men Who Have Sex with Men." In Peter Aggleton, Peter Davies, and Graham Hart, eds., *AIDS: Rights, Risk and Reason,* pp. 102–18. London: Falmer Press.

Kippax, Susan, June Crawford, Mark Davis, Pam Rodden, and Gary Dowsett. 1993. "Sustaining Safe Sex: A Longitudinal Study of a Sample of Homosexual Men." *AIDS* 7: 257–63.

Kippax, Susan, June Crawford, G. W. Dowsett, G. Bond, V. Sinnott, D. Baxter, R. Berg, R. W. Connell, and L. Watson. 1990. "Gay Men's Knowledge of HIV Transmission and 'Safe' Sex: A Question of Accuracy." *Australian Journal of Social Issues* 25, no. 3: 199–219.

Kippax, Susan, June Crawford, Pam Rodden, and Kim Benton. 1994. *Report on Project Male-Call: National Telephone Survey of Men Who Have Sex with Men* (Report to the Commonwealth Department of Human Services and Health). Canberra: Australian Government Publishing Service.

Kippax, Susan, June Crawford, and Cathy Waldby. 1990. "Women Negotiating Heterosex: Implications for AIDS Prevention." *Women's Studies International Forum* 13, no. 6: 533–42.

Kippax, Susan, G. W. Dowsett, Mark Davis, Pam Rodden, and June Crawford. 1991. *Social Aspects of the Prevention of AIDS 1991 Sustaining Safe Sex Survey—Technical Report to the Australian Federation of AIDS Organisations and the AIDS Council of New South Wales.* Sydney: Macquarie University, AIDS Research Unit.

Kippax, S., G. W. Dowsett, M. Davis, P. Rodden, and J. Crawford. 1992. "Sustaining Safe Sex or Relapse: Gay Men's Response to HIV." Paper presented to the Eighth International Conference on AIDS, Amsterdam, July.

Kippax, Susan, Susan Koenig, and Gary Dowsett. 1986. *Potential Arts Audiences: Attitudes and Practices*. Sydney: Australia Council Occasional Papers.

Kirby, Michael. 1989. "Annecy Revisited—Memoire of a Colloquium on AIDS." Paper presented at the Fondation Marcel Mérieux, Fondation Universitaire des Sciences et Techniques du Vivant, Pensieres Veyrier-Du-Luc, France, April.

Klein, Fritz, Barry Sepekoff, and Timothy J. Wolf. 1985. "Sexual Orientation: A Multi-Variable Dynamic Process." In Fritz Klein and Timothy J. Wolf, eds., *Two Lives to Lead: Bisexuality in Men and Women*, pp. 35-49. New York: Harrington Park Press.

Kramer, Larry. 1986. *Faggots*. London: Metheun.

Kuhn, T. S. 1962. *The Structure of Scientific Revolutions*. Chicago: University of Chicago Press.

Langfeldt, Thore. 1981. "Sexual Development in Children." In Mark Cook and Kevin Howells, eds., *Adult Sexual Interest in Children*, pp. 99-120. London: Academic Press.

Leslie, Charles. 1978. "The Prussian from Taormina." *Blueboy*, January, 37-40.

Lette, K., and G. Carey. 1979. *Puberty Blues*. Melbourne: McPhee Gribble.

Levine, Martin P. 1992. "The Life and Death of Gay Clones." In Gilbert Herdt, ed., *Gay Culture in America: Essays from the Field*, pp. 68-86. Boston: Beacon Press.

Lewes, Kenneth. 1988. *The Psychoanalytic Theory of Male Homosexuality*. New York: Simon & Schuster.

Li, C. K., D. J. West, and T. P. Woodhouse. 1990. *Children's Sexual Encounters with Adults*. London: Duckworth.

Lifson, Alan R., Paul M. O'Malley, Nancy A. Hessol, Susan P. Buchbinder, Lyn Cannon, and George W. Rutherford. 1990. "HIV Seroconversion in Two Homosexual Men After Receptive Oral Intercourse with Ejaculation: Implications for Counseling Concerning Safe Sexual Practices." *American Journal of Public Health* 80, no. 12: 1509-11.

Lloyd, Genevieve. 1990. "AIDS and Philosophy." *Australian Journal of Social Issues* 25, no. 3: 167-76.

Lupton, Deborah. 1994. *Moral Threats and Dangerous Desires: AIDS in the News Media*. London: Taylor & Francis.

Lynn, Lawrence S., Jane S. Spiegel, William C. Matthews, Barbara Leake, Robert Lien, and Scott Brooks. 1989. "Recent Sexual Behaviors Among Homosexual Men Seeking Primary Medical Care." *Archives of Internal Medicine* 149: 2685-90.

Maasen, Thijs. 1990. "Man-Boy Friendships on Trial: On the Shift in the Discourse on Boy Love in the Early Twentieth Century." *Journal of Homosexuality* 20, nos. 1/2: 47-70.

Macnair, Mike. 1989. "The Contradictory Politics of SM." In Simon Shepherd and Mick Wallis, eds., *Coming on Strong: Gay Politics and Culture*, pp. 147-62. London: Unwin Hyman.

Mantell, J. E. 1989. "AIDS Health Promotion Among New York Males Who Have Sex with Males." Paper presented at the World Health Organization Workshop on Health Promotion Activities Directed Towards Gay and Bisexual Men, Geneva, May.

Marcuse, Herbert. 1955. *Eros and Civilization*. Boston: Beacon Press.

Marr, David. 1991. *Patrick White: A Life*. Sydney: Random House Australia.

Marshall, Stuart. 1990. "Picturing Deviancy." In Tessa Boffin and Sunil Gupta, eds., *Ecstatic Antibodies: Resisting the AIDS Mythology*, pp. 19–36. London: Rivers Oram Press.

Masson, J. M. 1984. *Freud: The Assault on Truth. Freud's Suppression of the Seduction Theory*. London: Faber & Faber.

Masters, William H., and Virginia E. Johnson. 1966. *Human Sexual Response*. Boston: Little, Brown.

———. 1970. *Homosexuality in Perspective*. Boston: Little, Brown.

Masters, William, Virginia Johnson, and Robert Kolodny. 1988. *Crisis: Heterosexual Behavior in the Age of AIDS*. New York: Grove.

McDonald, Boyd. 1987. *Filth: An S.T.H. Chap-book*. New York: GPNY.

McIntosh, Mary. 1968. "The Homosexual Role." *Social Problems* 16: 182–92.

McWhirter, David P., and Andrew M. Mattison. 1984. *The Male Couple: How Relationships Develop*. Englewood Cliffs, N.J.: Prentice-Hall.

Merrick, Gordon. 1978. *The Quirk*. New York: Avon Books.

Michaels, Eric. 1990. *Unbecoming: An AIDS Diary*. Sydney: EMPress.

Mills, C. Wright. 1959. *The Sociological Imagination*. New York: Oxford University Press.

Moore, Oscar. 1991. *A Matter of Life and Sex*. London: Penguin.

Morlet, A., and J. Guinan. 1989. "Continued Risk Taking Behaviour and Seroconversion in HIV Antibody Tested Individuals." *Counselling Psychology Quarterly* 2, no. 1: 7–13.

National Centre in HIV Epidemiology and Clinical Research [NCHECR]. 1992. *Australian HIV Surveillance Report* 8, supplement 1 (January).

———. 1993. *Australian HIV Surveillance Report* 9, no. 2 (April).

———. 1994. *Australian HIV Surveillance Report* 10, no. 2 (April).

———. 1995. *Australian HIV Surveillance Report* 11, no. 4 (October).

New South Wales Health Department [AIDS Bureau]. 1990. *Report: Planning for HIV/AIDS Care and Treatment Services in New South Wales 1990–1994*. Sydney: State Health Publication (AIDS) 90-68.

O'Carroll, Tom. 1982. *Paedophilia: The Radical Case*. Boston: Alyson Publications.

O'Reilly, Chris. 1991. *Western Sydney Men Who Have Sex with Men Project* (Report on Initial Outreach Work to Non-Gay Identifying Men Who Have Sex with Men Living in Western Sydney). Sydney: Western Sydney Area Health Service, AIDS Unit, Education and Training Section.

Odijk, Michael. 1987. "Concepts of Homosexuality as Derivatives from Sex and Gender." Paper presented at the Homosexuality, Which Homosexuality? Conference, Amsterdam, December.

*Outrage*, March 1992, no. 106.

Parnell, Bruce. 1989. "Peer Education: Its Role in AIDS Prevention." *National AIDS Bulletin* 3, no. 5: 32–37.

Patton, Cindy. 1989. "Resistance and the Erotic." In Peter Aggleton, Graham Hart, and Peter Davies, eds., *AIDS: Social Representations, Social Practices*, pp. 237–51. London: Falmer Press.

———. 1990. *Inventing AIDS*. New York: Routledge.

Penny, R., R. Marks, J. Berger, D. Marriot, and D. Bryant. 1983. "Acquired Immune Deficiency Syndrome." *Medical Journal of Australia* 13: 554–57.

Peplau, Letitia Anne. 1988. "Research on Homosexual Couples: An Overview." In John P. De Cecco, ed., *Gay Relationships*, pp. 33–40. New York: Haworth Press.

Peters, Robert. 1973. "The First Kiss." In Ian Young, ed., *The Male Muse: A Gay Anthology*, p. 85. Trumansburg, N.Y.: Crossing Press.

Plummer, Ken, ed. 1981. *The Making of the Modern Homosexual*. London: Hutchinson.

———. 1983. *Documents of Life: An Introduction to the Problems and Literature of a Humanistic Method* (Contemporary Social Research: 7, Series editor: Martin Bulmer). London: George Allen & Unwin.

Pollak, Michaël. 1989. "AIDS Prevention Activities and Their Impact on Behaviour: The Case of French Homo- and Bisexuals." Paper presented at the World Health Organization Workshop on AIDS Health Promotion Activities Directed Towards Gay and Bisexual Men, Geneva, May.

Pollak, Michaël, R. Tielman, M. Bochow, M-A. Schiltz, and F. Dubios-Arber. 1992. "EC Concerted Action 'Assessment of the AIDS/HIV Prevention Strategies': Homo- Bisexual Men." Poster presented at the Seventh International Conference on AIDS, Amsterdam, July.

Preston, John. 1981. "Once I Had a Master." In François Peraldi, special ed., *Polysexuality. Semiotext(e)* 4, no. 1: 172–74.

Pringle, Rosemary. 1988. *Secretaries Talk: Sexuality, Power and Work*. Sydney: Allen & Unwin.

———. 1992. "Absolute Sex? Unpacking the Sexuality/Gender Relationship." In R. W. Connell and G. W. Dowsett, eds., *Rethinking Sex: Social Theory and Sexuality Research*, pp. 76–101. Melbourne: Melbourne University Press.

Randall, Richard S. 1989. *Freedom and Taboo: Pornography and the Politics of a Self Divided*. Berkeley and Los Angeles: University of California Press.

Rechy, John. 1977. *The Sexual Outlaw: A Documentary*. New York: Grove Weidenfeld.

Reid, Elizabeth. 1988. "National Strategy in Australia." In Commonwealth of Australia, ed., *Living with AIDS: Toward the Year 2000* (Report of the Third National Conference on AIDS, Hobart, August 4–6), pp. 106–12. Canberra: Australian Government Publishing Service.

Rich, Adrienne. 1980. "Compulsory Heterosexuality and Lesbian Existence." *Signs* 5: 631–60.

Rodgerson, Gillian, and Elizabeth Wilson, eds. 1991. *Pornography and Feminism: The Case Against Censorship* (by Feminists Against Censorship). London: Lawrence & Wishart.

Roffman, R. A., M. R. Gillmore, L. D. Gilchrist, S. A. Mathias, and L. Krueger.

1990. "Continuing Unsafe Sex: Assessing the Need for AIDS Counseling." *Public Health Reports* 105: 202–8.

Rosenthal, Doreen, Susan Moore, and Irene Brumen. 1990. "Ethnic Group Differences in Adolescents' Responses to AIDS." *Australian Journal of Social Issues* 25, no. 3: 220–39.

Rosenthal, Doreen, and Heidi Reichler. 1994. *Young Heterosexuals, HIV/AIDS, and STDs* (Report for the Commonwealth Department of Human Services and Health). Canberra: Australian Government Publishing Service.

Ross, M. W. 1988. "Prevalence of Risk Factors for Human Immunodeficiency Virus Infection in Australia." *Medical Journal of Australia* 149: 362–65.

Ross, M. W., B. Freedman, and R. Brew. 1989. "Changes in Sexual Behaviour Between 1986 and 1988 in Matched Samples of Homosexually Active Men." *Community Health Studies* 13, no. 3: 276–80.

Rubin, Gayle. 1981. "The Leather Menace: Comments on Politics and S/M." In Samois, ed., *Coming to Power: Writing and Graphics on Lesbian S/M*, pp. 192–227. Boston: Alyson Publications.

———. 1993. "Thinking Sex: Notes for a Radical Theory of the Politics of Sexuality." In Henry Abelove, Michèle Aina Barale, and David M. Halperin, eds., *The Gay and Lesbian Studies Reader*. pp. 3–44. New York and London: Routledge.

Rubin, Lillian B. 1976. *Worlds of Pain: Life in the Working Class Family*. New York: Basic Books.

Rumaker, Michael. 1982. *A Day and a Night at the Baths*. San Francisco: Grey Fox Press.

Ruse, Michael. 1988. *Homosexuality: A Philosophical Inquiry*. Oxford: Basil Blackwell.

Russo, Vito. 1981. *The Celluloid Closet*. New York: Harper & Row.

Sandfort, Theo. 1982. *The Sexual Aspect of Paedophile Relations: The Experience of Twenty-Five Boys*. Amsterdam: Pan/Spartacus.

———. 1987. "Pedophilia: Perversion, Parafilia, or Identity." Paper presented at the Homosexuality, Which Homosexuality? Conference, Amsterdam, December.

Sandfort, Theo, Edward Brongersma, and Alex van Naerssen, eds. 1990. *Male Intergenerational Intimacy: Historical, Socio-Psychological, and Legal Perspectives*. Special issue, *Journal of Homosexuality* 20, nos. 1/2.

Sargent, Dave. 1983. "Reformulating (Homo)sexual Politics: Radical Theory and Practice in the Gay Movement." In Judith Allen and Paul Patton, eds., *Beyond Marxism? Interventions After Marx*, pp. 163–82. Sydney: Intervention Publications.

Saslow, James M. 1986. *Ganymede in the Renaissance: Homosexuality in Art and Society*. New Haven and London: Yale University Press.

Saunders, Gill. 1989. *The Nude: A New Perspective*. London: Herbert Press.

Savin-Williams, Ritch C. 1989. "Coming Out to Parents and Self-Esteem Among Gay and Lesbian Youth." In Frederick W. Bozett, ed., *Homosexuality and the Family*, pp. 1–35. New York: Haworth Press.

Schecter, Stephen. 1990. *The AIDS Notebooks*. Albany, N.Y.: State University of New York Press.

Schippers, Jan. 1989. "Homosexual Identity: Essentialism and Constructionism." In Dennis Altman et al., *Homosexuality, Which Homosexuality? Essays from the International Scientific Conference on Gay and Lesbian Studies*, pp. 139–48. London: GMP Publishers; Amsterdam: Uitgeverij An Dekker/Schorer.

Schofield, M. 1965. *The Sexual Behaviour of Young People*. London: Longmans.

Scholder, Amy, and Ira Silverberg, eds. 1991. *High Risk: An Anthology of Forbidden Writings*. London: Serpent's Tail.

Schranzer, Kurt Joseph. 1991. "Time Likes His Toes Sucked." In Kerry Bashford et al., comp., *Pink Ink: An Anthology of Australian Lesbian and Gay Writers*, pp. 173–74. Sydney: Wicked Women Publications.

Scoville, John Wyeth. 1985. *Sexual Domination Today: Sado-Masochism and Domination-Submission*. New York: Irvington Publishers.

Sedgwick, Eve Kosovsky. 1990. *Epistemology of the Closet*. Berkeley and Los Angeles: University of California Press.

Segal, Lynne, and Mary McIntosh, eds. 1992. *Sex Exposed: Sexuality and the Pornography Debate*. London: Virago Press.

Sennett, Richard, and Jonathan Cobb. 1972. *The Hidden Injuries of Class*. New York: Vintage.

Sharp, Rachel. 1991. "Justice and Medical Practice: Misdiagnosis and Maltreatment of a Chronic Disorder." In Jan O'Leary and Rachel Sharp (The Social Justice Collective), eds., *Inequality in Australia: Slicing the Cake*, pp. 258–82. Melbourne: William Heinemann, Australia.

Sharp, R., M. Davis, G. W. Dowsett, Susan Kippax, K. Hewitt, S. Morgan, and W. Robertson. 1991. *Ways of Using: Functional Injecting Drug Users Project*. Sydney: Macquarie University, Centre for Applied Social Research.

Shilts, Randy. 1988. *And the Band Played On: Politics, People, and the AIDS Epidemic*. Harmondsworth: Penguin.

Silverstein, Charles. 1982. *Man to Man: Gay Couples in America*. New York: Quill.

Sinnott, V., and S. Todd. 1988. *Victorian AIDS Council Community Education Evaluation Project—Final Report*. Melbourne: Victorian AIDS Council.

Solomon, P. J., R. G. Attewell, E. B. Freeman, and S. R. Wilson. 1991. *AIDS in Australia: Reconstructing the Epidemic from 1980 to 1990 and Predicting Future Trends in HIV Disease*. Canberra: Australian National University, National Centre for Epidemiology and Population Health, Working Papers No. 29.

Spence, Christopher. 1986. *AIDS: Time to Reclaim Our Power*. London: Lifestory.

Stall, Ron, and Maria Ekstrand. 1989. "Implications of Relapse from Safe Sex." *Focus: A Guide to AIDS Research and Counseling* 4 (February): 3.

Stall, Ron, Maria Ekstrand, Mitchell E. Cohen, Gary Dowsett, Gottfried van Griensven, Graham Hart, and Jeffrey Kelly. 1992. "Maintenance of HIV Risk Reduction Among Gay-Identified Men." In Jonathan Mann, Daniel J. M. Tarantola, and Thomas W. Netter, eds., *AIDS in the World 1992*, pp. 653–57. Cambridge: Harvard University Press.

Stambolian, George. 1984. *Male Fantasies/Gay Realities. Interviews with Ten Men.* New York: Seahorse Press.

Stoller, Robert J. 1985. *Observing the Erotic Imagination.* New Haven: Yale University Press.

Strauss, A., and J. Corbin. 1990. *Basics of Qualitative Research: Grounded Theory Procedures and Techniques.* Newbury Park, Calif.: Sage Publications.

Strong, Philip, and Virginia Berridge. 1990. "No One Knew Anything: Some Issues in British AIDS Policy." In Peter Aggleton, Peter Davies, and Graham Hart, eds., AIDS: *Individual, Cultural, and Policy Dimensions,* pp. 233–52. London: Falmer Press.

*Sydney Star Observer,* June 7, 1981.

Symonds, John Addington. 1983. *Male Love: A Problem in Greek Ethics, and Other Writings,* ed. John Lauritsen. New York: Pagan Press.

Tabori, Paul. 1978. "Fetishism." In Bettina Arndt, ed., *Forum: Guide to Sexual Variety,* special ed., pp. 115–79. Sydney: Tinmin Enterprises.

Teal, Donn. 1971. *The Gay Militants.* New York: Stein & Day.

Terkel, Studs. 1972. *Working: People Talk About What They Do All Day and How They Feel About What They Do.* New York: Pantheon.

Tielman, R.A.P. 1989. "AIDS Health Promotion Activities in the Netherlands Among Men with Homosexual Contacts." Paper presented at the World Health Organization Workshop on Health Promotion Activities Directed Towards Gay and Bisexual Men, Geneva, May.

Timewell, Eric, Victor Minichiello, and David Plummer, eds. 1992. AIDS *in Australia.* Sydney: Prentice-Hall.

Treichler, Paula A. 1988. "AIDS, Homophobia, and Biomedical Discourse: An Epidemic of Signification." In Douglas Crimp, ed., AIDS: *Cultural Analysis, Cultural Activism,* pp. 31–70. Cambridge, Mass.: MIT Press.

Tsang, Daniel, ed. 1981. *The Age Taboo: Gay Male Sexuality, Power, and Consent.* Boston: Alyson Publications; London: Gay Men's Press.

Turtle, A. M., B. Ford, G. M. Habgood, J. Bekiaris, C. Constantinou, M. Mecek, and H. Polyzoidis, 1989. "AIDS-Related Beliefs and Behaviours of Australian University Students." *Medical Journal of Australia* 150: 371–76.

Tyler, Carole-Anne. 1991. "Boys Will Be Girls: The Politics of Gay Drag." In Diana Fuss, ed., *Inside/Out: Lesbian Theories, Gay Theories,* pp. 32–70. New York: Routledge.

Vadasz, Danny, and Jeffrey Lipp. 1990. *Feeling Our Way: Gay Men Talk About Relationships.* Melbourne: Designer Publications.

van Naerssen, Lex. 1987. "Social Networks of Men and Boys Involved in Sexual Relationships." Paper presented at the Homosexuality, Which Homosexuality? Conference, Amsterdam, December.

van Reyk, P. 1990. *On the Beat: A Report on an Outreach Program of AIDS Preventative Education for Men Who Have Sex with Men.* Sydney: AIDS Council of New South Wales.

Vance, Carole S. 1989. "Social Construction Theory: Problems in the History of Sexuality." In Dennis Altman et al., *Homosexuality, Which Homosexuality?*

*Essays from the International Scientific Conference on Gay and Lesbian Studies*, pp. 13–34. London: GMP Publishers; Amsterdam: Uitgeverij An Dekker/Schorer.

Vicinus, Martha. 1989. " 'They Wonder to Which Sex I Belong': The Historical Roots of the Modern Lesbian Identity." In Dennis Altman et al., *Homosexuality, Which Homosexuality? Essays from the International Scientific Conference on Gay and Lesbian Studies*, pp. 171–98. London: GMP Publishers; Amsterdam: Uitgeverij An Dekker/Schorer.

Virkkunen, Matti. 1981. "The Child as Participating Victim." In Mark Cook and Kevin Howells, eds., *Adult Sexual Interest in Children*, pp. 121–34. London: Academic Press.

von Gloeden, Wilhelm. 1984. *Taomina*. London: GMP Publishers.

Waddell, C. 1992. "Social Correlates of Unsafe Sexual Intercourse." *Australian and New Zealand Journal of Sociology* 28, no. 2: 192–207.

———. 1993. "Testing for HIV Infection Among Heterosexual, Bisexual and Gay Men." *Australian Journal of Public Health* 17, no. 1: 27–31.

Waddell, C., and D. Buchbinder. 1992. "A Ternary Structure of Male Bisexuality." *National AIDS Bulletin* 6, no. 4: 48–49.

Watney, Simon. 1986. "The Banality of Gender." *Oxford Literary Review* 8, nos 1/2: 13–21.

———. 1987a. "AIDS: The Cultural Agenda." Paper presented at the Homosexuality, Which Homosexuality? Conference, Amsterdam, December.

———. 1987b. *Policing Desire: Pornography, AIDS, and the Media*. London: Methuen.

———. 1988a. "AIDS, 'Moral Panic' Theory and Homophobia." In Peter Aggleton and Hilary Homans, eds., *Social Aspects of AIDS*, pp. 52–64. London: Falmer Press.

———. 1988b. "The Spectacle of AIDS." In Douglas Crimp, ed., *AIDS: Cultural Analysis, Cultural Activism*, pp. 71–86. Cambridge, Mass.: MIT Press.

———. 1992. "Antibody: The Killing Fields of Europe." *Outrage*, July, 44–47.

Weatherburn, P. 1989. "AIDS Health Promotion Activities Targeted at Homosexually Active Men in London (U.K.): A Briefing Document Prepared for the WHO Global Programme on AIDS." Paper presented to the World Health Organization Workshop on Health Promotion Activities Directed Towards Gay and Bisexual Men, Geneva, May.

Weeks, Jeffrey. 1985. *Sexuality and Its Discontents: Meanings, Myths, and Modern Sexualities*. London: Routledge & Kegan Paul.

———. 1988. "Love in a Cold Climate." In Peter Aggleton and Hilary Homans, eds., *Social Aspects of AIDS*, pp. 10–19. London: Falmer Press.

———. 1989. "AIDS: The Intellectual Agenda." In Peter Aggleton, Graham Hart, and Peter Davies, eds., *AIDS: Social Representations, Social Practices*, pp. 1–20. London: Falmer Press.

———. 1990. *Coming Out: Homosexual Politics in Britain from the Nineteenth Century to the Present*. Rev. ed. London: Quartet Books.

White, Edmund. 1986. *States of Desire: Travels in Gay America*. London: Pan Books.

Willis, Paul. 1977. *Learning to Labour: How Working Class Kids Get Working Class Jobs*. Westmead, Hants: Saxon House.

Wilson, Paul. 1981. *The Man They Called a Monster: Sexual Experiences Between Men and Boys*. Sydney: Cassell Australia.

Wilson, Rhonda. 1984. *Good Talk: The Extraordinary Lives of Ten Ordinary Australian Women*. Melbourne: McPhee Gribble/Penguin.

Wilton, Tamsin. 1991. "Feminism and the Erotics of Health Promotion." Paper presented at the Fifth Social Aspects of AIDS Conference, London, March.

Wittig, Monique. 1989. "On the Social Contract." In Dennis Altman et al., *Homosexuality, Which Homosexuality? Essays from the International Scientific Conference on Gay and Lesbian Studies*, pp. 239–49. London: GMP Publishers; Amsterdam: Uitgeverij An Dekker/Schorer.

Woods, Gregory. 1987. *Articulate Flesh: Male Homo-eroticism and Modern Poetry*. New Haven: Yale University Press.

Wotherspoon, Garry, ed. 1986. *Being Different*. Sydney: Hale & Iremonger.

———. 1991. *City of the Plain: History of a Gay Subculture*. Sydney: Hale & Iremonger.

Yeatman, Anna. 1990. *Bureaucrats, Technocrats, Femocrats. Essays on the Contemporary Australian State*. Sydney: Allen & Unwin.

Young, Ian, ed. 1973. *The Male Muse: A Gay Anthology*. Trumansburg, N.Y.: The Crossing Press.

———, ed. 1983. *The Son of the Male Muse: New Gay Poetry*. Trumansburg, N.Y.: The Crossing Press.

# Index

In this index "f" after a number indicates a separate reference on the next page, and "ff" indicates separate references on the next two pages. A continuous discussion over two or more pages is indicated by a span of page numbers. *Passim* is used for a cluster of references in close but not consecutive sequence.

Library of Congress Cataloging-in-Publication Data

Dowsett, G. W. (Gary W.)
    Practicing desire : homosexual sex in the era of AIDS / Gary W.
Dowsett.
        p.   cm.
    Includes bibliographical references and index.
    ISBN 0-8047-2711-2 (cloth : alk. paper). — ISBN 0-8047-2712-0
(pbk. : alk. paper)
    1. AIDS (Disease)—Social aspects.   2. Gays—Diseases.   3. Gay
libreration movement.   4. Homosexuality.   I. Title.
RA644.A25D69   1996
362.1'969792'008664—dc20                                    96-10879
                                                                CIP

⊗ This book is printed on acid-free, recycled paper.

Original printing 1996
Last figure below indicates year of this printing:
05   04   03   02   01   00   99   98   97   96